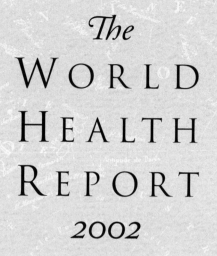

The

WORLD
HEALTH
REPORT
2002

Reducing Risks,

Promoting Healthy Life

WHO Library Cataloguing in Publication Data.

The World health report : 2002 : Reducing risks, promoting healthy life.

1.Risk factors 2.Risk assessment 3.Epidemiologic methods
4.Cost of illness 5.Risk management - methods 6.Public policy 7.Quality of life
8.World health - trends I.Title II.Title: Reducing risks, promoting life.

ISBN 92 4 156207 2 (NLM Classification: WA 540.1)
ISSN 1020-3311

Publications of the World Health Organization can be obtained from Marketing and Dissemination, World Health Organization, 20 Avenue Appia, 1211 Geneva 27, Switzerland (tel: +41 22 791 2476; fax: +41 22 791 4857; email: bookorders@who.int). Requests for permission to reproduce or translate WHO publications – whether for sale or for noncommercial distribution – should be addressed to Publications, at the above address (fax: +41 22 791 4806; email: permissions@who.int).

The designations employed and the presentation of the material in this publication do not imply the expression of any opinion whatsoever on the part of the World Health Organization concerning the legal status of any country, territory, city or area or of its authorities, or concerning the delimitation of its frontiers or boundaries. Dotted lines on maps represent approximate border lines for which there may not yet be full agreement.
  The mention of specific companies or of certain manufacturers' products does not imply that they are endorsed or recommended by the World Health Organization in preference to others of a similar nature that are not mentioned. Errors and omissions excepted, the names of proprietary products are distinguished by initial capital letters.
  The World Health Organization does not warrant that the information contained in this publication is complete and correct and shall not be liable for any damages incurred as a result of its use.

Information concerning this publication can be obtained from:
World Health Report
World Health Organization
1211 Geneva 27, Switzerland
Email: whr@who.int
Fax: (41-22) 791 4870

Copies of this publication can be ordered from: bookorders@who.int

This report was produced under the overall direction of Christopher Murray and Alan Lopez. The two principal authors were Anthony Rodgers (Chapters 2 & 4) and Patrick Vaughan (Chapters 3 & 6). The Overview and Chapter 1 were written by Thomson Prentice. All of the above contributed to Chapter 7. Chapter 5 was written by Tessa Tan-Torres Edejer, David Evans and Julia Lowe.

The writing team was greatly assisted by Michael Eriksen, Majid Ezzati, Susan Holck, Carlene Lawes, Varsha Parag, Patricia Priest and Stephen Vander Hoorn.

Valuable input was received from an internal advisory group and a regional reference group, the members of which are listed in the Acknowledgements. Additional help and advice were appreciated from regional directors, executive directors and members of their staff at WHO headquarters, and senior policy advisers to the Director-General.

The risk assessments in this report were coordinated by Majid Ezzati, Alan Lopez and Anthony Rodgers, with statistical analyses by Stephen Vander Hoorn. The assessments are the result of several years' work by many scientists worldwide. These scientists are listed in the Acknowledgements, as are the many WHO specialists who worked on the cost-effectiveness assessment section.

The report was edited by Barbara Campanini, with assistance from Angela Haden. The figures, maps and tables were coordinated by Michel Beusenberg. Translation coordination and other administrative and production support for the World Health Report team was provided by Shelagh Probst. Further assistance was given by Patrick Unterlerchner. The index was prepared by Liza Furnival.

Cover illustration by Laura de Santis
Design by Marilyn Langfeld. Layout by WHO Graphics
Printed in France
2002/14661 – Sadag – 25000

CONTENTS

Tables

Figures

BOXES

Message from the Director-General

*T*hese are dangerous times for the well-being of the world. In many regions, some of the most formidable enemies of health are joining forces with the allies of poverty to impose a double burden of disease, disability and premature death on many millions of people. It is time for us to close ranks against this growing threat.

Reducing risks to health, the subject of this year's *World health report*, has been a preoccupation of people and their physicians and politicians throughout history. It can be traced back at least 5000 years to some of the world's earliest civilizations. But it has never been more relevant than it is today.

Virtually every major advance in public health has involved the reduction or the elimination of risk. Improvements in drinking-water supplies and sanitation during the 19th and 20th centuries were directly related to the control of the organisms that cause cholera and other diarrhoeal diseases.

Mass immunization programmes eradicated the scourge of smallpox from the planet and have reduced the risk to individuals and whole populations of infectious diseases such as poliomyelitis, yellow fever, measles and diphtheria by providing protection against the causative agents. Countless millions of premature deaths have been avoided as a result.

Legislation enables risks to health to be reduced in the workplace and on the roads, whether through the wearing of a safety helmet in a factory or a seat belt in a car. Sometimes laws, education and persuasion combine to diminish risks, as with health warnings on cigarette packets, bans on tobacco advertising, and restrictions on the sale of alcohol.

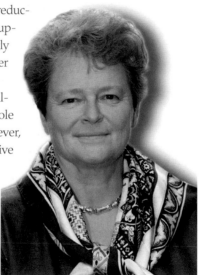

Dr Gro Harlem Brundtland

The result is that, in many ways, the world is a safer place today. Safer from what were once deadly or incurable diseases. Safer from daily hazards of waterborne and food-related illnesses. Safer from dangerous consumer goods, from accidents at home, at work or in hospital.

But in many other ways the world is becoming more dangerous. Too many of us are living dangerously – whether we are aware of that or not. I believe that this *World health report* is a wake-up call to the global community. In one of the largest research projects WHO has ever undertaken, it tries to quantify some of the most important risks to health and to assess the cost-effectiveness of some of the measures to reduce them. The ultimate goal is to help governments of all countries lower these risks and raise the healthy life expectancy of their populations.

The picture that is taking shape from our research gives an intriguing – and alarming – insight into current causes of disease and death and the factors underlying them. It shows how the lifestyles of whole populations are changing around the world, and the impact of these changes on the health of individuals, families, communities and whole populations.

These are issues that deeply concern us all. This was reflected in the in-depth discussions involving ministers of health from almost all of WHO's Member States during the World Health Assembly in Geneva in May of this year. These discussions helped shape this report, and are summarized in the opening chapter. They provided invaluable assessments of the risks to health that countries around the world today regard as most important.

These risks, and some additional ones, are systematically investigated in this report. They include some familiar enemies of health and allies of poverty, such as underweight, unsafe water, poor sanitation and hygiene, unsafe sex (particularly related to HIV/AIDS), iron deficiency, and indoor smoke from solid fuels.

The list also includes risks that are more commonly associated with wealthy societies, such as high blood pressure and high blood cholesterol, tobacco and excessive alcohol consumption, obesity and physical inactivity. These risks, and the diseases linked to them, are now dominant in all middle and high income countries. The real drama now being played out is that they are becoming more prevalent in the developing world, where they create a double burden on top of the infectious diseases that still afflict poorer countries.

In my address to the World Health Assembly in May of this year, I warned that the world is living dangerously, either because it has little choice or because it is making the wrong choices about consumption and activity.

I repeat that warning now. Unhealthy choices are not the exclusive preserve of industrialized nations. We all need to confront them.

Many of the risks discussed in this report concern consumption – either too little, in the case of the poor, or too much, in the case of the better-off.

Two of the most striking findings in this report are to be found almost side by side. One is that in poor countries today there are 170 million underweight children, over three million of whom will die this year as a result. The other is that there are more than one billion adults worldwide who are overweight and at least 300 million who are clinically obese. Among these, about half a million people in North America and Western Europe combined will have died this year from obesity-related diseases.

Could the contrast between the haves and the have-nots ever be more starkly illustrated?

WHO is determined to tackle specific nutrient deficiencies in vulnerable populations and to promote good health through optimal diets, particularly in countries undergoing rapid nutritional transition.

At the same time, we are developing new guidelines for healthy eating. When these are complete, key players in the food industry will be invited to work with us in combating the rising incidence of obesity, diabetes and vascular diseases in developing countries.

Our actions will be vital. The rapidly growing epidemic of noncommunicable diseases, already responsible for some 60% of world deaths, is clearly related to changes in global dietary patterns and increased consumption of industrially processed fatty, salty and sugary foods. In the slums of today's megacities, we are seeing noncommunicable diseases caused by unhealthy diets and habits, side by side with undernutrition.

As I said at the World Food Summit in Rome in June of this year, economic development and globalization need not be associated with negative health consequences. On the contrary, we can harness the forces of globalization to reduce inequity, to diminish hunger and to improve health in a more just and inclusive global society.

Whatever the particular risks to health, whether they are related to consumption or not, every country needs to be able to adapt risk reduction policies to its own needs.

The best health policies are those based on scientific evidence. The World Health Organization's mandate is to get the evidence right and ensure that it is properly used to make the world a healthier place.

This report contains that evidence. It shows the way forward. It helps every country in the world to see what are the most appropriate, most cost-effective measures it can take to reduce at least some risks and promote healthy life for its own population. I urge each and every one of these countries to consider urgently what actions are necessary and to commit themselves to carrying them out.

This report also explains the importance of communicating risks clearly and openly to the public, and of creating an atmosphere of trust and shared responsibility between the government, the public at large and the media.

This is essential. We know that most people will choose to adopt healthier behaviours – especially when they receive accurate information from authorities they trust, and when they are supported through sensible laws, good health promotion programmes and vigorous public debate.

Reducing risks to health is the responsibility of governments – but not only of governments. It rightly remains a vital preoccupation of all people, in all populations, and of all those who serve them. In this *World health report* there is a message for everybody.

Gro Harlem Brundtland
Geneva
October 2002

OVERVIEW

INTRODUCTION

*T*he *World Health Report 2002* represents one of the largest research projects ever undertaken by the World Health Organization. In collaborating with experts worldwide, WHO has collected and analyzed evidence that will have implications for global health for many years to come. Although the report carries some ominous warnings, it also opens the door to a healthier future for all countries – if they are prepared to act boldly now.

The report describes the amount of disease, disability and death in the world today that can be attributed to a selected number of the most important risks to human health. This is of great interest in itself but, more importantly, the report also calculates how much of this present burden could be avoided in the next couple of decades if the same risk factors were reduced from now onwards.

Furthermore, it shows how some of those possible reductions can be achieved in a range of cost-effective ways. The ultimate goal is to help governments of all countries to raise the healthy life expectancy of their populations. The report says that very substantial health gains can be made for relatively modest expenditures. It suggests that at least an extra decade of healthy life could be within the grasp of the populations of many of the world's poorest countries. Even the people of the most industrialized countries, such as the United States of America, the Western European nations and those of the Asian Pacific, stand to gain another five years or so of healthy life.

Although there are many possible definitions of the word "risk", it is defined in this report as *"a probability of an adverse outcome, or a factor that raises this probability"*. The number of such factors is countless and the report does not attempt to be comprehensive. For example, some important risk factors associated with infectious diseases, such as viruses, bacteria, and antimicrobial resistance, are not included. Instead the report concentrates on a selection of risk factors – real risks to health, and often the actual causes of major diseases – for which the means to reduce them are known, and produces some startling findings about their true impact.

From this selected group, the report identifies the top ten risks, globally and regionally, in terms of the burden of disease they cause. The ten leading risk factors globally are: *underweight; unsafe sex; high blood pressure; tobacco consumption; alcohol consumption; unsafe water, sanitation and hygiene; iron deficiency; indoor smoke from solid fuels; high cholesterol; and obesity.* Together, these account for more than one-third of all deaths worldwide.

The report shows that a relatively small number of risks cause a huge number of premature deaths and account for a very large share of the global burden of disease.

For example, at least 30% of all disease burden occurring in many developing countries, such as those in sub-Saharan Africa and South-East Asia, results from fewer than five of the ten risks listed above. Underweight alone accounts for over three million childhood deaths a year in developing countries.

In other, more developed, countries such as China and most countries in Central and South America, five risk factors cause at least one-sixth of their total disease burden. At the same time in the most industrialized countries of North America, Europe and the Asian Pacific, at least one-third of all disease burden is caused by tobacco, alcohol, blood pressure, cholesterol and obesity. Furthermore, more than three-quarters of cardiovascular disease – the world's leading cause of death – results from tobacco use, high blood pressure or cholesterol, or their combination. Overall, cholesterol causes more than 4 million premature deaths a year, tobacco causes almost 5 million, and blood pressure causes 7 million.

The report identifies a number of cost-effective interventions to counter some of the risk factors. In the report, an intervention is defined broadly as *"any health action – any promotive, preventive, curative or rehabilitative activity where the primary intent is to improve health"*. According to the report, the impact of many of the risk factors can be reversed quickly, and most benefits will accrue within a decade. Even modest changes in risk factor levels could bring about large benefits.

In order to know which interventions and strategies to use, governments must first be able to assess and compare the magnitude of risks accurately. The subject of risk assessment is thus a major component of this report. Risk assessment is defined as *"a systematic approach to estimating the burden of disease and injury due to different risks"*.

The report makes key recommendations to help countries develop risk reduction policies which, if implemented, will result in substantially more years of healthy life for many millions of people. At the same time, governments will need to strengthen the scientific and empirical bases for their policies. They will have to improve public dialogue and communications, and develop greater levels of trust for risk prevention among all interested parties. They will also have to develop sound strategies to manage risk uncertainties, and consider carefully a range of ethical and other issues.

Apart from the obvious health benefits, the report says that, overall, reducing major risks to health will promote sustainable development and reduce inequities in society.

ENEMIES OF HEALTH, ALLIES OF POVERTY

The findings of the report give an intriguing – and alarming – insight into not just the current causes of disease and death and the factors underlying them, but also into human behaviour and how it may be changing around the world. Most of all they emphasize the global gap between the haves and the have-nots by showing just how much of the world's burden is the result of undernutrition among the poor and of overnutrition among those who are better-off, wherever they live.

The contrast is shocking. According to the report, at the same time that there are 170 million children in poor countries who are underweight – and over three million of them die each year as a result – there are more than one billion adults worldwide who are overweight and at least 300 million who are clinically obese. Among these, about half a million people in North America and Western Europe die from obesity-related diseases every year.

So it is clear that at one end of the risk factor scale lies poverty, where underweight remains the leading cause of disease burden among hundreds of millions of the world's poorest people and a major cause of death, especially among young children. The report shows that underweight remains a massive and pervasive problem in developing countries, where poverty is a strong underlying determinant.

All ages are at risk, but underweight is most prevalent among children under five years of age, and WHO estimates that approximately 27% of children in this age group are underweight. This caused an estimated 3.4 million deaths in 2000, including about 1.8 million in Africa and 1.2 million in countries in Asia. It was a contributing factor in 60% of all child deaths in developing countries. In other words, the report says, deaths from underweight every year rob the world's poorest children of an estimated total of 130 million years of healthy life.

In terms of global risk factors, underweight is closely followed by unsafe sex, the main factor in the spread of HIV/AIDS, with a major impact in the poor countries of Africa and Asia. The report says HIV/AIDS is now the world's fourth biggest cause of death. Currently 28 million (70%) of the 40 million people with HIV infection are concentrated in Africa, but epidemics elsewhere in the world are growing rapidly. The rate of development of new cases is highest in Eastern Europe and central Asia. Life expectancy at birth in sub-Saharan Africa is currently estimated at 47 years; without AIDS it is estimated that it would be around 62 years.

Current estimates suggest that more than 99% of the HIV infections prevalent in Africa in 2001 are attributable to unsafe sex. In the rest of the world, the 2001 estimates for the proportion of HIV/AIDS deaths attributable to unsafe sex range from 13% in East Asia and the Pacific to 94% in Central America. Globally, about 2.9 million deaths are attributable to unsafe sex, most of these deaths occurring in Africa.

In both Africa and Asia, unsafe water, sanitation and hygiene, iron deficiency, and indoor smoke from solid fuels are among the ten leading risks for disease. All are much more common in poor countries and communities than elsewhere. As with underweight, these risks continue to be some of the most formidable enemies of health and allies of poverty.

About 1.7 million deaths a year worldwide are attributed to unsafe water, sanitation and hygiene, mainly through infectious diarrhoea. Nine out of ten such deaths are in children, and virtually all of the deaths are in developing countries.

Iron deficiency is one of the most prevalent nutrient deficiencies in the world, affecting an estimated two billion people, and causing almost a million deaths a year. Young children and their mothers are the most commonly and severely affected because of the high iron demands of infant growth and pregnancy. The report also considers the disease burdens associated with deficiencies in Vitamin A, iodine, and zinc. Vitamin A deficiency is the leading cause of acquired blindness in children. Iodine deficiency is probably the single most preventable cause of mental retardation and brain damage. Severe zinc deficiency causes short stature, impaired immune function and other disorders and is a significant cause of respiratory infections, malaria and diarrhoeal disease.

Half the world's population is exposed to indoor air pollution, mainly the result of burning solid fuels for cooking and heating. Globally, it is estimated to cause 36% of all lower respiratory infections and 22% of chronic obstructive pulmonary disease.

Most of the risk factors discussed in this report are strongly related to patterns of living, and particularly to consumption – where it can be a case of either too much or too little. At the other end of the scale from poverty lies "overnutrition" or, perhaps more accurately, "overconsumption".

Overweight and obesity are important determinants of health and lead to adverse metabolic changes, including increases in blood pressure, unfavourable cholesterol levels and increased resistance to insulin. They raise the risks of coronary heart disease, stroke, diabetes mellitus, and many forms of cancer. The report shows that obesity is killing about 220 000 men and women a year in the United States of America and Canada alone, and about 320 000 men and women in 20 countries of Western Europe.

High blood pressure and high blood cholesterol are closely related to excessive consumption of fatty, sugary and salty foods. They become even more lethal when combined with the deadly forces of tobacco and excessive alcohol consumption, which also cause a range of cancers as well as heart disease, stroke and other serious illnesses.

The report traces the rapid evolution of the tobacco epidemic by showing that the estimated number of attributable deaths in the year 2000 – 4.9 million – is over one million more than it was in 1990, with the increase being most marked in developing countries. However, most of the smoking-related disease burden is still found in industrialized countries.

Global alcohol consumption has increased in recent decades, with most or all of this increase occurring in developing countries, according to the report. Worldwide, alcohol caused 1.8 million deaths, equal to 4% of the global disease burden; the proportion was greatest in the Americas and Europe. Alcohol was estimated to cause, worldwide, 20–30% of oesophageal cancer, liver disease, epilepsy, motor vehicle accidents, and homicide and other intentional injuries.

Until recently, all of these factors – blood pressure, cholesterol, tobacco, alcohol and obesity, and the diseases linked to them – had been thought to be most common in industrialized countries. Unfortunately, as this report demonstrates, they are now becoming more prevalent in developing nations, where they create a double burden in addition to the remaining, unconquered infectious diseases that have always afflicted poorer countries.

In a number of ways, then, this report shows that the world is living dangerously – either because it has little choice, which is often the case among the poor, or because it is making the wrong choices in terms of its consumption and its activities.

Indeed, there is evidence that these risk factors are part of a "risk transition" showing marked changes in patterns of living in many parts of the world. In many developing countries, rapid increases in body weight are being recorded, particularly among children, adolescents and young adults. Obesity rates have risen threefold or even more in some parts of North America, Eastern Europe, the Middle East, the Pacific Islands, Australasia and China since 1980. Changes in food processing and production and in agricultural and trade policies have affected the daily diet of hundreds of millions of people.

The report says that while eating fruit and vegetables can help prevent cadiovascular diseases and some cancers, low intake of them as part of diet is responsible for almost three million deaths a year from those diseases. At the same time, changes in living and working patterns have led to less physical activity and less physical labour. The report finds that physical inactivity causes about 15% of some cancers, diabetes and heart disease.

Meanwhile, tobacco and alcohol are being marketed increasingly in low and middle income countries. Today, more people than ever before are exposed to such products and patterns, imported or adopted from other countries, which pose serious long-term risks to their health. For example, smokers of all ages have death rates two or three times higher than non-smokers.

The report warns that if global health is to be further improved and burdens of disease lowered, countries need to adopt control policies now. It says that risks such as unsafe sex and tobacco consumption could increase global deaths substantially in the next few decades and could decrease life expectancy in some countries by as much as 20 years unless they are brought under better control very soon.

RECOMMENDED ACTIONS

In general, the report suggests that priority should be given to controlling those risks that are well known, common, substantial and widespread, and for which effective and acceptable risk reduction strategies are available. These criteria apply to many of the risks in the report. The increasing level of tobacco consumption, particularly in Asia, is one clear example. The report says a substantial increase in government tobacco taxes would produce significant health benefits at very low cost.

Government action, in partnership with multiple stakeholders, to reduce the salt content of processed foods would also achieve substantial health benefits in all settings. The report suggests that this should be one component of a comprehensive strategy for the control of cardiovascular disease risks. The overall strategy would be based on a mix of community-wide interventions, such as salt reduction, and treatment-based interventions focusing on individuals whose risk of a cardiovascular event in the next ten years is assessed to be high.

For many of the main risk factors there is likely to be good agreement between the general public and public health experts on what needs to be done. In some countries, risk understanding may need to be strengthened among the general public, politicians and public health practitioners.

Recommended actions that governments can take in risk reduction have been tailored to suit high, middle and low income countries. More generally, the report makes the following recommendations.

- Governments, especially health ministries, should play a stronger role in formulating risk prevention policies, including more support for scientific research, improved surveillance systems and better access to global information.
- Countries should give top priority to developing effective, committed policies for the prevention of globally increasing high risks to health, such as tobacco consumption, unsafe sex in connection with HIV/AIDS, and, in some populations, unhealthy diet and obesity.
- Cost-effectiveness analyses should be used to identify high, medium and low priority interventions to prevent or reduce risks, with highest priority given to those interventions that are cost-effective and affordable.
- Intersectoral and international collaboration to reduce major extraneous risk to health, such as unsafe water and sanitation or a lack of education, is likely to have large health benefits and should be increased, especially in poorer countries.
- Similarly, international and interesectoral collaboration should be strengthened to improve risk management and increase public awareness and understanding of risks to health.
- A balance between government, community and individual action is necessary. For example, community action should be supported by nongovernmental organizations, local groups, the media and others. At the same time, individuals should be empowered and encouraged to make positive, life-enhancing health decisions for themselves on matters such as tobacco use, excessive alcohol consumption, unhealthy diet and unsafe sex.

SUMMARY OF CHAPTERS

Chapter One: Protecting the people sets the scene with a general introduction to the subject of measuring, communicating and reducing risks to health – people's exposure to them and the role of government in protecting the population from them. It shows how governments, particularly in the 20th century, have been instrumental in reducing some major risks to health. But it also explains how the current demographic transition is being accompanied by a "risk transition" and a double burden of disease on developing countries – the combination of long-established infectious diseases and the greater relative importance of chronic, noncommunicable diseases.

Chapter Two: Defining and assessing risks to health offers a detailed explanation of this report's approach to health risks. It points out that much scientific effort and most health resources today are directed towards treating disease, rather than preventing it. It argues that focusing on risks to health is the key to prevention. Population-based strategies aim to make healthy behaviour a social norm, thus lowering risk in the entire population. Small shifts in some risks in the population can translate into major public health benefits.

Thus, the chapter strongly advocates the assessment of population-wide risks as well as high-risk individuals in strategies for risk reduction. The key challenge, it says, is to find the right balance between the two approaches.

This chapter also describes how risk assessment has emerged in recent years from its roots in the study of environmental problems. It shows how the steps generally involved in environmental risk assessment can be adapted to apply more specifically to the analysis of health risks, and it explains the benefits of comparing different risks to health.

Chapter Three: Perceiving risks explains that both risks and benefits have to be considered when seeking to understand what drives some behaviours and why some interventions are more acceptable and successful than others. Perceptions of risk are often polarized between expert understanding and public views; between quantitative and qualitative assessments; and between analytical and emotive responses.

This chapter examines the roles of social, cultural and economic factors in shaping individuals' understanding of health risks. The structural factors which influence the adoption of risk control policies by government, and the impact of interventions, are considered. The importance of understanding and managing the risk perceptions of different groups in society, when seeking to reduce risks, is also discussed. The chapter concludes that reducing risk exposure has to be planned within the context of local society, and that prevention through interventions is only partly a matter of individual circumstances and education. It suggests a need for a concerted international research agenda to raise population awareness of major risks in developing countries, such as the tobacco epidemic.

The chapter says that information about risks and their consequences, presented in scientific terms and based on a risk assessment, has to be communicated with particular emphasis and care. It concludes by stressing that an atmosphere of trust and shared responsibility between the government and all interested parties, especially the media, is essential if interventions are to be adopted and successfully implemented.

Chapter Four: Quantifying selected major risks to health provides the main results of a major WHO-initiated project quantifying the health effects of selected major health risks, on a global scale and in a comparable fashion. Most of these results have been briefly referred to in this overview.

An introduction to the generic approach is provided, followed by a description of the major health risks in terms of their extent and the types of threat they pose. The key results of the analysis are summarized and discussed in terms of their potential to improve healthy life expectancy by focusing on causes of disease and injury. The overall aim of the analyses reported in this chapter has been to obtain reliable and comparable estimates of attributable burden of disease and injury on which to build the basis of a variety of policy-relevant measures.

The chapter points out that, very often, the greatest burden of health risks is borne by the poor countries, and by the disadvantaged in all societies. The vast majority of threats to health are more commonly found in the poor, in those with little education, and with low-status occupations. Studying exposure to risk factors among poor households and individuals, and the disease burden they cause, enables the design of policies most likely to reduce them.

Chapter Five: Some strategies to reduce risk puts forward the best available evidence on the cost and effectiveness of selected interventions to reduce some of the major risk factors discussed in Chapter 4. It looks at the extent to which these interventions are likely to improve population health, both singly and in combination. The analysis in this chapter is used to identify both actions that are very cost-effective and those that do not seem to be cost-effective in different settings. It illustrates how decision-makers can begin the policy debate about priorities with information about which interventions would yield the greatest possible improvements in population health for the available resources. It says this evidence will be a key input, but not the only one, to the final decision about the best combination of interventions.

The chapter examines a range of strategies to reduce different types of risk, and the possible impact of those strategies on costs and effectiveness. It considers individual behaviours related to risk, such as food intake, smoking and sexual behaviour. It also discusses individual factors, such as genetics, and environmental factors including water and sanitation. The chapter says that many risk reduction strategies involve a component of behaviour change. However, some types of behaviour change might require active government intervention to succeed. Different ways of attaining the same goal are discussed, for example, the population-wide versus the individual-based approach and prevention versus treatment. Combinations of these two approaches are likely to be the best ways of improving health.

With regard to policy implications, the chapter says that very substantial health gains can be made for relatively modest expenditures on interventions. However, the maximum possible gains for the resources that are available will be attained only through careful consideration of the costs and effects of interventions. A strategy to protect the environment of the child is cost-effective in all settings. The components include micronutrient supplementation, treatment of diarrhoea and pneumonia, and disinfection of water at the point of use as a way of reducing the incidence of diarrhoea. This last measure is particularly cost-effective in regions of high child mortality. A policy shift towards household water management appears to be the most attractive short-term water-related health intervention in developing countries.

Preventive interventions to reduce the incidence of HIV infections, including measures to encourage safer injection practices, are very cost-effective. The use of antiretroviral therapy in conjunction with preventive activities is cost-effective in most settings.

In all settings, at least one type of intervention to reduce the risks associated with cardiovascular disease was found to be cost-effective. Population-wide strategies to lower cholesterol by reducing salt intake are always very cost-effective both singly and in combination. In addition, governments would be well advised to consider taking steps to reduce the salt content of processed foods on a population-wide basis, either through regulation or self-regulation.

The chapter highlights the important role for government in encouraging risk reduction strategies. Taxes on cigarette products are very cost-effective globally, and higher tax rates result in larger improvements in population health. Even greater improvements would arise if higher taxes were combined with comprehensive tobacco advertising bans.

Chapter Six: Strengthening risk prevention policies argues that governments, in their stewardship role for better health, need to invest heavily in risk prevention, in order to contribute substantially to future avoidable mortality.

Substantial agreement on what needs to be done exists between the international scientific community and those charged with improving public health. Strategies to achieve these potential gains, particularly in developing countries, ought to involve a question of balance. It is a balance between the priority of sharply reducing the burden from exposures such as underweight and poor water and sanitation, which are largely confined to poorer populations, and the priority of reducing or preventing further population exposure to factors such as tobacco, elevated blood pressure and cholesterol.

Much is already known about how to reduce risks to health effectively. That reduction will require sustained policy action and commitment by governments and other partners. Key elements will be the creation or strengthening of national institutions to implement and evaluate risk reduction programmes, and more effective engagement of sectors such as transport, education and finance to capitalize on the potential for greatly reducing population exposures.

The chapter also highlights important considerations to be kept in mind when deciding on risk reduction measures. These include the criteria for choosing which key risks to tackle; the right balance between efforts targeted on primary, secondary or subsequent prevention; the management of uncertain risks; and the related issue of strengthening the evidence base for policy action. The ethical implications of various programme strategies, including their impact on inequities in population health, must also be taken into account.

Chapter Seven: Preventing risks and taking action contains the report's conclusions. It says that in order to protect and improve health globally, much more emphasis is needed on preventing the actual causes of important diseases as well as treating the diseases themselves. Prevention can best be achieved through concerted efforts to identify and reduce common, major risks and by taking advantage of the prevention opportunities they present. Tackling major risks could improve global health much more than is generally realized.

This chapter says the report offers a unique opportunity for governments. They can use it to take bold and determined actions against only a relatively few major risks to health, in the knowledge that the likely result within the next ten years will be large gains in healthy life expectancy for their citizens. The potential benefits apply equally to poor countries and rich countries, even if some of the risk factors are different.

Bold policies will be required. Governments can decide to aim for increased taxes on tobacco; legislation to reduce the proportion of salt and other unhealthy components in foods; stricter environmental controls and ambitious energy policies; and stronger health promotion and health safety campaigns.

This is undoubtedly a radical approach. It requires governments to see the value of shifting the main focus from the minority of high-risk individuals to include preventive measures that can be applied to the whole population.

There are compelling reasons for governments to play a greater role in tackling these major risks. Governments are the stewards of health resources and have a responsibility to protect their citizens. In addition, reducing risks will promote sustainable development and can also reduce inequities in society.

CHAPTER ONE

Protecting the People

This report deals with health risks, where risk is defined as a probability of an adverse outcome, or a factor that raises this probability. In order to protect people – and help them protect themselves – governments need to be able to assess risks and choose the most cost-effective and affordable interventions to prevent risks from occurring. Some risks have already been reduced, but changes in patterns of consumption, particularly of food, alcohol and tobacco, around the world are creating a "risk transition". Diseases such as cancers, heart disease, stroke and diabetes are increasing in prominence. This trend is particularly serious for many low and middle income countries which are still dealing with the traditional problems of poverty, such as undernutrition and infectious diseases.

1

PROTECTING THE PEOPLE

REDUCING THE RISKS

*P*eople everywhere are exposed all their lives to an almost limitless array of risks to their health, whether in the shape of communicable or noncommunicable disease, injury, consumer products, violence or natural catastrophe. Sometimes whole populations are in danger, at other times only an individual is involved. Most risks cluster themselves around the poor.

No risk occurs in isolation: many have their roots in complex chains of events spanning long periods of time. Each has its cause, and some have many causes.

In this report, risk is defined as "*a probability of an adverse outcome, or a factor that raises this probability*".

Human perceptions of and reactions to risk are shaped by past experience and by information and values received from sources such as family, society and government. It is a learning process that begins in childhood – when children learn not to play with fire – and is constantly updated in adulthood. Some risks, such as disease outbreaks, are beyond our individual control; others, such as smoking or other unhealthy consumptions, are within our power to either heighten or diminish.

The challenge and responsibility of reducing risks as much as possible, in order to achieve a long and healthy life, is shared by individuals, whole populations and their governments. For example, putting on a car seat belt is an individual action to reduce risk of injury; introducing a law to make wearing seat belts compulsory is a government action on behalf of the population.

Many people believe it is their government's duty to do all it reasonably can to reduce risks on their behalf, such as making sure that foods and medicines are safe. This is particularly important where individuals have little control over their exposure to risks. Such actions are commonly referred to as "interventions". In this report, an intervention means "*any health action – any promotive, preventive, curative or rehabilitative activity where the primary intent is to improve health*".

Although governments rarely can hope to reduce risks to zero, they can aim to lower them to a more acceptable level, and explain, through open communication with the public, why and how they are doing so. Governments must also develop high levels of public trust, because the public is quick to judge how well risks are being managed on its behalf. This applies whether the risk relates to a rapidly moving new epidemic or to a long-term exposure.

In order to protect the people – and help them protect themselves – governments need to be able to assess accurately how great the risks are. Until now, that has been a seriously neglected task. Without some quantitative approach to gauging the importance of specific risks, in terms of the likely size of their impact on populations, government policies might be driven exclusively by factors such as pressure groups or the emotive weight of individual cases.

A key purpose of this report is to provide governments with a strategy for that assessment as an avenue towards developing the best policies and an array of intervention options for risk reduction. It also offers a comprehensive approach to the definition and study of risks.

In this report, risk assessment is defined as "*a systematic approach to estimating the burden of disease and injury due to different risks*". It involves the identification, quantification and characterization of threats to human health. Risk assessment can provide an invaluable, overall picture of the relative roles of different risks to human health; it can illuminate the potential for health benefits by focusing on those risks, and it can help set agendas for research and policy action. The broader activity of risk analysis is a political activity as well as a scientific one and embraces public perception of risk, bringing in issues of values, process, power and trust.

THE RISK TRANSITION

In the general sense, many risks to health have, of course, already been reduced – and a few, such as smallpox, have been eliminated or eradicated. Much of the credit is due to the great progress in public health and medicine in the last century. Improvements in drinking-water and sanitation, the development of national health systems, the introduction of antibiotics and mass immunization against the causes of infectious diseases, and more recently, better nutrition, are outstanding examples. Governments, particularly in the last 100 years, have played the leading role in protecting and improving the health of their populations.

As the 20th century ended, *The World Health Report 1999* traced the revolutionary gains in life expectancy achieved in the previous few decades. These amounted to 30–40 years more life for people in some countries. Although the devastating impact of some diseases, such as HIV/AIDS, malaria and tuberculosis must be borne constantly in mind, it can still be said that a substantial proportion of the world's population faces relatively low risk from most infectious diseases. However, although the risk factors considered in this report do not include pathogens such as bacteria, viruses and parasites, these continue to be leading contributors to ill-health. Other risk factors related to infectious diseases should not be overlooked. These include the growing problem of antimicrobial resistance, chronic infections that are associated with certain cancers, and the deliberate use of microbial agents to cause harm through terrorism or warfare. More generally, the generation and application of new knowledge about diseases and their control has played a vital role in improving the quality as well as the duration of life.

Decades of scientific research into the causes of disease and injury has given the world a vast knowledge base – now more widely accessible than ever before, thanks to the Internet – and a huge potential for prevention and risk reduction. However, what is known, and what can be done, is not always reflected adequately in public health practice.

Meantime, while some risks to health have diminished, the very successes of the past few decades in infectious disease control and reduced fertility are inexorably generating a "demographic transition" from traditional societies where almost everyone is young to societies with rapidly increasing numbers of middle-aged and elderly people.

At the same time, researchers are observing marked changes in patterns of consumption, particularly of food, alcohol and tobacco, around the world. These changing patterns are identified in this report as being of crucial importance to global health. They amount to nothing less than a "risk transition" which is causing an alarming increase in risk factors in middle and low income countries.

Understanding why these changes are happening is vitally important. At a time when there is much discussion about globalization, it should be recognized that health itself has become globalized.

The rapid increases in international travel and trade and the mass movement of populations witnessed in the last few decades mean that infectious diseases can spread from one continent to another in a matter of hours or days, whether they are conveyed by individual travellers or in the cargo holds of aircraft or ships. However, the transition in which other forms of health risk appear to be shifting from one part of the world to another usually occurs much more slowly, more indirectly and less visibly, often requiring years to be detectable.

Nevertheless, as globalization continues to affect societies everywhere, the risk transition seems to be gaining speed. Today, more people than ever before are exposed to products and patterns of living imported or adopted from other countries that pose serious long-term risks to their health. The fact is that so-called "Western" risks no longer exist as such. There are only global risks, and risks faced by developing countries.

Increasingly, tobacco, alcohol and some processed foods are being marketed globally by multinational companies, with low and middle income countries their main targets for expansion. Changes in food processing and production and in agricultural and trade policies have affected the daily diet of hundreds of millions of people. At the same time, changes in living and working patterns have led to less physical activity and less physical labour. The television and the computer are two obvious reasons why people spend many more hours of the day seated and relatively inactive than a generation ago. The consumption of tobacco, alcohol and processed or "fast" foods fits easily into such patterns of life.

These changing patterns of consumption and of living, together with global population ageing, are associated with a rise in prominence of diseases such as cancers, heart disease, stroke, mental illness, and diabetes and other conditions linked to obesity. Already common in industrialized nations, they now have ominous implications for many low and middle income countries which are still dealing with the traditional problems of poverty such as undernutrition and infectious diseases.

Unfortunately, these latter countries are frequently unable to meet the health challenges confronting them. Demands on their health systems are increasing but resources for health remain scarce. Governments find themselves under pressure from the global demands of market forces and free trade. Such demands often imply the absence or reduction of appropriate laws, regulations and standards intended to protect the health and welfare of their citizens.

As *The World Health Report 1999* predicted, over a billion people entered the 21st century without having benefited from the health revolution: their lives remain short and scarred by predominantly "old" diseases. For many countries, this amounts to the notorious "double burden" – struggling to control the disease burden of the poor while simultaneously responding to rapid growth in noncommunicable diseases.

In short, while many risks have been reduced, others at least as serious have taken their place and are being added to those that still persist. And as the terrorist actions of 2001 showed, some previously unimaginable risks must now be confronted.

Meanwhile, large numbers of individuals, although not poor, fail to realize their full potential for better health because of a lack of enlightened policies and decisions in many sectors and the tendency of health systems to allocate resources to interventions of low quality or of low efficacy related to cost.

Increasing numbers of people forego or defer essential care or suffer huge financial burdens resulting from an unexpected need for expensive services. Altogether, the continuing challenges to reduce risks to health thus remain enormous.

However, there is growing national and international recognition of the risks themselves. During the World Health Assembly in Geneva in May 2002, WHO's Member States took part in organized round table discussions on risks to health *(1, 2)*. One after another, health ministers or their representatives spelt out the main risks confronting their country. Tobacco, alcohol, unhealthy diet and obesity featured prominently alongside chronic diseases and traffic injuries in many low income and middle income countries. Ministers clearly demonstrated their knowledge of the trends in major risks in their countries, and their willingness to take action to reduce them (see Box 1.1). This report is intended to help them choose the best risk reduction policies that will in turn promote healthy life in their populations.

Box 1.1 Countries endorse the focus on risks to health

Ministers of health attending the Fifty-fifth World Health Assembly in Geneva, Switzerland, in May 2002 participated in round table discussions on the major risks to health. Faced by the challenge of balancing preventive and treatment services, and the need to target prevention programmes where most health gain can be achieved, they supported the development of a scientific framework with consistent definitions and methods on which to build reliable, comparable assessments. There was support for an intersectoral approach to prevention strategies involving partnerships with communities, nongovernmental organizations, local government, and private sector organizations.

The number of potential risks to health is almost infinite, and the rapidly changing age structures of many populations will lead to changing risk profiles in the coming decades. Poverty is an underlying determinant of many risks to health and affects disease patterns between and within countries; other aspects of socioeconomic development, particularly education for women, also have a key role. Globalization has been hailed as a strategy to reduce poverty, but the liberalization of trade can lead to both benefits and harms for health. Tobacco is either an established or a rapidly emerging risk to health in all developing countries: the need for more stringent tobacco control is uniformly recognized – including increased taxation, bans on advertising, and the introduction or expansion of smoke-free environments and cessation programmes. Alcohol is another commonly cited and increasing risk to health in many countries; and conditions with important dietary components, such as diabetes, obesity and hypertension, are increasingly globalized, even in countries with coexistent undernutrition.

The chain of causes – from socioeconomic factors through environmental and community conditions to individual behaviour – offers many different entry points for prevention. Approaches can be combined so that interventions focus on background environmental (e.g. indoor air pollution) and distal (e.g. sanitation) risks, as well as more proximal risks such as physical inactivity and alcohol abuse.

Risk communication is an integral part of the risk management process. An open approach between governments and their scientific advisers and the public is recommended, even when there may be unpalatable messages or scientific uncertainty. How risks are described, who are the scientific spokespersons, how dialogue and negotiations take place, and whether uncertainties are adequately communicated all have substantial influence on maintaining trust.

International as well as national efforts are needed to combat the very widely distributed risks to health – high blood pressure, tobacco, alcohol, inactivity, obesity and cholesterol – that are now major threats throughout the world, and cause a large proportion of disease burden in industrialized countries. In middle income countries these risk factors already contribute to the double burden of risks to health, and they are also of growing importance in low income countries. With ageing populations and trends in disease rates, these exposure levels are likely to assume increasing importance. Unless prevention begins early, with initiatives such as those envisaged in the Framework Convention on Tobacco Control, then the low and middle income countries will suffer a vast increase in the number of premature deaths from noncommunicable diseases.

Every country has major risks to health that are known, definite and increasing, sometimes largely unchecked, for which cost-effective interventions are insufficiently applied. Once major risks to health have been identified, the key challenge is to increase the uptake of known cost-effective interventions. Where cost-effective options to reduce major risks are not yet available, an international research investment is needed. Some countries have had considerable success with risk factor interventions that have led, for example, to large reductions in the prevalence of HIV/AIDS and moderate but population-wide shifts in major cardiovascular risk factors, such as blood pressure and high cholesterol levels. Sharing other countries' successes and learning from their predicaments will improve prevention in many different settings, especially in rapidly developing countries.

REFERENCES

1. *Fifty-fifth World Health Assembly. Ministerial round tables: risks to health.* Geneva: World Health Organization; 2002. WHO document A55/DIV/5.
2. *Fifty-fifth World Health Assembly. Ministerial round tables: risks to health. Report by the Secretariat.* Geneva: World Health Organization; 2002. WHO document A55/DIV/6.

CHAPTER TWO

Defining and Assessing Risks to Health

This chapter offers a detailed explanation of the report's approach to health risks. It argues that while much scientific effort and most health resources today are directed towards treating disease, rather than preventing it, focusing on risks to health is the key to prevention. Such risks do not occur in isolation, so both proximal and distal causes of adverse health outcomes need to be considered. Population-based strategies aim to make healthy behaviour a social norm, thus lowering risk in the entire population. Small shifts in some risks in the population can translate into major public health benefits. Therefore this chapter strongly advocates the assessment of population-wide risks as well as high-risk individuals in strategies for risk reduction. The key challenge is to find the right balance between the two approaches. Risk assessment has emerged in recent years from its roots in the study of environmental problems, and the steps generally involved in environmental risk assessment can be adapted to apply more specifically to the analysis of health risks. This chapter explains the benefits of comparing different risks to health and defines and explains risk assessment.

2

DEFINING AND ASSESSING

RISKS TO HEALTH

WHAT ARE RISKS TO HEALTH?

*R*isk can mean different things to different people, as summarized in Box 2.1. The two most common meanings will be used in this report – risk as a probability of an adverse outcome, or a factor that raises this probability.

WHY FOCUS ON RISKS TO HEALTH?

Focusing on risks to health is key to preventing disease and injury. The most emotive and tangible images in health are of people suffering from disease, but preventing disease and injury occurring in the first place requires systematic assessment and reduction of their causes. Much scientific effort and most health resources are directed towards treating disease – the "rule of rescue" still dominates *(3)*. Data on disease or injury outcomes, such as death or hospitalization, tend to focus on the need for palliative or curative services. In contrast, assessments of burden resulting from risk factors will estimate the potential of prevention. One notable exception concerns communicable diseases, since treating infected individuals can prevent further spread of infection, and hence treatment can be a method of prevention in itself.

Even when the focus is on causes as well as disease outcomes, much scientific activity has been directed to assessing whether a risk exists at all. Does electromagnetic frequency radiation cause leukaemia? Do certain infections predispose to heart attacks? These assessments are usually accompanied by estimates of how much higher the risk is in individuals who are exposed compared with those who are not. It has been much less common to assess impact at a population level by asking "of all the disease burden in this population, how much could be caused by this risk?"

Many factors are relevant in prioritizing strategies to reduce risks to health: the extent of the threat posed by different risk factors, the availability of cost-effective interventions, and societal values and preferences are particularly important. These factors are also key for research priorities – if major threats exist without cost-effective solutions, then these must be placed high on the agenda for research. Governments are also likely to place particular value on ensuring their main efforts focus on the largest threats to health in their countries. Reliable, comparable and locally relevant information on the size of different risks to health is therefore crucial to prioritization, especially for governments setting broad directions for health policy and research. However, such information has typically been very limited, creating a gap in which interest groups may seek either to downplay or to overestimate some risks. In addition, there is an inherent imbalance in media information about risks: common, major threats to health are usually not reported because they are already known, whereas rare or unusual threats to health are highly newsworthy.

Stewardship is one of the key functions of government, necessitating a broad overview, a long-term horizon and an evidence-based approach, and requiring information from reliable, comparable assessments of the magnitude of different major risks to health. This report helps to redress the dearth of such information. The report recognizes that risk analysis is a political enterprise as well as a scientific one, and that public perception of risk also plays a role in risk analysis, bringing issues of values, process, power and trust into the picture. The roles and contributions of risk assessment, communication, risk management, cost-effectiveness and policy development form the focus of the report.

DEVELOPMENT OF RISK ASSESSMENT

People have been interested in risks to health throughout history. During the past several decades, this interest has intensified and has also begun to include many new perspectives. The field of risk analysis has grown rapidly, focusing on the identification, quantification and characterization of threats to human health and the environment – a set of activities broadly called risk assessment.

While clearly there has been very long interest in comparing risks posed by different threats to health, formal frameworks have been developed only relatively recently. Risk assessment has its roots in the environmental sector, where it was developed as a systematic way of comparing environmental problems that pose different types and degrees of health risk. Such environmental risk assessment exercises generally comprise four elements.

- *Hazard identification* identifies the types of health effect that can be caused, based on toxicological data from laboratory or epidemiological studies: for example, chemical X causes liver damage.
- *Exposure assessment* combines data on the distribution and concentrations of pollution in the environment with information on behaviour and physiology to estimate the amount of pollutant to which humans are exposed. Biomarkers have been used to gauge levels of some exposures, such as lead and dioxin.
- *Dose–response assessment* relates the probability of a health effect to the dose of pollutant or amount of exposure.
- *Risk characterization* combines the exposure and dose–response assessments to calculate the estimated health risks, such as the number of people predicted to experience a particular disease, for a particular population. This typically includes estimation and communication of uncertainties.

Environmental risk assessments of likely health effects, together with consideration of costs, technical feasibility and other factors, can be used to set priorities for environmental management. Environmental risk assessment has analogies to the strategies developed in epidemiology for assessing population attributable risks, that is, the proportion of disease in a population that results from a particular hazard. A more general approach based on these frameworks can be extended to many other areas. A key part of this report outlines such methods and provides an illustrative analysis of burden caused by a variety of different risks to health.

Risk assessment can be defined here as a systematic approach to estimating and comparing the burden of disease and injury resulting from different risks. The work pre-

---

Box 2.1 What does risk mean?

- Risk can mean a probability, for example, the answer to the question: "What is the risk of getting HIV/AIDS from an infected needle?"
- Risk can mean a factor that raises the probability of an adverse outcome. For example, major risks to child health include malnutrition, unsafe water and indoor air pollution.
- Risk can mean a consequence. For example, what is the risk from driving while drunk? (answer: being in a car crash).
- Risk can mean a potential adversity or threat. For example, is there risk in riding a motorcycle?

In this report, the first two meanings are used. Risk is defined as a probability of an adverse health outcome, or a factor that raises this probability. Other important risk-related definitions are outlined below.

- ***Prevalence of risk*** – the proportion of the population who are exposed to a particular risk. For example, the prevalence of smoking might be 25% in a particular population.

- ***Relative risk*** – the likelihood of an adverse health outcome in people exposed to a particular risk, compared with people who are not exposed. For example, if people who smoke for a certain time are, on average, 15 times more likely to develop lung cancer than those who do not smoke, their relative risk is 15.
- ***Hazard*** – an inherent property, for example of a chemical, that provides the potential for harm.
- ***Population attributable risk*** – the proportion of disease in a population that results from a particular risk to health.
- ***Attributable burden*** – the proportion of current disease or injury burden that results from past exposure.
- ***Avoidable burden*** – the proportion of future disease or injury burden that is avoidable if current and future exposure levels are reduced to those specified by some alternative, or counterfactual, distribution.

Sources: *(1, 2)*.

---

sented in this report builds on several similar estimates conducted in recent years. The first global estimates of disease and injury burden attributable to a set of different risk factors were reported in the initial round of the global burden of disease study *(4, 5)*. These estimates add to the many others made for selected risk factors in specific populations, for example, tobacco *(6)*, alcohol and other drugs *(7)*, environmental factors *(8)*, blood pressure *(9)*, and selected risk factors for certain regions *(10–12)*.

In the first round of the global burden of disease study, risk factors were assessed that were either exposures in the environment (for example, unsafe water), human behaviour (for example, tobacco smoking) or physiological states (for example, hypertension). However, in such early risk assessments, there was a lack of comparability between different risk factor assessments arising, in part, from a lack of standard comparison groups and different degrees of reliability in assessing risk factors. Also, the relevance of varying time lags between exposure and outcome – for example, short for alcohol and injuries and long for smoking and cancer – was not captured. A key aim of this analysis is therefore to increase comparability between the estimates of the impact of different risk factors and characterize the timing of these impacts.

Risk assessment estimates burden of disease resulting from different risk factors, each of which may be altered by many different strategies; it can provide an overall picture of the relative roles of different risks to human health. Specific strategies for identifying the appropriate sets of interventions, and the crucial roles of cost-effectiveness analyses in choosing from among them, are outlined in Chapter 5.

KEY GOALS OF GLOBAL RISK ASSESSMENT

An effective risk assessment must have a well-defined scope, which in turn depends on the purpose of the analysis. For example, an evaluation of emissions from a particular industrial facility is likely to concentrate on their health effects on local populations. In contrast, a project to set national environmental priorities may be much broader in scope, covering such factors as emissions of greenhouse gases and ozone-depleting substances. Some trade-offs will inevitably be required. Governments and ministries of health oversee overall population health and so, at the broadest level, need information from risk assessments that are comprehensive as well as being reliable, relevant and timely. Because the range of risks to health is almost limitless, it is essential for governments to have a quantitative approach to gauging their importance. Risks need to be defined and studied comprehensively irrespective of factors such as their place in a causal chain or the methods used (from the disciplines of the physical, natural, health, and social sciences) for their analysis. The following sections outline some of the different dimensions that should be considered.

STANDARDIZED COMPARISONS AND COMMON OUTCOME MEASURES

Ideally, the impact of each risk factor should be assessed in terms of a "common currency" that incorporates loss of quality of life as well as loss of life years. The principal metric used in this report is the DALY (disability-adjusted life year) – one DALY being equal to the loss of one healthy life year *(13)*.

A key initial question when assessing the impact of a risk to health is to ask "compared to what?" This report employs an explicit counterfactual approach, in which current distributions of risk factors are compared with some alternative, or counterfactual, distribution of exposure. Many different counterfactuals are potentially of interest. To enhance comparability across risk factors, the basis for the results in Chapter 4 is the theoretical minimum risk distribution, that is exposure levels that would yield the lowest population risk (for example, no tobacco use by any members of a population). For the analysis of the costs and effects of interventions to reduce risk in Chapter 5, a related counterfactual is used – based on the burden that would exist in the absence of relevant interventions. Risk factor distributions that are plausible, feasible and cost-effective will lie somewhere between the current risk factor levels and the related theoretical minimum. The envisaged shift from current to counterfactual scenarios has been termed the *distributional transition* (see Figure 2.1).

In many instances, the counterfactual of most relevance will involve small to moderate distributional transitions (for example, 10%, 20% or 30%), as these are most likely to be feasible and cost-effective. These estimates are also less susceptible to the influence of arbitrary choices of theoretical minima, and are likely to be the most reliable, as the dose–response is often least certain at low exposure levels.

Figure 2.1 Example of distributional transitions for blood pressure and for tobacco smoking

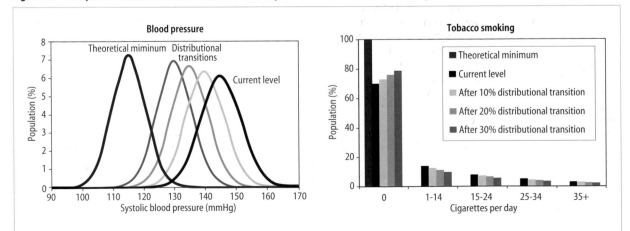

ASSESSING PROTECTIVE AS WELL AS HAZARDOUS FACTORS

Factors that affect risk of disease or injury are, of course, not all harmful. Risk factor does have a negative connotation, but ideally a risk assessment should include a range of protective as well as hazardous risk factors. For example, this report considers the protective benefits of fruit and vegetable intake and physical activity by assessing people with low levels of these factors. The important role of protective factors in adolescent health is outlined in Box 2.2.

INCLUDING PROXIMAL AND DISTAL CAUSES

Risks to health do not occur in isolation. The chain of events leading to an adverse health outcome includes both proximal and distal causes – proximal factors act directly or almost directly to cause disease, and distal causes are further back in the causal chain and act via a number of intermediary causes (see Figure 2.2). The factors that lead to someone developing disease on a particular day are likely to have their roots in a complex chain of environmental events that may have begun years previously, which in turn were shaped by broader socioeconomic determinants. For example, society and culture are linked to certain drinking patterns, which in turn influence outcomes such as coronary heart disease via physiological processes such as platelet aggregation. Clearly, there are risks over which an individual has at least some control (for example, inactivity) and risks that mostly or entirely rest at a population or group level (for example, ambient air pollution). It is essential that the whole of the causal chain is considered in the assessment of risks to health. Indeed, many risks cannot be disentangled in order to be considered in isolation, as they act at

---

Box 2.2 Protective factors

A growing body of cross-cultural evidence indicates that various psychological, social and behavioural factors are protective of health in adolescence and later life. Such protection facilitates resistance to disease, minimizes and delays the emergence of disabilities, and promotes more rapid recovery from illness.

Among the psychosocial factors that have been linked to protection in adults are: an optimistic outlook on life with a sense of purpose and direction, effective strategies for coping with challenge, perceived control over life outcomes, and expressions of positive emotion. Epidemiological studies have shown reduced morbidity and delayed mortality among people who are socially integrated. The quality of social relationships in the home (parent–child relations and spousal ties) and the workplace (employer–employee relations and coworker connections) are now recognized as key influences on physical and mental health. A growing literature underscores the protective health benefits associated with persistently positive and emotionally rewarding social relationships. Positive

health behaviours (e.g., proper diet and adequate exercise, and avoiding cigarettes, drugs, excessive alcohol and risky sexual practices) are also influenced by psychosocial factors.

The presence of psychosocial factors in understanding positive human health points to new directions for research and practice. The biological mechanisms through which psychosocial and behavioural factors influence health are a flourishing area of scientific inquiry: investigations in affective neuroscience are relating emotional experience to neural structures, function, dynamics and their health consequences. There is a need for greater emphasis in policy and practice on interventions built around the growing knowledge that psychosocial factors protect health.

Adolescence is a critical life stage when lifestyle choices are established, including health-related behaviours with impacts throughout life. Recent research has begun to focus on the role of protective factors in youth behaviour, complementing previous approaches concerned only with problems and risk taking.

Evidence from 25 developing countries, 25 European countries, Canada, Israel and the United States shows that adolescents who report having a positive connection to a trusted adult (parent or teacher) are committed to school, have a sense of spirituality and exhibit a significantly lower prevalence of risky behaviours. This is in addition to being more socially competent and showing higher self-esteem than adolescents without such a connection. Studies in the US have shown that these protective factors also predict positive outcomes (remaining connected to school, engaging in more exercise and having healthy diets) while diminishing negative behaviour (problem drinking, use of marijuana and other illicit drugs, and delinquent behaviour).

Protective factors promote positive behaviours and inhibit risk behaviours, hence mitigating the impacts of exposure to risk. Current efforts to reduce risks in the lives of adolescents should be broadened to include the strengthening of protective factors.

Sources: *(14–19).*

different levels, which vary over time. An appropriate range of policies can be generated only if a range of risks is assessed.

There are many trade-offs between assessments of proximal and distal causes. As one moves further from the direct, proximal causes of disease there can be a decrease in causal certainty and consistency, often accompanied by increasing complexity. Conversely, distal causes are likely to have amplifying effects – they can affect many different sets of proximal causes and so have the potential to make very large differences (20). In addition, many distal risks to health, such as climate change or socioeconomic disparity, cannot appropriately be defined at the individual level. A population's health may also reflect more than a simple aggregation of the risk factor profile and health status of its individual members, being a collective characteristic and a public good that in turn affects the health status of its members (21).

Research into the different levels of risks should be seen as complementary. There is considerable importance in knowing the population-level determinants of major proximal risks to health such as smoking. Similarly, there is value in knowing the mechanisms through which distal determinants operate. Understanding both proximal and distal risks requires contributions from different scientific traditions and different areas of health impact: environmental, communicable, noncommunicable, injury, and so on, and as a result different intellectual tools and methods, including those of health, physical and social sciences. This in turn requires consideration of the context of particular risks: some are likely always to have negative health effects (for example, tobacco use) while others may have a role that changes from setting to setting (for example, breastfeeding protects against diarrhoeal disease, to an extent that depends on the prevalent patterns of diarrhoea). Also, the same risk can be measured and quantified at various levels depending on measurement technology

Figure 2.2 Causal chains of exposure leading to disease

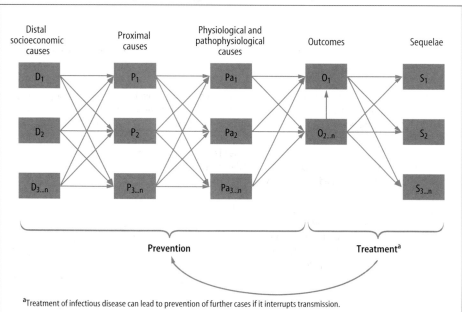

[a]Treatment of infectious disease can lead to prevention of further cases if it interrupts transmission.

An example:
Distal socioeconomic causes include income, education and occupation, all of which affect levels of proximal factors such as inactivity, diet, tobacco use and alcohol intake; these interact with physiological and pathophysiological causes, such as blood pressure, cholesterol levels and glucose metabolism, to cause cardiovascular disease such as stroke or coronary heart disease. The sequelae include death and disability, such as angina or hemiplegia.

and policy needs. For example, measuring iodine levels in food and in the environment requires different tools and the results have different implications.

When distal exposures operate through different levels of risk factors, their full impact may not be captured in traditional regression analysis methods in which both proximal and distal variables are included. More complex multilevel models and characterization of causal webs of interactions among risk factors may lead to more appropriate estimates, as well as facilitating estimation of the effect of simultaneous changes in two or more risk factor distributions. Some examples are shown later in the report.

Risk factors can also be separated from outcomes in time, sometimes by many decades. Box 2.3 shows how disadvantage can be accumulated across the life course.

ASSESSING POPULATION-WIDE RISKS AS WELL AS HIGH-RISK INDIVIDUALS

Many risks to health are widely distributed in the population, with individuals differing in the extent of their risk rather than whether they are at risk or not. Binary categorization into "exposed" and "unexposed" can substantially underestimate the importance of continuous risk factor–disease relationships. Consequently, much of this report estimates the effects of shifting distributions of exposures by applying a counterfactual approach, that is, by comparing the burden caused by the observed risk factor distribution with that expected from some alternative, or counterfactual, distribution. This approach allows assessment of population-wide interventions (see Box 2.4 and Figure 2.3).

INCLUDING RISKS THAT ACT TOGETHER TO CAUSE DISEASE

Many risks to health act jointly to cause disease or injury, and this has important implications for prevention opportunities, as outlined in Box 2.5. This report presents estimates of the individual effects of different selected risks to health, followed by analyses of the joint effect of selected clusters of risks.

Box 2.3 Risks to health across the life course

In recent years, a life-course approach to the study of health and illness – which suggests that exposure to disadvantageous experiences and environments accumulates throughout life and increases the risk of illness and premature death – has helped to explain the existence of wide socioeconomic differentials in adult morbidity and mortality rates.

Chronic illness in childhood, more common among children of manual workers, can have long-term consequences both for health and socioeconomic circumstances in later life. Slow growth in childhood (short stature for age and sex) is an indicator of early disadvantage. Early material and psychosocial disadvantage may also have an adverse impact on psychological and

cognitive development, which in turn may affect health and labour-market success later in life. The impact of living and working environments – and lifestyle factors such as smoking – on health inequalities has long been recognized. Cumulative differential lifetime exposure to health-damaging or health-promoting environments appears to be the main explanation for observed variations in health and life expectancy by socioeconomic status.

Disadvantage may begin even before birth: low birth weight is associated with increased rates of coronary heart disease, stroke, hypertension and non-insulin-dependent diabetes. These associations extend across the normal range of birth weight and depend on lower birth weights in relation to the duration of gestation rather than the

effects of premature birth. The associations may be a consequence of "programming", whereby a stimulus or insult at a critical, sensitive period of early life has permanent effects on structure, physiology and metabolism. Programming of the fetus may result from adaptations invoked when the maternal–placental nutrient supply fails to match the fetal nutrient demand. Although the influences that impair fetal development and programme adult cardiovascular disease remain to be defined, there are strong pointers to the importance of maternal body composition and dietary balance during pregnancy.

Sources: *(22–24).*

USING BEST AVAILABLE EVIDENCE TO ASSESS CERTAIN AND PROBABLE RISKS TO HEALTH

It is important in any risk assessment to review quantitatively the best available evidence for both "definite" and "probable" risks. Estimation of the potential impact of a health hazard can never wait until perfect data are available, since that is unlikely to occur. Timeliness is essential. This area can be a source of tension between scientists and policy-makers. However, arguments are often clouded by the use of dichotomies – assertions of uncertainty or certainty when, in fact, there are different degrees of uncertainty and disagreement about tolerable thresholds. Similarly, it may be asserted that there are no data when some indirect data are available, or at least the range of levels in other parts of the world is known. For example, in estimating fruit and vegetable intake for countries with no known surveys on this topic, upper and lower ranges can be estimated from surveys undertaken elsewhere, and food sales and agricultural data can be used to produce indirect estimates that occupy a narrower range. Internal consistency can help put ranges on uncertainty: for example, mortality rates, population numbers and birth rates should be internally consistent, and reliable estimates for some of these components will put bounds on the uncertainty of the others. However, as outlined earlier, the sum of causes is unbounded and so internal consistency checks cannot be performed in assessments of different risks to health. Strategies to minimize this problem include full documentation of data sources, methods and assumptions, extensive peer review, explicit assessments of causality, and quantitative estimates of other uncertainty.

Box 2.4 Population-wide strategies for prevention

"It makes little sense to expect individuals to behave differently from their peers; it is more appropriate to seek a general change in behavioural norms and in the circumstances which facilitate their adoption." – Geoffrey Rose, 1992.

The distribution and determinants of risks in a population have major implications for strategies of prevention. Geoffrey Rose observed, like others before and since, that for the vast majority of diseases "nature presents us with a process or continuum, not a dichotomy". Risk typically increases across the spectrum of a risk factor. Use of dichotomous labels such as "hypertensive" and "normotensive" are therefore not a description of the natural order, but rather an operational convenience. Following this line of thought, it becomes obvious that the "deviant minority" (e.g. hypertensives) who are considered to be at high risk are only part of a risk continuum, rather than a distinct group. This leads to one of the most fundamental axioms in preventive medicine: "a large number of people exposed to a small risk may generate many more cases than a small number exposed to high risk". Rose pointed out that wherever this axiom applies, a preventive strategy focusing on high-risk individuals will deal only with the margin of the problem and will not have any impact on the large proportion of disease occurring in the large proportion of people who are at moderate risk. For example,

people with slightly raised blood pressure suffer more cardiovascular events than the hypertensive minority. While a high-risk approach may appear more appropriate to the individuals and their physicians, it can only have a limited effect at a population level. It does not alter the underlying causes of illness, relies on having adequate power to predict future disease, and requires continued and expensive screening for new high-risk individuals.

In contrast, population-based strategies that seek to shift the whole distribution of risk factors have the potential to control population incidence. Such strategies aim to make healthy behaviours and reduced exposures into social norms and thus lower the risk in the entire population. The potential gains are extensive, but the challenges are great as well – a preventive measure that brings large benefits to the community appears to offer little to each participating individual. This may adversely affect motivation of the population at large (known as the "prevention paradox").

Although most often applied to cardiovascular disease prevention, a population-wide approach is often relevant in other areas. For example,

a high-risk strategy for melanoma prevention might seek to identify and target individuals with three or more risk factors (such as a number of moles, blonde or auburn hair, previous sunburn, and a family history of skin cancer). However, only 24% of cases of melanoma occur in this 9% of the population, so a targeted approach would succeed in identifying those at high risk but would do little for population levels of melanoma – 75% of cases occur in the 58% of the population with at least one risk factor. A population-wide strategy would seek to make sun protection a social norm, so that the whole population is less exposed to risk.

These approaches are complementary: a population approach can work to improve and extend the coverage of a high-risk approach. A key challenge is finding the right balance between population-wide and high-risk approaches. Rose concluded that this will require a wider world view of ill-health, its causes and solutions, and will lead to acknowledgement that the primary determinants of disease are mainly economic and social, and therefore remedies must also be economic and social.

Sources: *(20, 25, 26).*

Figure 2.3 The importance of population distributions of exposure

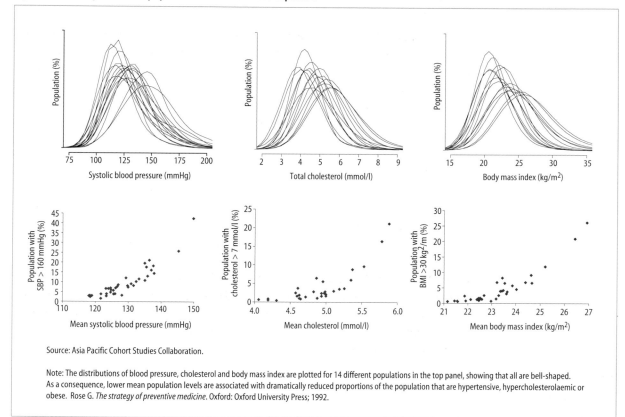

Source: Asia Pacific Cohort Studies Collaboration.

Note: The distributions of blood pressure, cholesterol and body mass index are plotted for 14 different populations in the top panel, showing that all are bell-shaped. As a consequence, lower mean population levels are associated with dramatically reduced proportions of the population that are hypertensive, hypercholesterolaemic or obese. Rose G. *The strategy of preventive medicine.* Oxford: Oxford University Press; 1992.

Extrapolations and indirect methods are often justified where there are implications in delaying estimates of health impacts and subsequent policy choices. If decisions await improved estimates, then not producing best current estimates (with appropriate indications of uncertainty) may mean inappropriate inaction. Alternatively, decisions may be made with other even more uncertain information, where the uncertainty will often be implicit. Nonetheless, there can be costs in making incorrect estimates and, ultimately, it is largely a matter of judgement to decide when data are adequate.

Whenever possible, the level of uncertainty should be reported explicitly in risk assessments. There is still considerable debate about how this is best done in a policy-relevant way, given the inevitable play of chance and uncertainties in both the likelihood of causality and the validity of the estimation methods. Major uncertainty should result in calls for more data. In particular, data are often absent or scanty in the developing countries, where many risks are highest and more information could produce the greatest gains in knowledge. The management of highly uncertain risks and the use of the precautionary principle are discussed in Chapter 6.

ASSESSING AVOIDABLE AS WELL AS ATTRIBUTABLE BURDEN

Risk assessments to date have typically used only attributable risk estimates, basically addressing the question "what proportion of current burden is caused by the accumulated effects of all prior exposure?" However, often a more policy-relevant question is "what are the likely future effects of partial removal of current exposure?" Two key developments are therefore needed: an explicit focus on future effects and on less-than-complete risk factor changes. This report presents estimates of attributable burden (current burden due to past exposure) and of avoidable burden (the proportion of future burden avoidable if current and future exposure levels are reduced to those specified by some alternative, or counterfactual, distribution). When the time between exposure and disease or death is short, the distinction between attributable and avoidable burden is not critical. However, for risk factors such as tobacco and some occupational exposures, a long time lag between exposure and health outcome may result in a major difference between attributable and avoidable burden. The distinction between attributable and avoidable burden is shown graphically in Figure 2.4.

OVERVIEW OF RISK ASSESSMENT METHODS

The overall aim of the analyses reported here was to obtain reliable and comparable estimates of attributable and avoidable burden of disease and injury, for selected risk factors. More specifically, the objectives were to estimate, by age, sex and region, for selected risk factors:

- attributable burden of disease and injury for 2000, compared to the theoretical minimum;
- avoidable burden of disease and injury in 2010, 2020 and 2030, for a standardized range of reductions in risk factors.

Box 2.5 Multiple causes of disease

The impact of a single risk factor on disease is often summarized as the proportion of disease caused by, or attributable to, that risk factor. The fact that diseases and injuries are caused by the joint action of two or more risk factors means that the sum of their separate contributions can easily be more than 100%. Consider a hypothetical situation of deaths from car crashes on a hazardous stretch of road. Studies may have shown that they could be reduced by 20% by using headlights in daytime, 40% by stricter speed limits, 50% by installing more traffic lights, and 90% by creating speed bumps.

As a further example consider a smoker, also a heavy drinker, who develops throat cancer. The cancer would not have developed on that particular day if the person had not smoked or drunk heavily: it was very likely caused by both tobacco and alcohol. There are three possible scenarios for throat cancer, each with a different set of causes that must be present for the disease to occur. In the first scenario, smoking and alcohol work together with other environmental and genetic causes to result in the disease ("environ-

mental" can be taken as all non-genetic causes). The second scenario is the same, except that throat cancer develops in a non-drinker. In the third, we do not know what caused the cancer, other than genetic and some unknown environmental causes. This simplified model illustrates the following important issues.

- Causes can add to more than 100%. If the scenarios were equally common, 66.6% of throat cancer would be attributable to smoking, 33.3% to alcohol, 100% to genetic causes, and 100% to unknown environmental causes, making a total of 300%. Causes can, and ideally should, total more than 100%; this is an inevitable result of different causes working together to produce disease, and reflects the extent of our knowledge of disease causation.
- Multicausality offers opportunities to tailor prevention. If these scenarios were numerically correct, throat cancer could be reduced by up to two-thirds with smoking cessation, by up to one-third with reduced alcohol intake, or by up to two-thirds with less marked decreases in both smoking and alcohol consumption. Fur-

ther reductions could also take place if research led to additional preventive strategies based on genetic or other environmental causes. The key message of multicausality is that different sets of interventions can produce the same goal, with the choice of intervention being determined by such considerations as cost, availability and preferences. Even the most apparently single-cause conditions are on closer inspection multicausal; the tubercle bacillus may seem to be the single cause of tuberculosis but, as improved housing has been shown to reduce the disease, living conditions must also be considered a cause.

- Prevention need not wait until further causes are elucidated. In the foreseeable future we will not know all the causes of disease, or how to avoid all the disease burden attributable to genetic causes. Nonetheless, multicausality means that in many cases considerable gains can be achieved by reducing the risks to health that are already known.

Sources: *(27, 28)*

Standard WHO age groups were chosen (0–4, 5–14, 15–24, 25–44, 45–59, 60–69, 70–79, and 80+ years) and epidemiological subregions were based on WHO regions, subdivided by mortality patterns (see the List of Member States by WHO Region and mortality stratum).

The methodology involved calculating population attributable risk, or where multi-level data were available, potential impact fractions. These measures estimate the proportional reduction in disease burden resulting from a specific change in the distribution of a risk factor. The potential impact fraction (PIF) is given by the following equation:

$$PIF = \frac{\sum\limits_{i=1}^{n} P_i\,(RR_i-1)}{\sum\limits_{i=1}^{n} P_i\,(RR_i-1) + 1}$$

where RR is the relative risk at a given exposure level, P is the population level or distribution of exposure, and n is the maximum exposure level.

Potential impact fractions require three main categories of data input, as summarized in Figure 2.5. The relationship between these key input variables and the basic methodology involved in calculating and applying population attributable fractions is summarized in Figure 2.6. It is clear from Figure 2.6 that risk factors that are more prevalent or that affect common diseases can be responsible for a greater attributable burden than other risk factors that have much higher relative risks.

Figure 2.4 Attributable and avoidable burdens

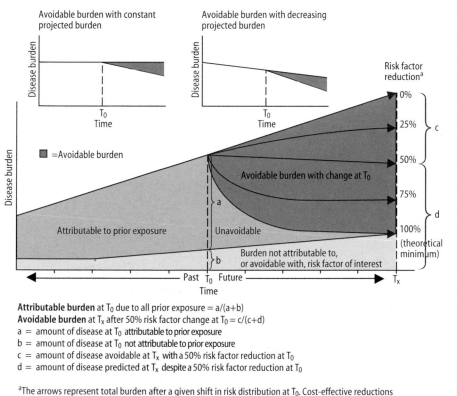

Attributable burden at T_0 due to all prior exposure = a/(a+b)
Avoidable burden at T_x after 50% risk factor change at T_0 = c/(c+d)
a = amount of disease at T_0 attributable to prior exposure
b = amount of disease at T_0 not attributable to prior exposure
c = amount of disease avoidable at T_x with a 50% risk factor reduction at T_0
d = amount of disease predicted at T_x despite a 50% risk factor reduction at T_0

[a]The arrows represent total burden after a given shift in risk distribution at T_0. Cost-effective reductions for age, sex and region groups can be chosen from the range of risk factor reductions that are evaluated.

CHOOSING AND DEFINING RISKS TO HEALTH

The risk factors assessed in this report were chosen with the following considerations in mind.

- Potential global impact: likely to be among leading causes of disease burden as a result of high prevalence and/or large increases in risk for major types of death and disability.
- High likelihood of causality.
- Potential modifiability.
- Neither too specific nor too broad (for example, environmental hazards as a whole).
- Availability of reasonably complete data on risk factor distributions and risk factor–disease relationships.

There is unavoidably an arbitrary component to any choice of risk factors for assessment, as time and resource constraints will always operate and trade-offs will be required. For example, some factors like global warming where data are substantially incomplete may nonetheless be of such potential importance that they should be included and their impact estimated based on possible scenarios and theoretical models. These trade-offs should be made clear when the data sources, methods and results are reported in detail, including estimation of uncertainty.

Clearly, one risk factor can lead to many outcomes, and one outcome can be caused by many risk factors. For each possible risk factor–burden relationship, a systematic and documented assessment of causality was performed. Many approaches have been proposed for the assessment of causality. One that is widely known and reasonably well accepted is the set of "standards" proposed by Hill *(29)*. These are not indisputable rules for causation, and Hill emphasized that they should not be taken directly as a score. It is, however, widely agreed that a judgement of causality should be increasingly confident with the accumulation of satisfied standards including the following.

Figure 2.5 Key inputs for assessment of attributable and avoidable burdens

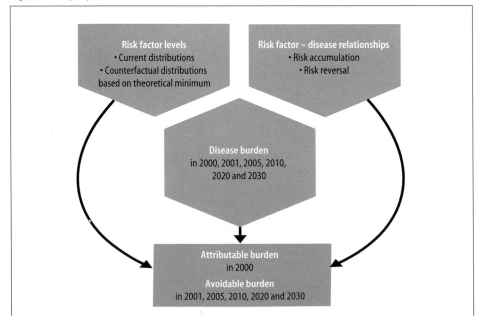

- **Temporality** – Cause must precede effect in time.
- **Strength** – Strong associations that are credible are more likely to be causal than weak associations, because if a strong association were wholly to result from some other factor, then it is more likely that other factor would be apparent. But a weak association does not rule out a causal connection.
- **Consistency** – Repeated observations of associations in different populations under different circumstances increase a belief that they are causal. But some effects are produced by their causes only under specific circumstances.
- **Biological gradient** – Presence of a dose–response curve suggests causality, although some causal associations do have a threshold, and for others the dose–response can arise from confounding factors.
- **Plausibility** – Biological plausibility is relevant, but can be subjective and is based on current level of knowledge and beliefs.
- **Experimental evidence** – Experimental evidence, in which some groups differ only with respect to the risk factor of interest, provides powerful evidence of causation. But evidence from human experiments is often not available.

Systematic assessments of causality, along with the other criteria listed above, led to the inclusion in this report of a number of risks to health and affected outcomes, which are discussed in Chapter 4.

Figure 2.6 Determination of attributable burden, taking account of prevalence and relative risk

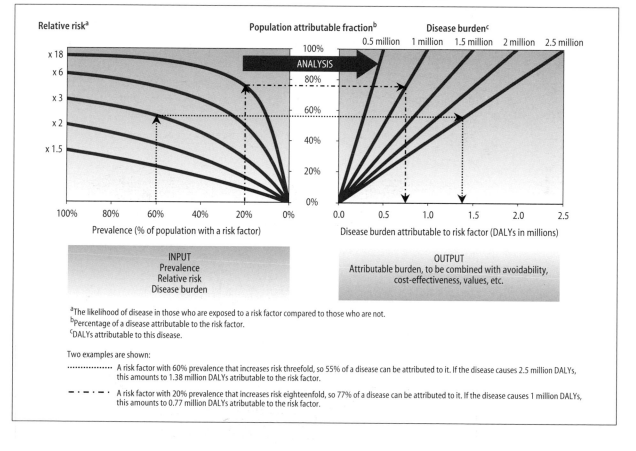

[a]The likelihood of disease in those who are exposed to a risk factor compared to those who are not.
[b]Percentage of a disease attributable to the risk factor.
[c]DALYs attributable to this disease.

Two examples are shown:

················· A risk factor with 60% prevalence that increases risk threefold, so 55% of a disease can be attributed to it. If the disease causes 2.5 million DALYs, this amounts to 1.38 million DALYs atributable to the risk factor.

— · — · — · A risk factor with 20% prevalence that increases risk eighteenfold, so 77% of a disease can be attributed to it. If the disease causes 1 million DALYs, this amounts to 0.77 million DALYs atributable to the risk factor.

ESTIMATING CURRENT RISK FACTOR LEVELS AND CHOOSING COUNTERFACTUALS

Risk factor levels in the population are the first main data input in estimating potential impact fractions. Extensive searches were required to estimate risk factor levels by the 224 age, sex and country groups used as the basis for analysis, particularly for data in economically developing countries. For all risk factors, there was a need to extrapolate data to some age, sex and country groups for which direct information was not available. Wherever possible, this extrapolation was based on generalizing from a particular subgroup that had similar health, demographic, socioeconomic or other relevant indicators.

The theoretical minimum was chosen as the counterfactual for all risk factors. For risk factors for which zero is not possible (for example, cholesterol), the theoretical minimum was the distribution associated with lowest overall risk. For some exposures (such as alcohol) there may be subgroups (by region, age or sex) for which zero exposure may not always be associated with the lowest risk. To maximize comparability, however, the theoretical minimum counterfactual was taken to be the same across population groups. This aided overall interpretation of the results, avoiding "shifting goal posts", yet still allowed for estimation of when minimum risks occurred at non-zero levels. Since policy-relevant reductions are likely to vary by, for example, age, sex or region, a range of estimates was made for counterfactual distributions at set intervals between the current situation and the theoretical minimum.

For the purposes of this report, risk factors were defined in light of data availability, the requirement for consistency, and a preference to assess multiple levels of exposure and hence the likely impact of shifting the risk factor distribution in the population.

ESTIMATING CURRENT AND FUTURE DISEASE AND INJURY BURDEN

The second data input into potential impact fractions is information on amounts of burden of disease and injury in the population, by age, sex and region. Current and future disease and injury burden was estimated as part of the ongoing global burden of disease project *(30)*.

ESTIMATING RISK FACTOR–BURDEN RELATIONSHIPS

The third data input into potential impact fractions comprised estimates of risk factor–burden relationships by age, sex and subregion. For most risks, direct information on such relationships came only from developed countries. This highlights the importance of assessing generalizability of data, in view of the need to extrapolate results to age, sex and region groups for which direct evidence is not available. For risk factor levels, there is often no particular reason to expect levels to be consistent between regions. Risk factor–disease relationships will, however, often be more generalizable, since they may, at least in part, be intrinsic biological relationships. Consistency between the results of reliable studies conducted in different settings is an indicator of causality and generalizability. While the representativeness of a study population is an essential component of extrapolating results for risk factor levels, study reliability and comparability will often be more important in assessing risk factor–disease relationships. Since relative risks tend to be the most generalizable entity, these were typically reported. When relative risk per unit exposure varied between populations, this was incorporated wherever possible. For example, the relative risk for current tobacco smoking and heart disease appears to be less in the People's Republic of China than in North America and Europe, principally because of a shorter history of smoking among the Chinese.

Estimates of avoidable burden

Current action to target risks to health can change the future but cannot alter the past. Future disease burden can be avoided but nothing can be done about attributable burden. For this analysis, avoidable burden was defined as the fraction of disease burden in a particular year that would be avoided with a specified alternative current and future exposure. Estimates of avoidable burden are particularly challenging, given that they involve all the uncertainty in the estimates of attributable burden plus those in a number of extra data inputs, described below.

- Projected global burden of disease.
- Risk factor levels under a "business as usual" scenario. Some projections were based on observed trends over the past few decades (for example, childhood malnutrition) and others based on models using exposure determinants and their expected trends (for example, physical inactivity, indoor smoke from solid fuels).
- Projected risk factor levels under a counterfactual scenario – for example, a 25% transition towards the theoretical minimum, starting from 2000 and remaining at 25% of the distance from business as usual and theoretical minimum exposure.
- Estimates of risk "reversibility". These may occur to different extents and over different time frames for various risk factor–burden relationships. After some time, the excess risk of a "previously exposed" group may reach that of the "never exposed" group, or may only be partially reversed. For all acute or almost-acute hazards, including injuries and childhood mortality risk factors, immediate reversibility was assumed. The impact of cessation of the use of alcohol and illicit drugs on neuropsychological diseases, while known to be delayed, was assumed to be fully reversed by 2010, the earliest reporting year. Thus ex-exposed in 2010 were assumed to have the same risk as never-exposed. For blood pressure *(31, 32)* and cholesterol *(33)*, most or all of the risks were assumed to be reversed within five years and all within 10 years. Since more distal risk factors such as obesity and physical inactivity operate in large part through these exposures, these data formed the basis of risk reversibility for other major causes of cardiovascular disease assessed here. For tobacco, data on risk reversibility after smoking cessation was obtained from the large American Cancer Society's Cancer Prevention Study *(34)*. This evidence shows that most excess risk for cancer, and almost all for vascular disease, is avoided within a decade of cessation. In the absence of similar studies for other risk factors, these data were also used to estimate the temporal relation between exposure reduction for other carcinogens and airborne particles and cause-specific disease outcomes. Lastly, a time-lag factor was used when appropriate, for example with childhood sexual abuse, reflecting the delay between cessation of abuse and the lower risks of adult mental health problems.

Estimating the joint effects of multiple risks

The main estimates presented in this report are for burden resulting from single risk factors, with the assumption that all others are held constant. Such estimates are valuable for comparative assessments, but there is also a need for estimates of the net effects of clusters of risk factors. When two risks affect different diseases, then clearly their net effects are simply the sum of their separate effects. However, when they affect the same disease or injury outcomes, then the net effects may be less or more than the sum of their separate effects. The size of these joint effects depends principally on the amount of prevalence overlap (for example, how much more likely people who smoke are to drink alcohol) and the biological effects of joint exposures (for example, whether the risks of alcohol are greater among those who smoke) *(27)*. However, these have very little influence on net effects when the population attributable fractions are high for individual risk factors, as was often the case in these analyses – for example, more than 80% of diarrhoeal disease was attributed to unsafe water, sanitation and hygiene. The data requirements for ideal assessment of joint effects are substantial and assumptions were made of multiplicatively independent relative risks, except for empirical assessments of joint effects for two main clusters – risk factors that are major causes of cardiovascular disease and those that are major causes of childhood mortality. An alternative approach is outlined in Box 2.6. This simulation method based on individual participant data from a single cohort is compatible with the joint effects estimated from aggregate data as described above.

ESTIMATES OF UNCERTAINTY

Confidence intervals for the attributable burden were estimated by a simulation procedure *(37)* incorporating sources of uncertainty from domains of the exposure distribution and the exposure–response relationships. Briefly, the method involved simultaneously varying all input parameters within their respective distributions and reiterating the calculation of the population attributable fraction. An uncertainty distribution around each estimate of population attributable fraction was obtained after 500 iterations of the simulation and, from this, 95% confidence intervals were derived. Each risk factor group provided data characterizing the uncertainty in the estimates of exposure distribution and exposure–response relationships. To the extent possible, the uncertainty estimates accounted for statistical uncertainty in available data as well as uncertainty in the methods used to extrapolate parameters across regions or countries.

Still further refinements would improve the current estimates and are not reflected in the reported uncertainty indicators. These include uncertainty in the burden of disease estimates; lack of data on prevalence among those with disease, such data ideally being

---

Box 2.6 Estimating the combined effects of cardiovascular disease risk factors

There are several major risk factors for cardiovascular disease, and the actions of some are mediated through others. For example, overweight and obesity increase the risk of coronary disease in part through adverse effects on blood pressure, lipid profile and insulin sensitivity. The causal web model of disease causation reflects the fact that risk factors often increase not only the risk of disease, but also levels of other risk factors.

Separate estimation of the effects of individual risk factors does not typically take into account the effect of changes on the levels of other risk factors. One way of achieving this is to use measured relationships between the levels of the different risk factors to simulate what would happen in a 'counterfactual cohort', if levels of one or more risk factors were altered. The relationship between levels of risk factors

Sources: *(35, 36)*.

and disease can then be used to determine the rate of disease in the simulated cohort. The proportion of people in the population that would develop coronary heart disease (CHD) under each intervention is a counterfactual (unobserved) quantity. The g-formula (Robins, 1986) is a general nonparametric method that allows estimation of the counterfactual proportions under the assumption of no unmeasured confounders. This approach was taken using data from the Framingham Offspring Study on the risk factors body mass index, smoking, alcohol consumption, diabetes, cholesterol and systolic blood pressure.

A formula for predicting risk of CHD, given risk factor history, was estimated, and also the history of the other risk factors was used to predict future values of each risk factor following changes in some. A simulated cohort was generated from the study by sampling with replacement and various

scenarios were applied to the cohort to assess the impact on 12-year CHD risk, taking into account the joint effects of all the risk factors. A combination of complete cessation of smoking, setting all individuals' body mass index to no more than 22, and a simulated mean cholesterol level of 2.3 mmol/l and corresponding variance was estimated to halve the 12-year risk of CHD in both women and men. The estimated effect of all three interventions – a 50% relative risk reduction in coronary disease – was less than a crude sum of the separate effects (19%, 9% and 31%, respectively). This is because some people suffered CHD resulting from the joint actions of two or more of the risk factors, and this model estimates the size of these joint effects.

required in population attributable fraction estimates that incorporate adjusted relative risks (38); and the likelihood that reduction of exposure to risks such as unsafe medical injections in 2000 would lead to less infection in subsequent years and also a smaller pool of infected people from whom transmission could be propagated. Finally, competing risks – for example, someone saved from a stroke in 2001 is then "available" to die from other diseases in ensuing years – have not been estimated, which is likely to lead to an overestimate of the absolute amount of attributable and avoidable disease burden, although it may not substantially affect the ranking of risk factors. However, competing risks are accounted for in the dynamic models that assessed the joint effects of risks on healthy life expectancy. This topic, along with appropriate discount rates, is considered in Chapter 5.

REFERENCES

1. Last JM, editor. *A dictionary of epidemiology*. New York: Oxford University Press; 2001.

2. Slovic P. Informing and educating the public about risk. *Risk Analysis* 1986; 6:403-15.

3. Hope T. Rationing and life-saving treatments: should identifiable patients have higher priority? *Journal of Medical Ethics* 2001; 3:179-85.

4. Murray CJL, Lopez AD. Quantifying the burden of disease and injury attributable to ten major risk factors. In: Murray CJL, Lopez AD, editors. *The global burden of disease: a comprehensive assessment of mortality and disability from diseases, injuries, and risk factors in 1990 and projected to 2020*. Cambridge (MA): Harvard University Press; 1996. p. 295-324.

5. Murray CJL, Lopez AD. Global patterns of cause of death and burden of disease in 1990, with projections to 2020. In: *Investing in health research and development. Report of the Ad Hoc Committee on Health Research Relating to Future Intervention Options*. Geneva: World Health Organization; 1996.

6. Peto R, Lopez AD, Boreham J, Thun M, Heath CW. Mortality from tobacco in developed countries: indirect estimates from national vital statistics. *Lancet* 1992; 339:1268-78.

7. English DR, Holman CDJ, Milne E, Winter MG, Hulse GK, Codde JP, et al. *The quantification of drug-caused morbidity and mortality in Australia, 1995*. Canberra: Commonwealth Department of Human Services and Health; 1995.

8. Smith KR, Corvalan CF, Kjellstrom T. How much global ill health is attributable to environmental factors? *Epidemiology* 1999; 10:573-84.

9. Rodgers A, Lawes C, MacMahon S. The global burden of cardiovascular disease conferred by raised blood pressure. Benefits of reversal of blood pressure-related cardiovascular risk in Eastern Asia. *Journal of Hypertension* 2000; 18 (Suppl):S3-S5.

10. *Determinants of the burden of disease in the European Union. Sweden 1997*. Stockholm: National Institute of Public Health Sweden; 1997.

11. Mathers C, Vos T, Stevenson C. *The burden of disease and injury in Australia*. Canberra: Australian Institute of Health and Welfare; 1999.

12. *Our health, our future. The health of New Zealanders 1999*. Wellington: Ministry of Health; 1999.

13. Murray CJL, Lopez AD, editors. *The global burden of disease: a comprehensive assessment of mortality and disability from diseases, injuries, and risk factors in 1990 and projected to 2020*. Cambridge (MA): Harvard University Press; 1996.

14. Cacioppo JT, Berntson GG, Sheridan JF, McClintock MK. Multi-level integrative analyses of human behavior. Social neuroscience and the complementing nature of social and biological approaches. *Psychological Bulletin* 2000; 126: 829-43.

15. Ryff CD, Singer B. Biopsychosocial challenges of the new millennium. *Psychotherapy and Psychosomatics* 2000; 69(4):170-7.

16. Ryff CD, Singer B. The role of emotions on pathways to positive health. In: Davidson RJ, Goldsmith HH, Scherer K, editors. *Handbook of affective science*. New York: Oxford University Press; 2002.

17. Jessor R, Van Den Bos J, Vanderryn J, Costa FM, Turbin M S. Protective factors in adolescent problem behaviours: moderator effects and developmental change. *Developmental Psychology* 1995; 31:923-33.

18. *Broadening the horizon: balancing protection and risk for adolescents*. Geneva: World Health Organization; 2002. WHO document WHO/FCH/CAH/01.20 (Revised).

19. Jessor R, Turbin MS, Costa FM. Risk and protection in successful outcomes among disadvantaged adolescents. *Applied Developmental Science* 1998; 2:194-208.

20. Rose G. *The strategy of preventive medicine*. Oxford: Oxford University Press; 1992.

21. McMichael AJ, Beaglehole R. The changing global context of public health. *Lancet* 2000; 356:495-99.

22. Winslow CEA. *The cost of sickness and the price of health*. Geneva: World Health Organization; 1951. WHO Monograph Series, No.7.

23. Barker DJP. *Mothers, babies and disease in later life*. 2nd ed. London: BMJ Publishing Group; 1998.

24. Ben-Shlomo Y, Kuh D. A life course approach to chronic disease epidemiology: conceptual models, empirical challenges and interdisciplinary perspectives. *International Journal of Epidemiology* 2002; 31:285-93.

25. Rose G. Sick individuals and sick populations. *International Journal of Epidemiology* 1985; 4:32-8.

26. Rose G, Day S. The population mean predicts the number of deviant individuals. *British Medical Journal* 1990; 301:1031-4.

27. Rothman KJ, Greenland S. *Modern epidemiology*. 2nd ed. Philadelphia: Lippincott-Raven Publishers; 1998.

28. Magnus P, Beaglehole R. The real contribution of the major risk factors to the coronary epidemics. Time to end the "only-50%" myth. *Archives of Internal Medicine* 2001; 161:2657-60.

29. Hill AB. The environment and disease: association or causation? *Proceedings of the Royal Society of Medicine* 1965;58:295-300.

30. Murray CJL, Lopez AD, Mathers CD, Stein C. *The Global Burden of Disease 2000 project: aims, methods and data sources*. Geneva: World Health Organization; 2001. Global Programme on Evidence for Health Policy Discussion Paper No. 36 (revised).

31. MacMahon S, Peto R, Cutler J, Collins R, Sorlie P, Neaton J, et al. Blood pressure, stroke, and coronary heart disease. Part 1. Prolonged differences in blood pressure: prospective observational studies corrected for the regression dilution bias. *Lancet* 1990; 335:765-74.

32. Collins R, Peto R, MacMahon S, Hebert P, Fiebach NH, Eberlein KA, et al. Blood pressure, stroke, and coronary heart disease. Part 2. Short-term reductions in blood pressure: overview of randomised drug trials in their epidemiological context. *Lancet* 1990; 335:827-38.

33. Law MR, Wald NJ, Thompson SG. By how much and how quickly does reduction in serum cholesterol concentration lower risk of ischaemic heart disease? *British Medical Journal* 1994; 308:367-73.

34. *Tobacco control country profiles*. Atlanta (GA): American Cancer Society; 2000. Also available at: URL: http://www1.worldbank.org/tobacco/countrybrief.asp

35. Robins JM. A new approach to causal inference in mortality studies with a sustained exposure period: applications to control of the healthy workers survivor effect. *Mathematical Modeling* 1986; 7:1393-512.

36. Wilson PWF, D'Agostino RB, Levy D, Belanger AM, Silbershatz H, Kannel WB. Prediction of coronary heart disease using risk factor categories. *Circulation* 1998; 97:1837-47.

37. King G, Tomz M, Wittenberg J. Making the most of statistical analysis: improving interpretation and presentation. *American Journal of Political Science* 2000; 44:341-55.

38. Rockhill B, Newman B, Weinberg C. Use and misuse of population attributable fractions. *American Journal of Public Health* 1998; 88:15-9.

CHAPTER THREE

Perceiving Risks

Both risks and benefits have to be considered when seeking to understand what drives some behaviours and why some interventions are more acceptable and successful than others. Social, cultural and economic factors are central to how individuals perceive health risks. Similarly, societal and structural factors can influence which risk control policies are adopted and the impact that interventions can achieve. Preventing risk factors has to be planned within the context of local society, bearing in mind that the success of preventive interventions is only partly a matter of individual circumstances and education. In designing intervention strategies, it cannot automatically be assumed that the diverse groups which make up the general public think in the same way as public health professionals and other risk experts. In addition, estimates of risk and its consequences, presented in scientific terms based on a risk assessment, have to be communicated with particular caution and care. The best way is for well-respected professionals, who are seen to be independent and credible, to make the communications. An atmosphere of trust between the government and all interested parties, in both the public and private sectors, is essential if interventions are to be adopted and successfully implemented.

3

PERCEIVING RISKS

CHANGING PERCEPTIONS OF RISK

*G*iven the research on the global burden of risks to health, together with the analysis that underpins the choice of cost-effective interventions, what lessons have been learned about risk perceptions? For high priority risks, how can we implement more effective risk avoidance and reduction policies in the future?

This chapter starts with an overview of how the study of risk analysis has developed since the 1970s. It then draws attention to the need to have a broad perspective on how risks are defined and perceived in society, both by individuals and by different groups. Next, emphasis is given to the importance of improving communications about health risks if successful strategies are to be adopted to control them. However, risk perceptions all over the world are increasingly being influenced by three other trends. First, by the power and influence of special interest groups connected to corporate business interests and the opposition being organized by many advocacy and public health groups. Second, by the increasing influence of the global mass media. And third, by the increase in risk factors within many middle and low income countries as a consequence of the effects of globalization.

Until recently, risks to health were defined largely from the scientific perspective, even though it has been recognized for some time that risks are commonly understood and interpreted very differently by different groups in society, such as scientists, professionals, managers, the general public and politicians. Assessment and management of risks to health is a relatively new area of study that has been expanding steadily since the early 1970s. It began by focusing on developing scientific methods for identifying and describing hazards and for assessing the probability of associated adverse outcome events and their consequences. Particular attention has been given to the type and scale of the adverse consequences, including any likely mortality. In the early years, risk analysis, as it was then called, was seen mainly as a new scientific activity concerned with environmental and other external threats to health, such as chemical exposures, road traffic accidents, and radiation and nuclear power disasters. The early study of risk developed mainly in the USA and Europe *(1)*.

During the early 1980s, risk analysis evolved into the two main phases of risk assessment and risk management, as more attention was given to how hazards or risk factors could be controlled at both the individual level and by society as a whole. The emphasis moved from determining the probability of adverse events for different risk factors to assessing the scale and range of possible consequences. Deaths are commonly seen as one of the most important consequences. Attempts were also made to reduce any uncertainties in making the scientific estimates *(2)*. An important consequence of this change was that individual people were now seen as being mainly responsibility for handling their own risks to health, since many risks were characterized as behavioural in origin and, therefore, largely under individual control. This in turn led to the lifestyles approach in health promotion. For instance, a great deal of attention was paid to combating coronary heart disease through health promotion aimed at high-risk individuals, such as increasing exercise and lowering dietary cholesterol, while policies for combating cigarette smoking also emphasized the importance of individual choice.

The need for stronger government regulatory controls also became more apparent, with two other important developments. First, governments in many industrialized countries saw their role as law enforcers and passed legislation to establish new and powerful public regulatory agencies, such as the Food and Drug Administration (FDA) in the USA and the Health and Safety Executive (HSE) in the United Kingdom. Second, increased attention was given to deriving minimum acceptable exposure levels and the adoption of many new international safety standards, particularly for environmental and chemical risks. This included, for example, risks associated with air pollutants, vehicle emissions, foods and the use of agricultural chemicals.

QUESTIONING THE SCIENCE IN RISK ASSESSMENT

The so-called scientific or quantitative approach to health risk assessment aims to produce the best possible numerical estimates of the chance or probability of adverse health outcomes for use in policy-making. Although high credibility is usually given to this approach, how valid is this assumption? Why is this approach often seen as more valid than the judgements made by the public or social scientists?

Although risk assessment appears to follow a scientifically logical sequence, in practice there are considerable difficulties in making "objective" decisions at each step in the calculations. Thus the risk modeller has to adopt a specific definition of risk and needs to introduce into the model a series of more subjective judgements and assumptions *(3, 4)*. Many of these include implicit and subjective values, such as the numerical expression for risk, weighting the value of life at different ages, the discount rates and choice of adverse health outcomes to be included. For instance, scientific judgements may be needed on the effects of different levels of exposure or which outcomes to include, particularly which disease episodes should be counted among the adverse events.

During the 1980s, scientific predictions were seen to be rational, objective and valid, while public perceptions were believed to be largely subjective, ill-informed and, therefore, less valid. This led to risk control policies that attempted to "correct" and "educate" the public in the more valid scientific notions of risk and risk management. However, this approach was increasingly challenged by public interest and pressure groups, which asked scientists to explain their methods and assumptions. These critical challenges often revealed the high levels of scientific uncertainty that were inherent in many calculations. Such groups then became more confident, enabling them to argue strongly for the validity of their own assessments and interpretation of risks.

EMERGING IMPORTANCE OF RISK PERCEPTIONS

By the early 1990s, particularly in North America and Europe, it became apparent that relying mainly on the scientific approaches to risk assessment and management was not always achieving the expected results. It also became clear that risk had different meanings to different groups of people and that all risks had to be understood within the larger social, cultural and economic context *(5–7)*. In addition, people compare health risks with any associated benefits and they are also aware of a wide array of other relevant risks. In fact, it has been argued that concepts of risk are actually embedded within societies and their cultures, which largely determines how individuals perceive risks and the autonomy they may have to control them *(8)*. In addition, it became apparent that public perceptions of risks to health did not necessarily agree with those of the scientists, whose authority was increasingly being questioned by both the general public and politicians. Although there was considerable agreement between the public and scientists on many risk assessments, there were also some, such as nuclear power and pesticides, where there were large differences of opinion (see Box 3.1). These differences of perception often led to intense public controversy.

At the same time, there was also increasing disillusionment with the "lifestyles" approach to health promotion and education strategies, that relied on improving the health knowledge and beliefs of individuals. These approaches were not achieving sufficient behavioural change for the interventions to be judged cost-effective. For instance, the rapid emergence of HIV/AIDS demonstrated that relying on the health beliefs model for behavioural change was largely ineffective in reducing the high-risk sexual behaviours that increased transmission in the epidemic. In addition, as the general public and special interest groups, particularly those in the environmental movements, became better organized they also began challenging the motives of the large corporate businesses, such as the tobacco industry *(10)*.

By the mid-1990s, improving risk communications was seen as essential for resolving the differences between these various positions, as it became more widely accepted that both the scientific approaches and public perceptions of risk were valid. It was also generally accepted that differences in perceptions of risk had to be understood and resolved. This in turn led to the conclusion that governments and politicians had a major role to play in handling conflicts over risk policies by promoting open and transparent dialogue within society, in order to have high levels of public trust in such dialogue. A very important lesson is that high levels of trust between all parties are essential if reductions in the future global burden of risks to health are to be achieved *(11, 12)*.

Box 3.1 Perceptions of risk by scientists and the general public

"Perhaps the most important message from this research is that there is wisdom as well as error in public attitudes and perceptions. Lay people sometimes lack certain information about hazards. However, their basic conceptualisation of risk is much richer than that of experts and reflects legitimate concerns that are typically omitted from expert risk assessments. As a result, risk communication and risk management efforts are destined to fail unless they are structured as a two-way process. Each side, expert and public, has something valid to contribute. Each side must respect the insights and intelligence of the other."

Source: *(9)*. p.285.

RISK PERCEPTIONS

The assumption made in this report is that risk factors, risk probabilities and adverse events can be defined and measured. This is a valid starting point for the quantification of the adverse effects of a range of risk factors and for health advocacy. However, as we have seen above, when interpreting the global burden of risks to health and using this to design intervention strategies, wider perspectives are needed. Evaluating these risks must take place within a much broader context.

People's risk perceptions are based on a diverse array of information that they have processed on risk factors (sometimes called hazards) and technologies, as well as on their benefits and contexts. For instance, people receive information and form their values based on their past experience, communications from scientific sources and the media, as well as from family, peers and other familiar groups. This transfer and learning from experience also occurs within the context of a person's society and culture, including references to beliefs and systems of meaning. It is through the organization of all this knowledge, starting in early childhood, that individuals perceive and make sense of their world. In a similar way, perceptions of risks to health are embedded within different economic, social and cultural environments.

Much of the original impetus for research on perceptions came from the pioneering work of Starr *(13)* in trying to weigh the risks from technologies against their perceived benefits. Empirical studies of individual risk perceptions had their origins mainly in psychological studies conducted in the USA *(4, 14)*. A major early discovery was of a set of mental strategies or rules, also called heuristics, that people use to understand risks *(15)*. An early approach to study and map people's understanding of risks was to ask them to estimate the number of deaths for 40 different hazards and to compare these with known statistical estimates *(16, 17)*. This showed that people tend to overestimate the number of deaths from rarer and infrequent risks, while underestimating considerably those from common and frequent causes, such as cancers and diabetes. This finding has obvious implications for control strategies that are focused on many common and widely distributed risks to health. In addition, rare but vivid causes are even more overestimated. Familiarity and exposure through the mass media tend to reinforce these perceptions. However, people's rank ordering by the total number of deaths does usually correspond well overall with the rank order of official estimates.

Risk factors have many dimensions, including a variety of benefits, and certainly risk means far more to most people than just the possible number of deaths. Another pioneering research study, which is relevant to the present analysis of global risks to health, used psychometric testing to measure perceptions of 90 different hazards using 18 separate qualitative characteristics *(18)*. Following factor analysis these hazards were scaled depending on their degree of "dread" and their degree of "unknown risk" (see Figure 3.1, which shows 20 risks selected from the original 90). A third factor (not shown in the figure) related to the number of people involved. Figure 3.1 clearly shows that the most highly uncertain risks, such as nuclear power and pesticides, are the most dreaded, while risks associated with many health interventions and clinical procedures have more acceptable values. For instance, antibiotics, anaesthetics, childbirth and surgery are perceived as being much safer. The higher the dread factor levels and the higher the perceived unknown risks, the more people want action to reduce these risks, including through stricter government regulation and legislative controls. It appears that people often do not make a simple trade-off of benefits against perceived risks. Rather, they want stronger controls against many risks.

Risks that are both highly uncertain and highly dreaded are also clearly the most difficult to predict and control. Two very important factors for dread were found to be global catastrophe and risks that involve members of future generations. The advent of global terrorism and the development of genetically modified foods are two recent examples. Less dreaded risks tend to be those that are individual, controllable and easily reduced. The more acceptable risks are those that are known, observable and have immediate effects. In addition, the more equitable the risks, the more likely they are to be generally accepted.

It is useful to consider perceptions of dread and unknown risk in relation to public health interventions for reducing risks. If risk factors are to be controlled, the interventions should be perceived to have low dread and a low risk of adverse events. Higher risks from such interventions will normally only be accepted by individuals in the higher risk groups. However, population-wide interventions to reduce risk typically have to cover all people, even those at low risk. Thus interventions used in public health programmes need to have low dread and known low and acceptable levels of risk, combined with high safety levels. Typically, vaccination and screening programmes fall into this category, particularly as they are usually targeted at whole populations and involve many healthy people who are at low risk of getting ill and dying. The favourable perception of the public to prescribed medicines, for example, has been attributed to the direct benefits of such medicines and to the trust people place in their safety, achieved through research and testing carried out by medical and pharmaceutical professionals.

Figure 3.1 Hazards for dread and risk[a]

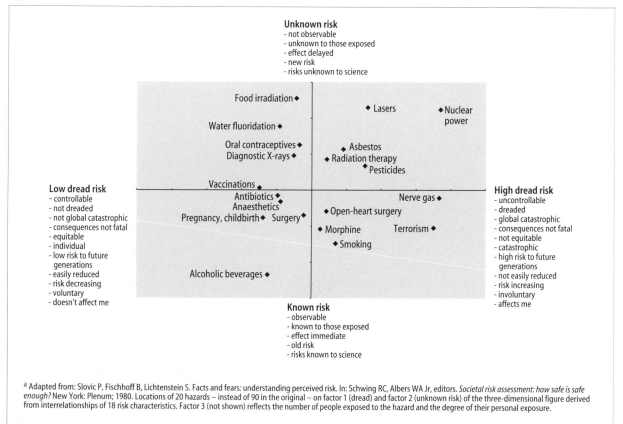

[a] Adapted from: Slovic P, Fischhoff B, Lichtenstein S. Facts and fears: understanding perceived risk. In: Schwing RC, Albers WA Jr, editors. *Societal risk assessment: how safe is safe enough?* New York: Plenum; 1980. Locations of 20 hazards – instead of 90 in the original – on factor 1 (dread) and factor 2 (unknown risk) of the three-dimensional figure derived from interrelationships of 18 risk characteristics. Factor 3 (not shown) reflects the number of people exposed to the hazard and the degree of their personal exposure.

DEFINING AND DESCRIBING RISKS TO HEALTH

Risk assessment and management is a political as well as a scientific process, and public perceptions of risk and risk factors involve values and beliefs, as well as power and trust. For policy-makers who are promoting intervention strategies to lower risks to health, it is obviously important, therefore, to understand the different ways in which the general public and health professionals perceive risks *(19)*. As described in Chapter 2, use of the term "risk" has many different meanings and this often causes difficulties in communication. This report uses the notions of the probability of a subsequent adverse health event, followed by its consequence which is mainly either morbidity or mortality.

While many scientists often assume that risks can be objectively verified, many social scientists argue that risk measures are inherently much more subjective. In addition, other members of the public have yet other notions of risk. How do people define and describe risk factors? How do they estimate risks? Answers to such questions obviously alter people's perceptions. Such information is needed, therefore, to improve communications and to predict public responses to public health interventions, including the introduction of new health technologies and risk factor and disease prevention programmes. Box 3.2 illustrates male perceptions of sexual health risks and the need to use preventive measures against HIV infection and pregnancy.

A complicated question is how the mortality outcome associated with a particular risk factor should be expressed. Even choosing or framing the end-point as death is surprisingly complex and can make large differences in the way risk is both perceived and evaluated. The following is a well-known example from occupational health, which shows how the choice of risk measure can make a technology appear less or more risky to health *(21)*. Between 1950 and 1970, coal mining in the USA became much less risky if the measure of risk was taken to be accident deaths per million tons of coal produced, but it became more risky if risk was described in terms of accident deaths per 1000 miners employed. Which measure is more appropriate for decision-making? From a national perspective, and given the need to produce coal, deaths of miners per million tons of coal produced appears to be the more appropriate measure of risk. However, from the point of view of individual miners and their trade unions the death rate per thousand miners employed is obviously far more relevant. Since both measures for framing the risks in this industry are relevant, both should be considered in any risk management decision-making process.

Each way of summarizing deaths embodies its own set of inherent and subjective values *(7)*. For example, an estimate based on reduction in life expectancy treats deaths of young people as more important than deaths of older people, who have less life expectancy to lose. However, counting all fatalities together treats all deaths of the young and old as equivalent. This approach also treats equally deaths immediately after mishaps and deaths that follow painful and lengthy debilitating diseases. Such choices all involve subjective value judgements. For instance, using "number of deaths" may not distinguish deaths of people who engage in an activity by choice and benefit from it directly, from those of people who are exposed to a hazard involuntarily and who get no direct benefits. Each approach may be justifiable but uses value judgements about which deaths are considered to be the most undesirable. To overcome such problems, information should be framed in a variety of different ways so that such complexities are revealed to decision-makers.

Box 3.2 Men's sexual behaviour related to risk of HIV infection and pregnancy

A greater understanding of men's perceptions of sexual risk and their risk-taking behaviour is necessary if interventions are to be more successful in improving the reproductive health of both men and women. In a questionnaire survey of reproductive risk behaviours in the capital cities of Argentina, Bolivia, Cuba and Peru, young adult males (aged 20–29 years) were asked whether they would take measures to prevent HIV infection and pregnancy during sexual intercourse with different categories of female partners. Samples of 750–850 men were selected randomly in each city. The percentages who reported having taken preventive measures – usually the use of condoms – to reduce the risk of HIV transmission or pregnancy are shown below.

The findings were very similar in all four cities, though the men clearly perceived the risks as being different with different partners. Preventive measures against HIV infection were believed to be highly necessary for sexual intercourse with prostitutes, strangers and lovers, but considerably less so with married partners. However, just over half the young men said they would use such measures when having intercourse with a virgin or a fiancée. The need for measures to prevent pregnancy was perceived, however, to be higher than that for HIV infection. To avoid pregnancy, such measures were commonly used with all sexual partners and even with about half the spouses.

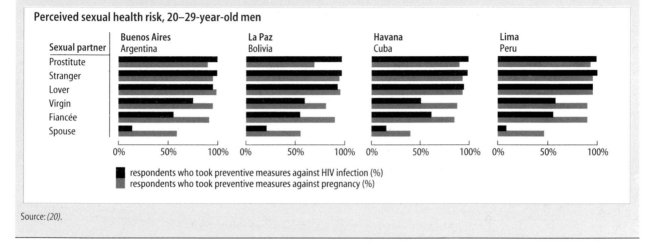

Perceived sexual health risk, 20–29-year-old men

legend:
- respondents who took preventive measures against HIV infection (%)
- respondents who took preventive measures against pregnancy (%)

Source: *(20)*.

INFLUENCES ON RISK PERCEPTIONS

Two important factors that influence risk perception are gender and world views, with affiliation, emotional affect and trust also being strongly correlated with the risk judgements of experts as well as lay persons. The influence of gender has been well documented, with men tending to judge risks as smaller and less problematic than do women. Explanations have focused mainly on biological and social factors. For example, it has been suggested that women are more socialized to care for human health and are less likely to be familiar with science and technology. However, female toxicologists were found to judge the same risks as higher than do male toxicologists *(22, 23)*. In another study dealing with perception of 25 hazards, males produced risk-perception ratings that were consistently much lower than those of females *(24)*. To the extent that sociopolitical factors shape public perception of risks, gender differences appear to have an important effect on interpreting risks.

The influence of social, psychological and political factors can also be seen in studies on the impact of world views on risk judgements. World views are general social, cultural and political attitudes that appear to have an influence over people's judgements about complex issues *(25)*. World views include feelings such as fatalism towards control over risks to health, belief in hierarchy and leaving decisions to the experts, and a conviction that individualism is an important characteristic of a fair society, or that technological developments are important for improving our health and social well-being. These world views have been found to be strongly linked to public perceptions of risk *(26)*. These views have also been the subject of a few international studies, for example comparing perceptions of risks to nuclear power in the USA with those in other industrialized countries *(27)*.

FRAMING THE INFORMATION ON RISKS

After defining a particular risk problem, determining which people are at risk, measuring exposure levels and selecting the risk outcomes, all this information has to be presented to decision-makers. How the information is presented usually depends on whether it is meant to influence individuals or national policy-makers. The way the information is presented is often referred to as "framing" (see Box 3.3).

Numerous research studies have demonstrated that different but logically equivalent ways of presenting the same risk information can lead to different evaluations and decisions. A famous example is the study which asked people to imagine that they had lung cancer and had to choose either surgery or radiation therapy *(29)*. The choices were strikingly different, depending on whether the results of treatment were framed as the probability of surviving for varying lengths of time after the treatment or in terms of the probability of dying. When the same results were framed in terms of dying, the choice of radiation therapy over surgery increased from 18% to 44%. The effect was just as strong for physicians as for lay persons.

All presentations of risk information use frames that can exert a strong influence on decision-makers. However, if all information is equally correct, there are really no "right" or "wrong" frames – just different frames. How risk information is framed and communicated to individuals or policy-makers, scientists or the general public can be of crucial importance in achieving maximum influence over public perceptions. It can also be very important in convincing the public health community and high-level policy-makers about the importance of risks to health and the value of adopting different interventions.

SOCIAL AND CULTURAL INTERPRETATIONS OF RISK

While the cognitive psychological approach has been very influential, it has also been criticized for concentrating too much on individual perceptions and interpretations of risk. Some psychologists, anthropologists and sociologists have argued that, since individuals are not free agents, risks can best be understood as a social construct within particular historical and cultural contexts and within groups and institutions, not only at the individual level *(8)*. These disciplines start from the belief that risks should not be treated independently and separately from the complex social, cultural, economic and political circumstances in

---

Box 3.3 Framing risks to health: choosing presentations

- Positive or negative framing? Striking changes in preference can result from framing the risk in either positive or negative terms, such as lives saved or lives lost, rates of survival or mortality, improving good health or reducing risks of disease.
- Relative or absolute risks? Although relative risks are usually better understood, it can be very important to present absolute changes as well.
- Percentages or whole numbers? Probabilities are better understood as percentage changes than by comparison of whole numbers.

- Whole numbers or an analogy? Whole numbers may be less well understood than an example or analogy for the size of an adverse event.
- Small or large numbers? A small number of deaths is more easily understood than a large number, which is often incomprehensible.
- Short or long periods? A few deaths at one time or over a short period, as in a tragic accident, often have more impact than a larger number of deaths occurring discretely over a longer period of time.

Source: *(28)*.

which people experience them *(30, 31)*. Different groups of people appear to identify different risks, as well as different attributes, depending on the form of social organization and the wider political culture to which they belong *(32)*.

Although it is widely accepted that the political and economic situation at a macrolevel is a strong determinant for many risk factors, microlevel studies can examine how such factors are perceived and interpreted rationally within a given local context. Microlevel studies can also be very useful in explaining certain apparent behaviours that do not appear to be rational to the "external" public health observer. For instance, although lay people may be well aware of risk factors for coronary heart disease, they also have their own "good" and rational reasons for not following expert advice on prevention *(33)*. Thus the context in which people find themselves also largely determines the constraints they face in trying to avoid risks and the length of time over which risk can be discounted. It is an irony, however, that people living in wealthy and safer societies, with their high living standards and longer life expectancy, appear to be even more highly concerned about risks to health than people living in poorer and less safe communities. This is particularly the case with highly uncertain and highly dreaded risks.

From the cultural perspective, therefore, the type and kind of risks, as well as a person's ability to cope with them, will vary according to the individual's wider context. For instance, risk perceptions and their importance can vary between developing and developed countries, as well as with such variables as sex, age, household income, faith and cultural groups, urban and rural areas, and geographical location and climate (for example, see Box 3.4).

PERCEPTIONS OF HEALTH RISKS IN DEVELOPING COUNTRIES

Risks to health, as an area for further study, have only recently begun to receive attention in developing countries. The need to view such risks in their local context is obvious when analysing perceptions of risk in these countries, especially when risk factors are considered alongside life-threatening diseases such as tuberculosis, malaria and HIV/AIDS. There are also other daily threats, such as poverty, food insecurity and lack of income. In addition, families may face many other important "external" risks, such as political instability, violence, natural disasters and wars. Thus every day there is a whole array of risks that have to be considered by individuals and families.

Models of individual risk perception and behaviour were, however, mainly developed in industrialized countries where people have considerably higher personal autonomy and freedom to act, better access to health information, and more scope for making choices for better health. These models may be less appropriate in low and middle income countries, where illnesses and deaths are closely associated with poverty and infectious and communicable diseases *(35)*. In industrialized countries, studies of HIV/AIDS and, to a lesser extent, noncommunicable diseases such as cancer *(5)* and coronary heart disease *(33)* have been carried out using the perspectives of applied medical anthropology and sociology *(36)*. However, in developing countries where communicable diseases still cause a high proportion of the avoidable mortality, these disciplines have most frequently been coopted to help evaluate the effectiveness of disease control programmes. Perceptions of disease, use of health services and reasons for non-compliance are some areas often studied *(37)*.

For communicable diseases, it is important to differentiate perceptions of the risk of a disease from those concerned with the risk of acquiring the infection, particularly as not all infections, such as sexually transmitted infections and tuberculosis, will develop into symptomatic disease. Interrupting transmission of infections, for example through the use of measles vaccine or bednets in malaria control, is the main way in which control programmes reduce risk. In such situations, risks are often determined from the point of view of whether an effective response exists in practice. Thus effectiveness evaluation is based on such indicators as early recognition of signs for severe illness (for example, acute respiratory infections), symptoms requiring self-referral for treatment (for example, leprosy and schistosomiasis), or use of impregnated bednets to prevent malaria transmission. Much of this anthropological research for effectiveness evaluation has been supported by multilateral agencies and bilateral donors, including WHO and UNAIDS.

Because of the effects of the demographic and epidemiological transitions, many middle and low income developing country populations face existing risks from communicable diseases, as well as rapid increases in risks to health from many risk factors and noncommunicable diseases. Although avoidance of risks of infection, often perceived as risk of disease, are implicit in most biomedical and public health models of disease control in developing countries, more research from the anthropological point of view is clearly needed to place these risks in perspective among a whole array of other risks to life. Given competing risks, it cannot be assumed that if people are better informed on their exposures to risk factors they will necessarily act to change their health behaviours.

IMPORTANCE OF RISK COMMUNICATIONS

As previously discussed in this chapter, risks and risk factors can be defined more narrowly by using technical means or more broadly by using sociopolitical parameters. Experts tend to prefer a focused and narrower approach, while public groups often prefer more comprehensive definitions. How risks and risk factors are defined therefore needs to be determined by the purpose of the risk communication. Risk communication can be seen as having six main components: the aims and objectives; framing of the content and messages;

Box 3.4 Perceptions of risk in Burkina Faso

Social scientists frequently argue that risks can not be considered "real" outside their sociocultural context. However, research on health risk perceptions and behaviours has often focused only on a particular disease, such as HIV/AIDS, tuberculosis or malaria, and has only rarely looked across several domains and development sectors. For example, as well as risks from diseases, inhabitants in rural Burkina Faso live constantly with risks from drought, food insecurity, endemic poverty, and lack educational facilities and health services.

A study in 40 villages examined risk perceptions in relation to health, health care, economics, agriculture and climate. Subsistence agriculture and pastoralism were the main economic activities of the mixed ethnic population. Using qualitative research methods

and focus group discussions, 12 important risks were identified; their perceived severity and people's vulnerability, i.e. the chance of their happening during the coming year, were assessed.

As one focus group participant said: "We have two main sources of risk: hunger and illness. In the dry season, November–February, we face soumaya (malaria) which is due to the wind and cold. Cough is due to the Harmattan winds and dust. In the hot season, March–April, we face headache due to the heat. In the rainy season, May–October, we face diarrhoea and stomach-ache due to hunger."

HIV infection was ranked as the most severe risk but it was placed twelfth in terms of personal vulnerability. In terms of perceived severity, the next four risks were a lack of rain, becoming mentally ill, being struck by lightening, and a lack of funds to buy medicines. Malaria was ranked

lowest for severity but first for the chances of it happening during the next year. After malaria, the next four perceptions of vulnerability were a lack of funds for medicines, snake-bite, becoming ill from tobacco smoking, and a lack of rain.

The study found an elaborate knowledge of risks in a number of domains for which the local people felt themselves to be personally at risk. Given the complexity of living conditions in the African Sahel, health risks cannot be seen in isolation from other domains such as climate, the economy and society. These all form part of a larger local discourse on the problems, difficulties, dangers and risks related to life in general.

Source: *(34)*.

population and target audiences; sources and presentation of information; the distribution and flow of communications; and mechanisms for dialogue and conflict resolution. Risk communication has come to mean much more than the mere passing on of information, as in the older style health education messages. It should also include the promotion of public dialogue between different stakeholders, resolution of conflicts, and agreement on the need for interventions to prevent the risks *(38)*.

The topic of risk communications became prominent in the mid-1980s, when it was realized that the risk management policies proposed by experts and specialized agencies were not necessarily acceptable to the wider public *(9)*. Efforts to prevent risks therefore expanded to include the improved handling of risks through better risk communication. The term "risk communication" is, however, still often used to refer to the narrower role it has played in conventional risk management, specifically relating to the communications emanating from scientists who wish to convey their technical recommendations. In this more restricted interpretation, risk communication is frequently designed for a health programme that is to be implemented by an expert regulatory body and directed at a particular population or target group, and which aims to achieve certain specified, often behavioural, outcomes *(39)*. Experience has shown that this expert-driven approach often did not live up to expectations. In addition, such communication approaches were not possible for some of the newer technologies, such as genetically modified foods, for which there was limited scientific knowledge on the potential risks and consequences. Such new technologies have revealed the importance of being more cautious and, if necessary, adopting the so-called "precautionary principle". (A fuller explanation of this principle is given in Chapter 6.) This has been found to be particularly true when the potential risks and future consequences are highly uncertain, when there are high levels of public dread and when future generations could be affected.

It is now generally accepted that if risk communication is to be more successful there has to be better dialogue and trust between all parties, particularly government officials, recognized experts and other legitimate groups in society and the general public *(6, 7)*. This change in perspective has meant that risk communication has had to become more integrated into the democratic and political processes, which in turn has forced decision-making on risks, particularly by governments, to become more open, transparent and democratic. This change acknowledges that success in handling risks needs to involve many more groups in society, the wider sharing of political power and more public accountability for the use of government and private resources. This in turn has raised such important issues as public trust in governments and expert agencies, freedom and availability of information in the public domain, mechanisms for public consultation, and roles of scientific experts and advisory committees (see Box 3.5).

INFLUENCE OF SPECIAL INTEREST GROUPS ON RISK PERCEPTIONS

Perception, understanding and framing of risks are affected, both positively and adversely, by the influences of powerful interest groups outside of government, including private for-profit corporations and public health campaigning organizations. Since scientific data do not "speak for themselves", special interest groups can play a critical role in interpreting the scientific information and hence in the framing of public perceptions of risks and risk factors. In this way such groups aim to influence public debate and government policies against or for the control and prevention of known risks.

Box 3.5 The Bovine Spongiform Encephalopathy (BSE) Inquiry, United Kingdom

"Our experience over this lengthy Inquiry has led us to the firm conclusion that a policy of openness is the correct approach. When responding to public or media demand for advice, the government must resist the temptation of attempting to appear to have all the answers in a situation of uncertainty. We believe that food scares and vaccine scares thrive on the belief that the Government is withholding information. If doubts are openly expressed and publicly explored, the public are capable of responding rationally and are more likely to accept reassurance and advice if and when it comes."

Source: *(40)*. p. 263.

While communicating accurate information on risks is essential to risk perception and better risk management, it is scientific information and research findings that provide the basis for risk assessment. Such information or "known facts" are nevertheless subject to interpretation and the social construction of the evidence, which largely determines how the risks are defined, perceived, framed and communicated in society *(30, 41)*. In addition, scientific uncertainties allow for widely different understandings of the same data, including distorting their interpretation in order to suit the interests of special groups. Although private for-profit and public health campaigning organizations often use similar tactics, businesses commonly promote public controversy as a means of avoiding greater government controls over risks. This strategy can be costly, as evidenced by the large financial resources that corporate interest groups commonly allocate to such activities. The tactics of industrial special interest groups, such as in the asbestos and tobacco industries, largely came to light when companies were forced to release a large number of internal documents after legal challenges by groups attempting to show that they had suffered because of these industries *(42, 43)* (see Box 3.6).

Special interest groups, whether public or private or for-profit or not-for-profit, are basically organized to promote and protect their own interests and it should be expected, therefore, that they will construct the evidence about health risks so as to support their position and interests *(44)*. Industrial special interest groups are primarily motivated to protect profitable products or services and thus tend to frame and communicate associated risks by hiding or minimizing their harm. They therefore do not in any way support such actions as increased regulation or greater import–export restrictions. Disputes about the regulation of risks, particularly environmental and industrial risks, frequently involve legal

Box 3.6 Strategies for fuelling public controversy

Policy-making is facilitated by building consensus in society, while scientific research is often characterized by uncertainties. Thus scientific debates on risks to health, particularly focusing on any assumptions and uncertainties, usually slow down policy decision-making after risk assessments have been carried out. Corporate and private-for-profit special interest groups can often benefit, therefore, by generating public controversy so as to prevent or delay regulation and control of their products. This is commonly done by emphasizing uncertainties in the original data, the methods, or the quality of the scientific conclusions.

On the other hand, public health groups campaigning for greater control of risks tend to emphasize ethical considerations and the need for stronger government policies and regulation. Both kinds of special interest groups use a number of strategies to support their position, for example by:
- setting up independent but sympathetic policy think-tanks and research funding organizations;
- encouraging and supporting experts who are sympathetic to their position;
- funding and publishing research that supports the interest group's position;
- disseminating supportive research studies in scientific publications;

- criticizing and suppressing research that is unfavourable to their cause;
- disseminating positive or negative interpretations of the risk data in the mass media, particularly the lay press;
- using lobbying groups and advertising campaigns to encourage greater public support;
- communicating favourable conclusions directly to politicians, government officials and bureaucrats;
- drawing attention to political and economic benefits, such as electoral support, employment and export opportunities.

Source: *(43)*.

proceedings at national level *(45)*, while many risks related to international trade may come under the jurisdiction of the disputes procedure of the World Trade Organization.

By comparison, public health interest groups have the difficult task of trying to achieve greater consensus in society in order to make government risk control policies more acceptable. These groups tend to communicate and frame risks by emphasizing their harm and hence encourage policies and strategies that aim to reduce risk, including better regulation. Although public health groups tend to act independently, they are often less well coordinated at national and international levels than corporate groups; they are also more accountable to the public than are private businesses. In addition, they usually have fewer financial resources to support their activities.

The tobacco industry is a prime example of how global business operations can be promoting cigarette consumption while at the same time distorting public perceptions of the risks involved *(42, 46)*. However, many anti-smoking groups also oppose both the tobacco industry and the coordinated international action contained in the Framework Convention for Tobacco Control (FCTC) promoted by the World Health Organization (see Box 3.7).

Besides private industry and public health campaigning groups, there are many other kinds of special interest groups that aim to influence policies to control risks. With the rapid growth in global media and communications, particularly those using the Internet, many informal global networks now exist, including links between specialist groups and community-based organizations. A constant danger is that private organizations may attempt to coopt and divert such public groups and networks. Although special interest groups are often better organized in industrialized countries, similar groups in developing countries can now benefit from faster international links, easier access to published information, and membership of related trade or professional organizations. For instance, the multinational pharmaceutical companies attempt to control the development, licensing, availability and costs of many patented drugs; national family planning associations and the International Planned Parenthood Federation (IPPF) disseminate information on risks to reproductive health and promote modern methods to control fertility; special groups exist to protect people with particular diseases, such those suffering from HIV/AIDS, diabetes and cancers; and other special groups aim to avoid new risks, such as those from greatly increased global trade in manufactured products, for example, food and pesticides.

Another important aspect of policy-making occurs at the international level. Besides special interest groups that can operate on a global basis, there are a number of

Box 3.7 Junking science to promote tobacco

"The goal of the tobacco industry's "scientific strategy" was not to reveal the truth but to protect the industry from loss of revenue and to prevent governments from establishing effective tobacco control measures. The industry's goals of creating doubt and controversy and placing the burden of proof on the public health community in policy forums have, therefore, met with a certain degree of success. Tobacco control policies are not being implemented worldwide at the rate that current scientific knowledge about the dangers of tobacco warrants. But this scenario is changing as the negotiations for the Framework Convention on Tobacco Control continue to advance. The convention marks the first time that WHO has used its treaty-making right to support Member States in developing a legally binding instrument in the service of public health. Negotiations are progressing well, and it is likely that Member States will vote on ratification of the convention in mid-2003.

"What do the revelations about tobacco company actions mean for public health policy? In general terms, they call for policy-makers to demand complete transparency about affiliations and linkages between allegedly independent scientists and tobacco companies. Academic naivety about tobacco companies' intentions is no longer excusable. The extent of the tobacco companies' manipulations needs to be thoroughly exposed, and students of many disciplines (public health, public policy, ethics, and law, to name a few) should be provided with the evidence that is increasingly available through the tobacco industry documents [in the Minnesota and Guildford archives]."

Source: *(46)*. p.1747.

international organizations that clearly aim to be influential in public health, including the World Health Organization, other multilateral and specialized agencies of the United Nations, and bilateral donor agencies. In addition, many international nongovernmental organizations do play a major role in gathering evidence, disseminating information and advocating risk control policies in such areas as child labour, dangerous chemicals and the dumping of waste products.

IMPORTANCE OF MASS MEDIA IN RISK PERCEPTIONS

Understanding common risks to health is crucial for the future well-being of many people in all countries, but information on risks, risk factors and uncertainty are inherently difficult to communicate. However, the mass media clearly do have a powerful influence on people's perceptions of risks and, in a global world, information on risks can be disseminated very rapidly through satellite technologies. Although newspapers, magazines, radio and television are often criticized for inaccurate and biased reporting, in industrialized countries they remain the most influential sources for everyday information on risks to health *(12)*. The rapid spread of these media in developing countries, together with improvements in literacy, means that this is also increasingly true in low and middle income countries.

How should the media evaluate and communicate the information on health risks such as HIV/AIDS or new vaccines, particularly if these are associated with scientific and ethical controversies? Such situations challenge the media to be responsible when dealing with complicated scientific issues and conflicting political goals *(47)*. What information should be conveyed? How fully should uncertainties and controversies be explained to the public?

With regard to health matters, the media perform two major functions – they can interpret scientific information and government policies to the public, and at the same time they reflect the concerns of the general public to a wider national audience. Media are also very much a part of the larger society in which they operate *(47)*. The way the different media outlets report risks to health reflects their biases and organizational constraints, such as whether they are private entities or government agencies and whether they are a free press or allied with particular political or business interests.

Since the media are organized to cover newsworthy events, they often seek out sensational and dramatic health episodes such as chemical accidents, exciting research discoveries, epidemics of communicable diseases, and safety defects in new medicines. Other controversial debates, such as those between the pharmaceutical industry and the medical profession over access to treatment for HIV/AIDS, often gain international attention. Media coverage tends to focus on human interest stories and news about dreaded diseases. In contrast, attention is not often given to common, chronic and low-level risks to health, such as passive exposure to tobacco smoke or poor levels of physical exercise. In addition, the media tend to avoid issues that may threaten prevailing social and cultural norms or moral and economic values.

Given the complex nature of many risks to health, media reporting has to rely on a variety of expert sources as well as on representatives of government ministries, private companies and special interest groups. Government press releases, national scientists and international scientific journals are often the main sources of information for the media. Journalists tend to use the best organized sources and those which provide technical information simply in the form of non-technical press releases. In addition, international news organizations frequently syndicate risk stories around the world. Special interest and advocacy groups aim to influence risk perceptions and are, therefore, often well organized to "help" the media in such complex areas as alcohol and tobacco use. A checklist of questions to use as a guide to the media understanding of risk issues has been published *(28)*.

IMPORTANCE OF PERCEPTIONS IN SUCCESSFUL RISK PREVENTION

Discussions of risk perceptions are often still bedevilled by a number of simplistic and polarized views, such as between expert (scientific) understanding and general public (lay) perceptions; between quantitative (objective) and qualitative (subjective) assessment of risks; and between rational analytical and "irrational" emotive responses. Such stereotyping, reflected in the debates about nuclear power in the 1970s and 1980s, is unhelpful today in considering risks to health and how risk factors can be prevented. In addition, policy recommendations are likely to be resisted if they attempt to define the "correct" definitions of risk and support only the so-called "true" and objective measures of risk factors. Risk acceptability depends upon many different aspects of perceived risks of technologies and interventions, as well as any perceived benefits. Both risks and benefits have to be considered when seeking to understand what drives some risk behaviours and why some interventions are more acceptable and successful than others.

Moreover, social, cultural and economic factors are central to how individuals perceive and understand health risks. Similarly, structural factors can influence which risk control policies are adopted and what impact interventions for risk factor prevention can finally achieve. A focus on individual perceptions, particularly when considering communicable diseases in the developing world, essentially considers the risk from the point of view of personal health services and individual people. This approach ignores, however, the constraints on the autonomy or control that individuals have to act in their societies. Preventing risk factors thus has to be planned within the context of the local society, and prevention through interventions is only partly a matter of the individuals' circumstances and education. In addition, because of the great lack of risk research in developing country populations, the transferability of research findings on risk perceptions from developed nations should also be treated with caution. This suggests a need for a concerted agenda for international research.

It is widely agreed that before interpreting risks and planning any communications or health interventions, people's basic perceptions and frames of reference for interpreting risks must be well understood. It cannot be assumed that the general public thinks in the same terms and categories that are routinely used by public health professionals and other risk experts. Although obvious, this is a common mistake in designing intervention strategies. The boundary between "experts" and "public" is not as straightforward as it might at first seem. The general public in fact consists of many different "publics", such as young and old, women and men, and poor and vulnerable. Each group can hold valid and different risk perceptions and frames of reference for similar risks factors.

Estimates of numerical risk and its consequences, presented in scientific terms based on a risk assessment, therefore have to be communicated with particular caution and care. Communicating information on risk frames and perceptions, and risk prevention, is best done by independent and creditable senior professionals. They can help create the atmosphere of trust between the government and all interested parties, in both the public and private sectors, that is essential if interventions are to be adopted and successfully implemented.

REFERENCES

1. Kates RW, Kasperson JX. Comparative risk analysis of technological hazards: a review. *Proceedings of the National Academy of Sciences* 1983; 80:7027-38.

2. Royal Society. *Risk analysis, perception and management.* London: Royal Society; 1992.

3. Carter S. Boundaries of danger and uncertainty: an analysis of the technological culture of risk assessment. In: Gabe J, editor. *Medicine, health and risk: sociological approaches.* Oxford: Blackwell; 1995. Chapter 7, p. 133-50.

4. Slovic P. *The perception of risk.* London: Earthscan; 2000. p. 473.

5. Gifford S. The meaning of lumps: a case study of the ambiguities of risk. In: Stall R, Janes C, Gifford S, editors. *Anthropology and epidemiology. Interdisciplinary approaches to the study of health and disease.* Dordrecht: Reidel Publishing; 1986. p. 213-46.

6. Pidgeon N. Risk perception. In: Royal Society. *Risk analysis, perception and management.* London: Royal Society; 1992. p. 89-134.

7. National Research Council, Committee on Risk Characterisation. Stern PC, Fineberg HV, editors. *Understanding risk. Informing decisions in a democratic society.* Washington (DC): National Academy Press; 1996.

8. Douglas M, Wildavsky A. *Risk and culture. An essay on the selection of technological and environmental dangers.* Los Angeles and London: University of California Press; 1982.

9. Slovic P. Perception of risk. *Science* 1987; 236:280-85.

10. Saloojee Y, Dagli E. Tobacco industry tactics for resisting public policy on health. *Bulletin of the World Health Organization* 2000; 78:902-10.

11. Fischhoff B. Managing risk perception. *Issues in Science and Technology* 1985; 2:83-96.

12. Slovic P. Informing and educating the public about risk. *Risk Analysis* 1986; 6:403-15.

13. Starr C. Social benefit versus technological risk. *Science* 1969; 165:1232-8.

14. Slovic P. Understanding perceived risk. Geneva: World Health Organization; 2001. Unpublished background paper for *The World Health Report 2002.*

15. Kahneman D, Slovic P, Tversky A, editors. *Judgement under uncertainty: heuristics and biases.* New York: Cambridge University Press; 1982.

16. Lichtenstein S, Slovic P, Fischhoff B, Layman M, Combs B. Judged frequency of lethal events. *Journal of Experimental Psychology: Human Learning and Memory* 1978; 4:551-78.

17. Fischhoff B, Lichtenstein S, Slovic P, Derby SL, Keeney RL. *Acceptable risk.* New York: Cambridge University Press; 1981.

18. Slovic P, Fischhoff B, Lichtenstein S. Facts and fears: understanding perceived risk. In: Schwing RC, Albers WA, editors. *Societal risk assessment: how safe is safe enough?* New York: Plenum; 1980. p. 181-214.

19. Fischhoff B, Watson S, Hope C. Defining risk. *Policy Sciences* 1984; 17:123-39.

20. Pantelides EA. Convergence and divergence: reproduction-related knowledge, attitudes and behaviour among young urban men in four Latin American cities. 2001 (unpublished paper).

21. Crouch EAC, Wilson R. *Risk-benefit analysis.* Cambridge (MA): Ballinger; 1982.

22. Barke R, Jenkins-Smith H, Slovic P. Risk perceptions of men and women scientists. *Social Science Quarterly* 1997; 78:167-76.

23. Slovic P, Malmfors T, Mertz CK, Neil N, Purchase IF. Evaluating chemical risks: results of a survey of the British Toxicology Society. *Human and Experimental Toxicology* 1997; 16:289-304.

24. Flynn J, Slovic P, Mertz CK. Gender, race and perception of environmental health risks. *Risk Analysis* 1994; 14:1101-8.

25. Dake K. Orienting dispositions in the perception of risk: an analysis of contemporary worldviews and cultural biases. *Journal of Cross-Cultural Psychology* 1991; 22:61-82.

26. Peters E, Slovic P. The role of affect and worldviews as orienting dispositions in the perception and acceptance of nuclear power. *Journal of Applied Social Psychology* 1996; 26:1427-53.

27. Jasper JM. *Nuclear politics: energy and the state in the United States, Sweden and France.* Princeton (NJ): Princeton University Press; 1990.

28. Fischhoff B. Risk perception and communication unplugged: 20 years of experience. *Risk Analysis* 1995; 15:137-45.

29. McNeil BJ, Pauker SG, Sox HC, Tversky A. On the elicitation of preferences for alternative therapies. *New England Journal of Medicine* 1982; 306:1259-62.

30. Nelkin D. Communicating technological risk: the social construction of risk perception. *Annual Review of Public Health* 1989; 10:95-113.

31. Ogden J. Psychosocial theory and the creation of the risky self. *Social Science and Medicine* 1995; 40:409-15.

32. Douglas M *Risk and blame: essays in cultural theory*. London and New York: Routledge; 1992.

33. Davison C, Davey Smith G, Frankel S. Lay epidemiology and the prevention paradox. *Sociology of Health and Illness* 1991; 13:1-19.

34. Sommerfeld J, Sanon M, Kouyate BA, Sauerborn R. Perceptions of risk, vulnerability and disease prevention in rural Burkina Faso: implications for community-based health care and insurance. *Human Organization* 2002:in press.

35. Manderson L. *Reducing health risks in resource-poor settings: The relevance of an anthropological perspective*. Geneva: World Health Organization; 2001. Unpublished background paper for *The World Health Report 2002*.

36. Manderson L, Tye LC. Condom use in heterosexual sex: a review of research, 1985-1994. In: Sherr L, Catalan J, Hedge B, editors. *The impact of AIDS: psychological and social aspects of HIV infection*. Chur, Switzerland: Harwood Academic Press; 1997. p. 1-26.

37. Pelto PJ, Pelto GH. Studying knowledge, culture and behaviour in applied medical anthropology. *Medical Anthropology Quarterly* 1997; 11:147-63.

38. Renn O. The role of risk communication and public dialogue for improving risk management. *Risk Decision and Policy* 1998; 3:5-30.

39. Plough A, Krimsky S. The emergence of risk communication studies: social and political context. *Science, Technology and Human Values* 1987; 12:4-10.

40. Phillips, Lord, Bridgeman J, Fergusan-Smith M. *The Bovine Spongiform Encephalopathy (BSE) Inquiry (the Phillips Inquiry): findings and conclusions (Volume 1)*. London: The Stationery Office; 2000. p. 263.

41. Krimsky S, Golding D, editors. *Societal theories of risk.* New York: Praeger; 1992.

42. Ong EK, Glantz AG. Constructing "sound science" and "good epidemiology": tobacco, lawyers and public relations firms. *American Journal of Public Health* 2001; 91:1749-57.

43. Bero L. *The role of special interest groups in influencing data on risk*. Geneva: World Health Organization; 2001. Unpublished background paper for *The World Health Report 2002*.

44. Jasanoff S. Is science socially constructed: and can it still inform public policy? *Science and Engineering Ethics* 1996; 2:263-76.

45. Jasanoff S. Science at the Bar: law, science and technology in America. Cambridge: Harvard University Press; 1995. p. 69-92.

46. Yach D, Bialous SA. Junking science to promote tobacco. *American Journal of Public Health* 2001; 91:1745-8.

47. Nelkin D. AIDS and the news media. *The Milbank Quarterly* 1991; 69:293-307.

CHAPTER FOUR

Quantifying Selected Major Risks to Health

In attempting to reduce risks to health and, in particular, to redress the imbalance that leaves the poor and the disadvantaged with the greatest burden of disease, the first steps are to quantify health risks and to assess the distribution of risk factors by poverty levels. The analysis in this report covers selected risk factors, grouped as follows: childhood and maternal undernutrition; other diet-related risk factors and physical inactivity; sexual and reproductive health; addictive substances; environmental risks; occupational risks; and other risks to health (including unsafe health care practices, and abuse and violence). These risk factors are responsible for a substantial proportion of the leading causes of death and disability. This chapter ranks them globally and within major world regions and goes on to estimate how much of the burden each of them causes is avoidable between now and the year 2020. The potential benefits are huge, but they will depend on effective and cost-effective interventions if they are to be realized.

4

Quantifying Selected Major Risks to Health

Risks to health and socioeconomic status

*T*he greatest burden of health risks is very often borne by the disadvantaged in our societies. The vast majority of threats to health are more commonly found among poor people, in people with little formal education, and those with lowly occupations. These risks cluster and they accumulate over time. In attempting to reduce risks to health, the focus of WHO and many other international organizations and governments is on trying to redress this imbalance – by directly tackling poverty, by concentrating on the risks to health amongst the impoverished, or by improving population health and hence overall economic growth *(1)*. An important component of the strategy is first to assess how much more prevalent risks are among the disadvantaged. While this provides information relevant to the targeting of interventions, it should be borne in mind that poverty and socioeconomic status are also of themselves key determinants of health status. This report seeks to shed further light on the mechanisms through which poverty acts, by assessing the distribution of risk factors by poverty levels.

Unfortunately, data are particularly scanty where they are required most – in the poorest countries of the world. Nonetheless, this report attempts to stratify global levels of selected risks by levels of absolute income poverty (<US$ 1, US$ 1–2 and >US$ 2 per day), as well as by age, sex and region. These analyses were conducted using individual-level data, not just comparisons of regional characteristics. The mapping of risk factors by poverty was conducted for:

- childhood protein–energy malnutrition;
- water and sanitation;
- lack of breastfeeding;
- unsafe sex;
- alcohol;
- tobacco;
- overweight;
- indoor air pollution;
- urban air pollution.

In addition, available research findings are summarized on the links between poverty and high blood pressure, cholesterol, physical inactivity, exposure to lead, and use of illicit drugs.

RATES OF POVERTY ACROSS THE WORLD

Approximately one-fifth of the world's population live on less than US$ 1 per day and nearly a half live on less than US$ 2 per day. Of the 14 world subregions (derived by dividing the six WHO regions into mortality strata – see the List of Member States by WHO Region and mortality stratum) three (EUR-A, AMR-A and WPR-A) had negligible levels of absolute poverty and were excluded from analyses. In the EMR-B subregion, 9% of people live on less than $2 per day (2% less than $1 per day), but the estimates for this subregion were based on sparse data. There were, however, more data supporting estimates for the remaining 10 subregions, where the corresponding percentages ranged from 18% (3%) for EUR-B to 85% (42%) for SEAR-D and 78% (56%) for AFR-D.

RELATIONSHIPS BETWEEN RISK FACTOR LEVELS AND POVERTY

For all subregions, there was a strong gradient of increasing child underweight with increasing absolute poverty (see Figure 4.1). The strength of the association varies little across regions, people living on less than $1 per day generally being at two- to three-fold higher relative risk compared with people living on more than $2 per day.

Unsafe water and sanitation, and indoor air pollution are also strongly associated with absolute poverty. For unsafe water and sanitation, the relative risks for those in households with an income of less than $1 per day, as compared to households with an income greater than $2 per day ranged from 1.7 (WPR-B) to 15.1 (EMR-D), with considerable variation between regions. For the association between indoor air pollution and poverty, there is considerable variation between subregions in the average level and in the relative differences within subregions. In the subregions of Africa, there is both a high prevalence of exposure to indoor air pollution and little relative difference between the impoverished and non-impoverished.

The associations of poverty with tobacco and alcohol consumption, lack of breastfeeding, and unsafe sex (unprotected sex with non-marital partner) are weaker and more variable between subregions. There is considerable variation between subregions in tobacco consumption, and a relatively weak association, within subregions, of tobacco consumption with individual-level poverty. Similarly, there is a more marked variation in alcohol consumption between WHO regions than within WHO regions by individual-level absolute poverty. In none of the subregions analysed was there a suggestion of increased alcohol

Figure 4.1 Prevalence of moderate underweight in children by average daily household income (<US$ 1, US$ 1-2 and >US$ 2 per day), by subregion[a]

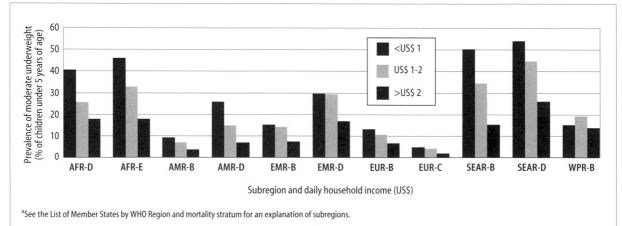

[a]See the List of Member States by WHO Region and mortality stratum for an explanation of subregions.

consumption among the more impoverished. But in two subregions, AFR-E (South Africa data only) and AMR-B (Panama data only), impoverished people had approximately half the alcohol consumption of non-impoverished people. However, these results were based on household survey data recording expenditure on alcohol (not consumption) that may not have fully captured individual consumption and consumption of non-manufactured sources, such as alcohol distilled locally. Findings were also consistent with the higher socioeconomic groups in the developing world having more adverse lipid profiles, high blood pressure and overweight than the poor. However, if the trends seen in the industrialized world are repeated, these patterns will reverse with increasing economic development. These cross-sectional analyses were consistent with differing stages of progression of tobacco, obesity and other key noncommunicable disease determinants in poorer regions of the world as they undergo economic development. For example, obesity and tobacco consumption are initially found among the non-impoverished within regions, and later these risks are given up by the non-impoverished but taken up among the impoverished. These findings were consistent with regions being at different stages of such a transition. In the absence of major public health initiatives, these risk factors are likely to become increasingly concentrated among poor people in the poorer regions of the world. Public health action is required now to prevent this progression.

POTENTIAL IMPACT ON RISK FACTOR LEVELS OF SHIFTING POVERTY DISTRIBUTIONS

In addition to estimating the associations of risk factor prevalence with poverty, population impact fractions of poverty on the risk factors were estimated. If people living on less than $2 per day had the same risk factor prevalence as people living on more than $2 per day, then protein–energy malnutrition, indoor air pollution and unimproved water and sanitation would be reduced by approximately 37%, 50% and 51%, respectively (see Table 4.1). These total population impact fractions would be reduced to 23%, 21% and 36% if the impoverished had the same risk factor prevalence as people living on exactly $2 per day.

Other risks present a more variable pattern, although data gaps particularly limit certainty of conclusions. Nonetheless, these analyses suggest that the prevalence of alcohol consumption and being overweight would increase by approximately 20% to 60% in Africa

Table 4.1 Population impact fractions by subregion for counterfactual scenario of population moving from living on <US$ 2 per day to >US$ 2 per day

Subregion	Protein–energy malnutrition (%)	Unsafe water, sanitation and hygeine (%)	Unsafe sex men (%)	women (%)	Indoor air pollution (%)	Tobacco (%)	Alcohol (%)	Body weight (%)
AFR-D	44	84	-17	-34	10	5	-19	-58
AFR-E	42	65	19	-9	38	-15	-38	-39
AMR-B	24	68	3	-5	58	4	-13	-3
AMR-D	43	69	3	-0.4	77	-16	-6	-5
EMR-B	8	17	...	...	...	...	...	0
EMR-D	32	85	...	...	60	24	...	-17
EUR-B	10	24	...	...	4	-4	-5	-3
EUR-C	24	68	...	-18	9	1	-5	0
SEAR-B	40	26	...	...	...	...	...	0
SEAR-D	43	75	...	...	65	...	...	-65
WPR-B	13	19	...	...	...	0.4	-8	0.7
Total	37	51	5	-13	50	0.5	-9	-9

Note: The 'total' population impact fractions apply only to subregions with population impact fraction estimates.
See the List of Member States by WHO Region and mortality stratum for an explanation of subregions.

overall if prevalence among the poor matched those amongst the better-off. The population impact fractions for breastfeeding, unsafe sex and tobacco were more moderate, and even varied in direction across subregions.

BURDEN OF DISEASE AND INJURY ATTRIBUTABLE TO SELECTED RISK FACTORS

The next sections of the chapter describe selected major health risk factors, grouped as follows: childhood and maternal undernutrition; other diet-related risk factors and physical inactivity; sexual and reproductive health; addictive substances; environmental risks; occupational risks; and other risks to health (including unsafe health care practices, and abuse and violence). Each risk is briefly described, along with its main causes, its extent in the world and what health problems it causes. The main results in terms of attributable mortality, years of life lost and DALYs as well as attributable fractions are summarized in Annex Tables 6–13. All these results should be considered in the context of likely uncertainty levels, indicated in the Statistical Annex Explanatory Notes.

CHILDHOOD AND MATERNAL UNDERNUTRITION

Many people in the developing world, particularly women and children, continue to suffer from undernutrition. The poor especially often suffer from a basic lack of protein and energy, the adverse health effects of which are frequently compounded by deficiencies in micronutrients, particularly iodine, iron, vitamin A and zinc. Another important risk factor is lack of breastfeeding.

The theoretical minimum exposure and measured adverse outcomes for this group of risk factors are shown in Table 4.2. Each of these factors is discussed separately below and some summary results are shown graphically in Figure 4.2.

UNDERWEIGHT

Undernutrition, defined in public health by poor anthropometric status, is mainly a consequence of inadequate diet and frequent infection, leading to deficiencies in calories, protein, vitamins and minerals. Underweight remains a pervasive problem in developing

Table 4.2 Selected major risks to health: childhood and maternal undernutrition

Risk factor	Theoretical minimum exposure	Measured adverse outcomes of exposure
Underweight	Same percentage of children under 5 years of age with <1 standard deviation weight-for-age as the international reference group; all women of childbearing age with BMI >20 kg/m^2	Mortality and acute morbidity from diarrhoea, malaria, measles, pneumonia, selected other Group 1 (infectious) diseases. Perinatal conditions from maternal underweight.
Iron deficiency	Haemoglobin distributions which halve anaemia prevalence, estimated to occur if all iron deficiency were eliminated (g/dl)	Anaemia, maternal and perinatal causes of death
Vitamin A deficiency	Children and women of childbearing age consuming sufficient vitamin A to meet physiological needs	Diarrhoea, malaria, maternal mortality, vitamin A deficiency disease
Zinc deficiency	The entire population consuming sufficient dietary zinc to meet physiological needs, taking into account routine and illness-related losses and bioavailability	Diarrhoea, pneumonia, malaria

countries, where poverty is a strong underlying determinant, contributing to household food insecurity, poor child care, maternal undernutrition, unhealthy environments, and poor health care. All ages are at risk, but underweight is most prevalent among children under five years of age, especially in the weaning and post-weaning period of 6–24 months. WHO has estimated that approximately 27% (168 million) of children under five years of age are underweight *(2)*. Underweight is also common among women of reproductive age, especially in Africa and South Asia, where some prevalence estimates of undernutrition are as high as 27–51% *(3)*.

Underweight children are at increased risk of mortality from infectious illnesses such as diarrhoea and pneumonia *(4)*. The effects of undernutrition on the immune system are wide-ranging, and infectious illnesses also tend to be more frequent and severe in underweight children. A child's risk of dying from undernutrition is not limited to those children with the most severe undernutrition. There is a continuum of risk such that even mild undernutrition places a child at increased risk. Since mild and moderate undernutrition are more prevalent than severe undernutrition, much of the burden of deaths resulting from undernutrition is associated with less severe undernutrition. These analyses indicate that 50–70% of the burden of diarrhoeal diseases, measles, malaria and lower respiratory infections in childhood is attributable to undernutrition. Chronic undernutrition in the first two to three years of life can also lead to long-term developmental deficits *(5)*. Among adolescents and adults, undernutrition is also associated with adverse pregnancy outcomes and reduced work capacity.

Figure 4.2   Burden of disease attributable to childhood and maternal undernutrition (% DALYs in each subregion)

A. Underweight

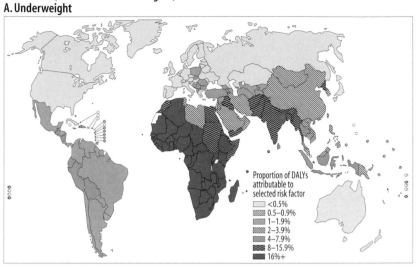

B. Iron deficiency

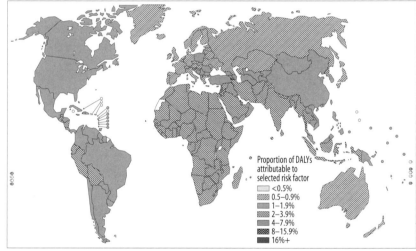

C. Vitamin A deficiency

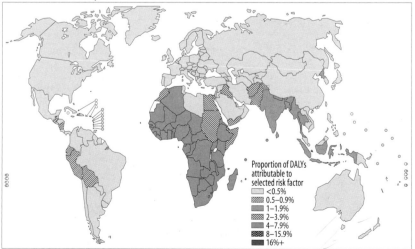

The values presented here are averages by subregion; variations occur within these subregions but are not shown here. For an explanation of subregions see the List of Member States by WHO Region and mortality stratum.

Underweight was estimated to cause 3.7 million deaths in 2000. This accounted for about 1 in 15 deaths globally. About 1.8 million deaths occurred in Africa, 1.2 million in SEAR-D and 0.5 million in EMR-D, accounting for 10–20% of deaths in these regions. The disease burden occurred about equally among males and females. Since deaths from undernutrition almost all occur among young children, the loss of healthy life years is even more substantial: about 138 million DALYs, 9.5% of the global total, were attributed to underweight. These estimates of burden resulting from underweight, together with those given below for micronutrient deficiences, are consistent with previous estimates of over half of childhood deaths in developing countries being caused by undernutrition *(6)*.

IODINE DEFICIENCY

Iodine deficiency is likely to be the single most common preventable cause of mental retardation and brain damage. "Endemic cretinism", the form of profound mental retardation most closely identified with iodine deficiency, represents the severe end of a broad spectrum of abnormalities collectively referred to as iodine deficiency disorders. Iodine deficiency has also been associated with lower mean birth weight and increased infant mortality, hearing impairment, impaired motor skills, and neurological dysfunction. Iodine deficiency is controlled through direct supplementation with oral or intramuscular iodized oil, addition of iodine to a vehicle such as irrigation water, or most commonly iodization of salt. Over 2.2 billion people in the world may be at risk for iodine deficiency, and recent estimates suggest over one billion experience some degree of goitre *(7–9)*. Globally, iodine deficiency disorders were estimated to result in 2.5 million DALYs (0.2% of total). Approximately 25% of this burden occurred in AFR-E, 17% in SEAR-D and 16% in EMR-D.

IRON DEFICIENCY

Iron is required in all tissues of the body for basic cellular functions, and is critically important in muscle, brain and red blood cells. Anaemia is simple to measure and has been used as the hallmark of iron deficiency severe enough to affect tissue functions. However, iron deficiency is not the sole cause of anaemia in most populations. Even in an individual, anaemia may be caused by multiple factors.

Iron deficiency is one of the most prevalent nutrient deficiencies in the world, affecting an estimated two billion people *(10)*. Young children and pregnant and postpartum women are the most commonly and severely affected because of the high iron demands of infant growth and pregnancy. Iron deficiency may, however, occur throughout the life span where diets are based mostly on staple foods with little meat intake or people are exposed to infections that cause blood loss (primarily hookworm disease and urinary schistosomiasis).

About one-fifth of perinatal mortality and one-tenth of maternal mortality in developing countries is attributable to iron deficiency. There is also a growing body of evidence indicating that iron deficiency anaemia in early childhood reduces intelligence in midchildhood. In its most severe form, this will cause mild mental retardation. There is also evidence that iron deficiency decreases fitness and aerobic work capacity through mechanisms that include oxygen transport and respiratory efficiency within the muscle.

In total, 0.8 million (1.5%) of deaths worldwide are attributable to iron deficiency, 1.3% of all male deaths and 1.8% of all female deaths. Attributable DALYs are even greater, amounting to the loss of about 35 million healthy life years (2.4% of global DALYs). Of these DALYs, 12.5 million (36%) occurred in SEAR-D, 4.3 million (12.4%) in WPR-B, and 10.1 million (29%) in Africa.

Vitamin A deficiency

Vitamin A is an essential nutrient required for maintaining eye health and vision, growth, immune function, and survival *(11)*. Several factors, often acting together, can cause Vitamin A deficiency: low dietary intake, malabsorption, and increased excretion associated with common illnesses. Severe vitamin A deficiency can be identified by the classic eye signs of xerophthalmia, such as corneal lesions. Milder vitamin A deficiency is far more common. While its assessment is more problematic, it can be gauged by serum retinol levels and reports of night blindness.

Vitamin A deficiency causes visual impairment in many parts of the developing world and is the leading cause of acquired blindness in children. Children under five years of age and women of reproductive age are at highest risk of this nutritional deficiency and its adverse health consequences. Globally, approximately 21% of all children suffer from vitamin A deficiency (defined as low serum retinol concentrations), with the highest prevalence of deficiency, and the largest number affected, in parts of Asia (30% in SEAR-D and 48% in SEAR-B) and in Africa (28% in AFR-D and 35% in AFR-E). There is a similar pattern for women affected by night blindness during pregnancy, with a global prevalence of approximately 5% and the highest prevalence among women living in Asia and Africa where maternal mortality rates are also high.

This analysis estimated that Vitamin A deficiency also caused about 16% of worldwide burden resulting from malaria and 18% resulting from diarrhoeal diseases. Attributable fractions for both diseases were 16–20% in Africa. In South-East Asia, about 11% of malaria was attributed to vitamin A deficiency. About 10% of maternal DALYs worldwide were attributed to vitamin A deficiency, again with the proportion highest in South-East Asia and Africa. Other outcomes potentially associated with vitamin A deficiency are fetal loss, low birth weight, preterm birth and infant mortality.

In total, about 0.8 million (1.4%) of deaths worldwide result from vitamin A deficiency, 1.1% in males and 1.7% in females. Attributable DALYs are higher: 1.8% of global disease burden. Over 4–6% of all disease burden in Africa was estimated to result from vitamin A deficiency.

Zinc deficiency

Zinc deficiency is largely related to inadequate intake or absorption of zinc from the diet, although excess losses of zinc during diarrhoea may also contribute. The distinction between intake and absorption is important: high levels of inhibitors (such as fibre and phytates) in the diet may result in low absorption of zinc, even though intake of zinc may be acceptable. For this reason, zinc requirements for dietary intake are adjusted upward for populations in which animal products – the best sources of zinc – are limited, and in which plant sources of zinc are high in phytates.

Severe zinc deficiency was defined in the early 1900s as a condition characterized by short stature, hypogonadism, impaired immune function, skin disorders, cognitive dysfunction, and anorexia *(12)*. Using food availability data, it is estimated that zinc deficiency affects about one-third of the world's population, with estimates ranging from 4% to 73% across subregions. Although severe zinc deficiency is rare, mild-to-moderate zinc deficiency is quite common throughout the world *(13)*.

Worldwide, zinc deficiency is responsible for approximately 16% of lower respiratory tract infections, 18% of malaria and 10% of diarrhoeal disease. The highest attributable fractions for lower respiratory tract infection occurred in AFR-E, AMR-D, EMR-D and

SEAR-D (18–22%); likewise, the attributable fractions for diarrhoeal diseases were high in these four subregions (11–13%). Attributable fractions for malaria were highest in AFR-D, AFR-E and EMR-D (10–22%).

In total, 1.4% (0.8 million) of deaths worldwide were attributable to zinc deficiency: 1.4% in males and 1.5% in females. Attributable DALYs were higher, with zinc deficiency accounting for about 2.9% of worldwide loss of healthy life years. Of this disease burden, amounting to 28 million DALYs worldwide, 34.2% occurred in SEAR-D, 31.1% in AFR-E and 18.0% in AFR-D.

LACK OF BREASTFEEDING

Breast milk provides optimal nutrition for a growing infant, with compositional changes that are adapted to the changing needs of the infant. Human milk contains adequate minerals and nutrients for the first six months of life. Breast milk also contains immune components, cellular elements and other host-defence factors that provide various antibacterial, antiviral and antiparasitic protection. Breast-milk components stimulate the appropriate development of the infant's own immune system. On the basis of the current evidence, WHO's public health recommendation is that infants should be exclusively breastfed during the first six months of life and that they should continue to receive breast milk throughout the remainder of the first year and during the second year of life *(14)*. "Exclusive breastfeeding" means that no water or other fluids (or foods) should be administered. In almost all situations, breastfeeding remains the simplest, healthiest and least expensive method of infant feeding, which is also adapted to the nutritional needs of the infant.

In general, exclusive breastfeeding rates are low. The proportion of infants less than 6 months of age that are exclusively breastfed ranges from about 9% in EUR-C and AFR-D, respectively, to 55% in WPR-B (excluding EUR-A and WPR-A for which sufficient information was not available). On the other hand, the proportion of infants less than six months old that are not breastfed at all ranges from 35% in EUR-C to 2% in SEAR-D (again, excluding all A subregions). In Africa, however, where breastfeeding is nearly universal, exclusive breastfeeding remains rare. For infants aged 6–11 months, the proportion not breastfed ranges from 5% in SEAR-D to 69% in EUR-C. In all the subregions in Africa and South-East Asia, over 90% of infants aged 6–11 months are still breastfed.

Lack of breastfeeding – and especially lack of exclusive breastfeeding during the first months of life – are important risk factors for infant and childhood morbidity and mortality, especially resulting from diarrhoeal disease and acute respiratory infections in developing countries. For example, in a study in Brazil *(15)*, infants less than 12 months of age who received only powdered milk or cow's milk had approximately 14 times the risk of death from diarrhoeal disease and about 4 times the risk of death from acute respiratory infection compared with those who were exclusively breastfed. Furthermore, those who received powdered milk or cow's milk in addition to breast milk were found to be at 4.2 times the risk of diarrhoeal death and 1.6 times the risk of death from acute respiratory infection, compared with infants exclusively breastfed. Breastfeeding has also been demonstrated to be important for neurodevelopment, especially in premature, low-birth-weight infants and infants born small for gestational age.

OTHER DIET-RELATED RISK FACTORS AND PHYSICAL INACTIVITY

As well as undernutrition, substantial disease burden is also attributable to risks that are related to overconsumption of certain foods or food components. This section includes estimates of burden of disease attributable to suboptimal blood pressure, cholesterol and overweight, as well as low fruit and vegetable intake and physical inactivity (see Table 4.3). Some summary results are shown graphically in Figure 4.3.

HIGH BLOOD PRESSURE

Blood pressure is a measure of the force that the circulating blood exerts on the walls of the main arteries. The pressure wave transmitted along the arteries with each heartbeat is easily felt as the pulse – the highest (systolic) pressure is created by the heart contracting and the lowest (diastolic) pressure is measured as the heart fills. Raised blood pressure is almost always without symptoms. However, elevated blood pressure levels produce a variety of structural changes in the arteries that supply blood to the brain, heart, kidneys and elsewhere. In recent decades it has become increasingly clear that the risks of stroke, ischaemic heart disease, renal failure and other disease are not confined to a subset of the population with particularly high levels (hypertension), but rather continue among those with average and even below-average blood pressure *(16–18)* (see Figure 4.4).

The main modifiable causes of high blood pressure are diet, especially salt intake, levels of exercise, obesity, and excessive alcohol intake. As a result of the cumulative effects of these factors blood pressure usually rises steadily with age, except in societies in which salt intake is comparatively low, physical activity high and obesity largely absent. Most adults have blood pressure levels that are suboptimal for health. This is true for both economically developing and developed countries, but in the European subregions blood pressure levels are particularly high. Across WHO regions, the range between the highest and lowest age-specific mean systolic blood pressure levels is estimated at about 20 mmHg. Globally, these analyses indicate that about 62% of cerebrovascular disease and 49% of ischaemic heart disease are attributable to suboptimal blood pressure (systolic >115 mmHg), with little variation by sex.

Table 4.3 Selected major risks to health: other diet-related factors and inactivity

Risk factor	Theoretical minimum exposure	Measured adverse outcomes of exposure
Blood pressure	115; SD 11 mmHg	Stroke, ischaemic heart disease, hypertensive disease, other cardiac disease
Cholesterol	3.8; SD 1 mmol/l (147 SD 39 mg/dl)	Stroke, ischaemic heart disease
Overweight	21; SD 1 kg/m²	Stroke, ischaemic heart disease, diabetes, osteoarthritis, endometrial cancer, postmenopausal breast cancer.
Low fruit and vegetable intake	600; SD 50 g intake per day for adults	Stroke, ischaemic heart disease, colorectal cancer, gastric cancer, lung cancer, oesophageal cancer
Physical inactivity	All taking at least 2.5 hours per week of moderate exercise or 1 hour per week of vigorous exercise	Stroke, ischaemic heart disease, breast cancer, colon cancer, diabetes

Figure 4.3 Burden of disease attributable to diet-related risk factors and physical inactivity (% DALYs in each subregion)

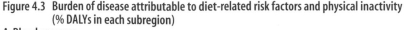

A. Blood pressure

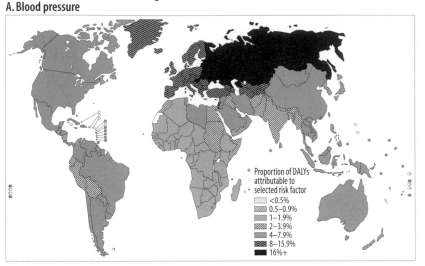

Proportion of DALYs attributable to selected risk factor
- <0.5%
- 0.5–0.9%
- 1–1.9%
- 2–3.9%
- 4–7.9%
- 8–15.9%
- 16%+

B. Cholesterol

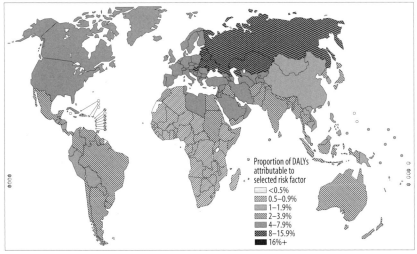

Proportion of DALYs attributable to selected risk factor
- <0.5%
- 0.5–0.9%
- 1–1.9%
- 2–3.9%
- 4–7.9%
- 8–15.9%
- 16%+

C. Overweight (high body mass index)

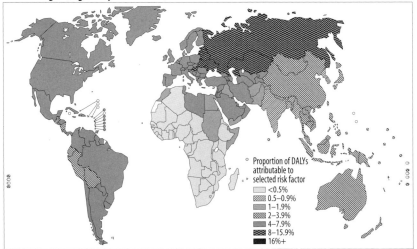

Proportion of DALYs attributable to selected risk factor
- <0.5%
- 0.5–0.9%
- 1–1.9%
- 2–3.9%
- 4–7.9%
- 8–15.9%
- 16%+

The values presented here are averages by subregion; variations occur within these subregions but are not shown here. For an explanation of subregions see the List of Member States by WHO Region and mortality stratum.

Worldwide, high blood pressure is estimated to cause 7.1 million deaths, about 13% of the total. Since most blood pressure related deaths or nonfatal events occur in middle age or the elderly, the loss of life years comprises a smaller proportion of the global total, but is nonetheless substantial (64.3 million DALYs, or 4.4% of the total). Of this disease burden, 20% occured in WPR-B, 19% in SEAR-D and 16% in EUR-C.

HIGH CHOLESTEROL

Cholesterol is a fat-like substance, found in the bloodstream as well as in bodily organs and nerve fibres. Most cholesterol in the body is made by the liver from a wide variety of foods, especially from saturated fats, such as those found in animal products. A diet high in saturated fat content, heredity, and various metabolic conditions such as diabetes mellitus influence an individual's level of cholesterol. Cholesterol levels usually rise steadily with age, more steeply in women, and stabilize after middle age. Mean cholesterol levels vary moderately between regions, although never more than 2.0 mmol/l in any age group.

Cholesterol is a key component in the development of atherosclerosis, the accumulation of fatty deposits on the inner lining of arteries. Mainly as a result of this, cholesterol increases the risks of ischaemic heart disease, ischaemic stroke and other vascular diseases. As with blood pressure, the risks of cholesterol are continuous and extend across almost all levels seen in different populations, even those with cholesterol levels much lower than those seen in North American and European populations.

High cholesterol is estimated to cause 18% of global cerebrovascular disease (mostly nonfatal events) and

56% of global ischaemic heart disease. Overall this amounts to about 4.4 million deaths (7.9% of total) and 40.4 million DALYs (2.8% of total). Of this total disease burden, 27% occurred in SEAR-D, 18% in EUR-C and 11% in WPR-B. In AMR-A and Europe, 5–12% of DALYs were attributable to suboptimal cholesterol levels. In most regions, the proportion of female deaths attributable to cholesterol is slightly higher than that for men.

Figure 4.4 Nine examples of continuous associations between risks and disease

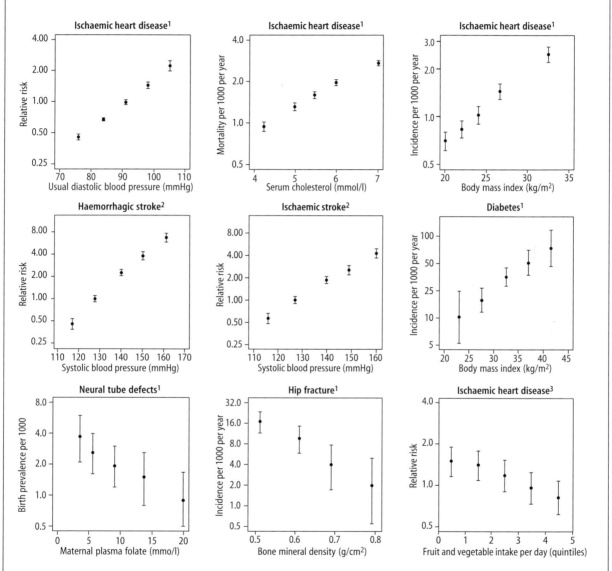

The figure shows continuous dose–response associations for a number of risk factor–outcome combinations. Lack of thresholds to these associations suggests there is no biological justification for typical binary categorizations, such as "hypertension" or "hypercholesterolaemia".

[1] Law MR, Wald NJ. Risk factor thresholds: their existence under scrutiny. *BMJ* 2002; 324:1570-6.
[2] Eastern Stroke and Coronary Heart Disease Collaborative Group. Blood pressure, cholesterol and stroke in eastern Asia. *Lancet* 1998; 352:1801-07.
[3] Joshipura KJ, Hu FB, Manson JE, Stampfer MJ, Rimm EB, Speizer FE, Colditz G, Ascherio A, Rosner B, Spiegelman D, Willett WC. The effect of fruit and vegetable intake on risk for coronary heart disease. *Annals of Internal Medicine* 2001; 134(12):1106-14.

OBESITY, OVERWEIGHT, AND HIGH BODY MASS

The prevalence of overweight and obesity is commonly assessed using body mass index (BMI), a height/weight formula with a strong correlation to body fat content. WHO criteria define overweight as a BMI of at least 25 kg/m^2 and obesity as a BMI of at least 30 kg/m^2. These markers provide common benchmarks for assessment, but the risks of disease in all populations increase progressively from BMI levels of 20–22 kg/m^2.

Adult mean BMI levels of 20–23 kg/m^2 are found in Africa and Asia, while levels are 25–27 kg/m^2 across North America and Europe. BMI increases among middle-aged and elderly people, who are at greatest risk of health complications. Increases in free sugar and saturated fats, combined with reduced physical activity, have led to obesity rates that have risen three-fold or more since 1980 in some areas of North America, the United Kingdom, Eastern Europe, the Middle East, the Pacific Islands, Australasia and China. A new demographic transition in developing countries is producing rapid increases in BMI, particularly among the young. The affected population has increased to epidemic proportions, with more than one billion adults worldwide overweight and at least 300 million clinically obese *(19)*.

Overweight and obesity lead to adverse metabolic effects on blood pressure, cholesterol, triglycerides and insulin resistance. Risks of coronary heart disease, ischaemic stroke and type 2 diabetes mellitus increase steadily with increasing BMI. Type 2 diabetes mellitus – confined to older adults for most of the 20th century – now affects obese children even before puberty. Modest weight reduction reduces blood pressure and abnormal blood cholesterol and substantially lowers risk of type 2 diabetes. Raised BMI also increases the risks of cancer of the breast, colon, prostate, endometrium, kidney and gallbladder. Although mechanisms that trigger these increased cancer risks are not fully understood, they may relate to obesity-induced hormonal changes. Chronic overweight and obesity contribute significantly to osteoarthritis, a major cause of disability in adults.

In the analyses carried out for this report, approximately 58% of diabetes mellitus globally, 21% of ischaemic heart disease and 8–42% of certain cancers were attributable to BMI above 21 kg/m^2. This amounted to about 13% of deaths in EUR-B and EUR-C and 9–10% of deaths in AMR-A, AMR-B and EUR-A. High BMI causes 8–15% of DALYs in Europe and AMR-A, but less than 3% in Africa, AMR-D, South-East Asia, EMR-D and WPR-A. The proportions of DALYs caused by high BMI are slightly higher for women than for men.

LOW FRUIT AND VEGETABLE INTAKE

Fruit and vegetables are important components of a healthy diet. Accumulating evidence suggests that they could help prevent major diseases such as cardiovascular diseases *(20)* and certain cancers principally of the digestive system *(21)*. There are several mechanisms by which these protective effects may be mediated, involving antioxidants and other micronutrients, such as flavonoids, carotenoids, vitamin C and folic acid, as well as dietary fibre. These and other substances block or suppress the action of carcinogens and, as antioxidants, prevent oxidative DNA damage.

Fruit and vegetable intake varies considerably among countries, in large part reflecting the prevailing economic, cultural and agricultural environments. The analysis assessed the levels of mean dietary intake of fruit and vegetables (excluding potatoes) in each region, measured in grams per person per day. The estimated levels varied two-fold around the world, ranging from about 189 g/day in AMR-B to 455 g/day in EUR-A.

Low intake of fruit and vegetables is estimated to cause about 19% of gastrointestinal cancer, and about 31% of ischaemic heart disease and 11% of stroke worldwide. Overall,

2.7 million (4.9%) deaths and 26.7 million (1.8%) DALYs are attributable to low fruit and vegetable intake. Of the burden attributable to low fruit and vegetable intake, about 85% was from cardiovascular diseases and 15% from cancers. About 43% of the disease burden occurred in women and 15% in EUR-C, 29% in SEAR-D and 18% in WPR-B.

PHYSICAL INACTIVITY

Opportunities for people to be physically active exist in the four major domains of their day-to-day lives: at work (especially if the job involves manual labour); for transport (for example, walking or cycling to work); in domestic duties (for example, housework or gathering fuel); or in leisure time (for example, participating in sports or recreational activities). In this report, physical inactivity is defined as doing very little or no physical activity in any of these domains.

There is no internationally agreed definition or measure of physical activity. Therefore, a number of direct and indirect data sources and a range of survey instruments and methodologies were used to estimate activity levels in these four domains. Most data were available for leisure-time activity, with fewer direct data available on occupational activity and little direct data available for activity relating to transport and domestic tasks. Also, this report only estimates the prevalence of physical inactivity among people aged 15 years and over. The global estimate for prevalence of physical inactivity among adults is 17%, ranging from 11% to 24% across subregions. Estimates for prevalence of some but insufficient activity (<2.5 hours per week of moderate activity) ranged from 31% to 51%, with a global average of 41% across the 14 subregions.

Physical activity reduces the risk of cardiovascular disease, some cancers and type 2 diabetes. These benefits are mediated through a number of mechanisms *(22)*. In general, physical activity improves glucose metabolism, reduces body fat and lowers blood pressure; these are the main ways in which it is thought to reduce the risk of cardiovascular diseases and diabetes. Physical activity may reduce the risk of colon cancer by effects on prostaglandins, reduced intestinal transit time, and higher antioxidant levels. Physical activity is also associated with lower risk of breast cancer, which may be the result of effects on hormonal metabolism. Participation in physical activity can improve musculoskeletal health, control body weight, and reduce symptoms of depression. The possible effects on musculoskeletal conditions such as osteoarthritis and low back pain, osteoporosis and falls, obesity, depression, anxiety and stress, as well as on prostate and other cancers are, however, not quantified here.

Overall physical inactivity was estimated to cause 1.9 million deaths and 19 million DALYs globally. Physical inactivity is estimated to cause, globally, about 10–16% of cases each of breast cancer, colon and rectal cancers and diabetes mellitus, and about 22% of ischaemic heart disease. Estimated attributable fractions are similar in men and women and are highest in AMR-B, EUR-C and WPR-B. In EUR-C, the proportion of deaths attributable to physical inactivity is 8–10%, and in AMR-A, EUR-A and EUR-B it is about 5–8%.

SEXUAL AND REPRODUCTIVE HEALTH

Risk factors in the area of sexual and reproductive health can affect well-being in a number of ways (see Table 4.4). The largest risk by far is that posed by unsafe sex leading to infection with HIV/AIDS. Other potentially deleterious outcomes, such as other sexually transmitted infections, unwanted pregnancy or the psychological consequences of sexual violence are considered elsewhere in this report (see Figure 4.5).

ADDICTIVE SUBSTANCES

Humans consume a wide variety of addictive substances. The addictive substances assessed quantitatively in this report included tobacco, alcohol and illicit drugs (see Table 4.5). Some summary results are shown in Figure 4.6.

SMOKING AND ORAL TOBACCO USE

Tobacco is cultivated in many regions around the world and can be legally purchased in all countries. The dried leaf of the plant *nicotiana tabacum* is used for smoking, chewing or snuff. Comparable data on the prevalence of smoking are not widely available and are often inaccurate, especially when age-specific data are required. More importantly, current prevalence of smoking is a poor proxy for the cumulative hazards of smoking, which depend on several factors including the age at which smoking began, duration of smoking, number of cigarettes smoked per day, degree of inhalation, and cigarette characteristics such as tar and nicotine content or the type of filter. To overcome this problem the smoking impact ratio, which estimates excess lung cancer, is used as a marker for accumulated smoking risk.

There were large increases in smoking in developing countries, especially among males, over the last part of the 20th century *(24, 25)*. This contrasts with the steady but slow decreases, mostly among men, in many industrialized countries. Smoking rates remain relatively high in most former socialist economies. While prevalence of tobacco use has declined in some high income countries, it is increasing in some low and middle income countries, especially among young people and women.

Smoking causes substantially increased risk of mortality from lung cancer, upper aerodigestive cancer, several other cancers, heart disease, stroke, chronic respiratory disease and a range of other medical causes. As a result, in populations where smoking has been common for many decades, tobacco use accounts for a considerable proportion of mortality, as illustrated by estimates of smoking-attributable deaths in industrialized countries *(26)*. The first estimates of the health impacts of smoking in China and India have also shown substantially increased risk of mortality and disease among smokers *(27–30)*. Smoking also harms others – there are definite health risks from passive smoking (see Box 4.1) and smoking during pregnancy adversely affects fetal development. While cigarette smoking causes the majority of the adverse health effects of tobacco, chewing is also hazardous, causing oral cancer in particular, as does tobacco smoking via cigars or pipes.

Among industrialized countries, where smoking has been common, smoking is estimated to cause over 90% of lung cancer in men and about 70% of lung cancer among women. In addition, in these countries, the attributable fractions are 56–80% for chronic

Table 4.5 Selected major risks to health: addictive substances

Risk factor	Theoretical minimum exposure	Measured adverse outcomes of exposure
Tobacco	No tobacco use	Lung cancer, upper aerodigestive cancer, all other cancers, chronic obstructive pulmonary disease, other respiratory diseases, all vascular diseases
Alcohol	No alcohol use	Stroke, ischaemic heart disease, other cardiac diseases, hypertensive disease, diabetes mellitus, liver cancer, cancer of mouth and oropharynx, breast cancer, oesophagus cancer, other neoplasms, liver cirrhosis, epilepsy, alcohol use, falls, motor accidents, drownings, homicide, other intentional injuries, self-inflicted injuries, poisonings
Illicit drugs	No illicit drug use	HIV/AIDS, overdose, drug use disorder, suicide, trauma

respiratory disease and 22% for cardio-vascular disease. Worldwide, it is estimated that tobacco causes about 8.8% of deaths (4.9 million) and 4.1% of DALYs (59.1 million). The rapid evolution of the tobacco epidemic is illustrated by comparing these estimates for 2000 with those for 1990: there are at least a million more deaths attributable to tobacco, with the increase being most marked in developing countries. The extent of disease burden is consistently higher among groups known to have smoked longest – for example, attributable mortality is greater in males (13.3%) than females (3.8%). Worldwide, the attributable fractions for tobacco were about 12% for vascular disease, 66% for trachea bronchus and lung cancers and 38% for chronic respiratory disease, although the pattern varies by subregion. Approximately 16% of the global attributable burden occurred in WPR-B, 20% in SEAR-D and 14% in EUR-C.

ALCOHOL USE

Alcohol has been consumed in human populations for millennia, but the considerable and varied adverse health effects, as well as some benefits, have only been characterized recently (*39, 40*). Alcohol consumption has health and social consequences via intoxication (drunkenness), dependence (habitual, compulsive, long-term heavy drinking) and other biochemical effects. Intoxication is a powerful mediator for acute outcomes, such as car crashes or domestic violence, and can also cause chronic health and social problems. Alcohol dependence is a disorder in itself. There is increasing evidence that patterns of drinking are relevant to health as well as volume of alcohol consumed, binge drinking being hazardous.

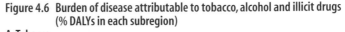

Figure 4.6 Burden of disease attributable to tobacco, alcohol and illicit drugs (% DALYs in each subregion)

A. Tobacco

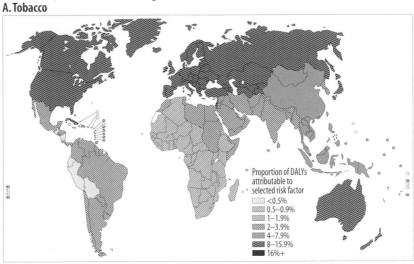

Proportion of DALYs attributable to selected risk factor
- <0.5%
- 0.5–0.9%
- 1–1.9%
- 2–3.9%
- 4–7.9%
- 8–15.9%
- 16%+

B. Alcohol

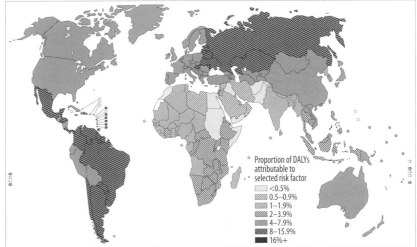

Proportion of DALYs attributable to selected risk factor
- <0.5%
- 0.5–0.9%
- 1–1.9%
- 2–3.9%
- 4–7.9%
- 8–15.9%
- 16%+

C. Illicit drugs

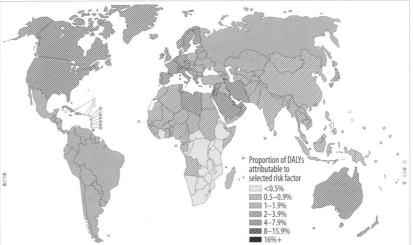

Proportion of DALYs attributable to selected risk factor
- <0.5%
- 0.5–0.9%
- 1–1.9%
- 2–3.9%
- 4–7.9%
- 8–15.9%
- 16%+

The values presented here are averages by subregion; variations occur within these subregions but are not shown here. For an explanation of subregions see the List of Member States by WHO Region and mortality stratum.

Global alcohol consumption has increased in recent decades, with most or all of this increase occurring in developing countries. Both average volume of alcohol consumption and patterns of drinking vary dramatically between subregions. Average volume of drinking is highest in Europe and North America, and lowest in the Eastern Mediterranean and SEAR-D. Patterns are most detrimental in EUR-C, AMR-B, AMR-D and AFR-E. Patterns are least detrimental in Western Europe (EUR-A) and the more economically established parts of the Western Pacific region (WPR-A).

Overall, there are causal relationships between average volume of alcohol consumption and more than 60 types of disease and injury. Most of these relationships are detrimental, but there are beneficial relationships with coronary heart disease, stroke and diabetes mellitus, provided low-to-moderate average volume of consumption is combined with non-binge patterns of drinking. For example, it is estimated that ischaemic stroke would be about 17% higher in AMR-A, EUR-A and WPR-A subregions if no-one consumed alcohol.

Worldwide, alcohol causes 3.2% of deaths (1.8 million) and 4.0% of DALYs (58.3 million). Of this global burden, 24%occurs in WPR-B, 16% in EUR-C, and 16% in AMR-B. This proportion is much higher in males (5.6% of deaths, 6.5% of DALYs) than females (0.6% of deaths, 1.3% of DALYs). Within subregions, the proportion of disease burden attributable to alcohol is greatest in the Americas and Europe, where it ranges from 8% to 18% of total burden for males and 2% to 4% for females. Besides the direct effects of intoxication and addiction resulting in alcohol use disorders, alcohol is estimated to cause about 20–30% of each of the following worldwide: oesophageal cancer, liver cancer, cirrhosis of the liver, homicide, epilepsy, and motor vehicle accidents. For males in EUR-C, 50–75% of drownings, oesophagus cancer, epilepsy, unintentional injuries, homicide, motor vehicle crashes and cirrhosis of the liver are attributed to alcohol.

ILLICIT DRUG USE

Illicit drug use includes the non-medical use of a variety of drugs that are prohibited by international law. The current analysis focuses on the burden attributable to the injection of amphetamines and opioids, including cocaine and heroin. Other illegal drugs, such as ec-

Box 4.1 Environmental tobacco smoke

Environmental tobacco smoke (ETS) is a combination of exhaled smoke from active smokers and the smoke coming from smouldering tobacco between puffs. Also known as second-hand smoke or passive (involuntary) smoking, ETS causes disease in non-smokers; it contains all the same toxic components as mainstream tobacco smoke, although in somewhat different relative amounts.

ETS exposure is primarily dependent on the prevalence of smoking, including both commercial and non-commercial forms of tobacco. In addition, smoking intensity (the amount of tobacco smoked per smoker), differences in ventilation, and differences in places where people smoke affect the amount of ETS exposure that results per smoker.

Most studies on the health effects of ETS have focused on household and occupational exposures. People are also exposed in other environments, such as schools, transport systems, bars and restaurants. Exposure to ETS has been associated with lower respiratory infections, sudden infant death syndrome, asthma, ischaemic heart disease, otitis media, lung cancer and nasal-sinus cancer. In the United States, for example, several thousand lung cancer deaths are associated with ETS exposure each year. There is increasing evidence that ETS causes heart disease and in the United States alone it has been estimated to cause tens of thousands of premature deaths each year. There is evidence that even short-term exposures to ETS can increase the risk of coronary thrombosis by increasing blood platelet aggregation.

In addition, maternal smoking during pregnancy results in passive smoke exposure for the fetus (sometimes referred to as tertiary smoke), resulting in an increased risk of low birth weight and sudden infant death syndrome. The risk of sudden infant death syndrome is doubled when mothers smoke.

Protecting people from ETS exposure has a large role in policy debates about controlling active smoking, since ETS exposures affect not only smokers but also others around them, most importantly young children who are not in a position to protect themselves. Without major efforts to bring smoking and ETS exposure under control, the burden of disease from ETS will continue to increase in the future.

Sources: *(31–38).*

stasy, solvents and cannabis have not been included because there is insufficient research to quantify their health risks globally.

Because the use of these drugs is illicit and often hidden, it is difficult to estimate the prevalence of their use and the occurrence of adverse health consequences. Despite these difficulties, it is apparent that illicit drugs cause considerable disease burden and their use is increasing in many countries, including those with little past history of such use *(41, 42)*.

The estimated prevalence of illicit drug use varies considerably across WHO regions. For example, estimates from the United Nations Drug Control Programme of the prevalence of opioid use in the past 12 months among people over the age of 15 years varies by an order of magnitude or more, from 0.02–0.04% in the Western Pacific region to 0.4–0.6% in the Eastern Mediterranean region. Cocaine use varies to a similar extent, but the prevalence of amphetamine use is estimated to be 0.1%–0.3% in most regions.

The mortality risks of illicit drugs increase with frequency and quantity of use *(43, 44)*. The most hazardous patterns are found among dependent users who typically inject drugs daily or near daily over periods of years. Studies of treated injecting opioid users show this pattern is associated with increased overall mortality, including that caused by HIV/AIDS, overdose, suicide and trauma. Other adverse health and social effects that could not be quantified include other bloodborne diseases such as hepatitis B and hepatitis C, and criminal activity associated with the drug habit.

Globally, 0.4% of deaths (0.2 million) and 0.8% of DALYs (11.2 million) are attributed to overall illicit drug use. Attributable burden is consistently several times higher among men than women. Illicit drugs account for the highest proportion of disease burden among low mortality, industrialized countries in the Americas, Eastern Mediterranean and European regions. In these areas illicit drug use accounts for 2–4% of all disease burden among men.

ENVIRONMENTAL RISKS

The environment in which we live greatly affects our health. The household, workplace, outdoor and transportation environments pose risks to health in a number of different ways, from the poor quality of the air many people breathe to the hazards we face as a result of climate change (see Table 4.6). A range of selected environmental risk factors is assessed here and some summary results are shown in Figure 4.7.

Table 4.6 Selected major risks to health: environmental factors

Risk factor	Theoretical minimum exposure	Measured adverse outcomes of exposure
Unsafe water, sanitation and hygiene	Absence of transmission of diarrhoeal disease through water, sanitation and hygiene practices	Diarrhoea
Urban air pollution	7.5 µg/m^3 for PM$_{2.5}$	Cardiovascular mortality, respiratory mortality, lung cancer, mortality from acute respiratory infections in children
Indoor smoke from solid fuels	No solid fuel use	Acute respiratory infections in children, chronic obstructive pulmonary disease, lung cancer
Lead exposure	0.016 µg/dl blood lead levels	Cardiovascular disease, mild mental retardation
Climate change	1961–1990 concentrations	Diarrhoea, flood injury, malaria, malnutrition

UNSAFE WATER, SANITATION AND HYGIENE

Adverse health outcomes are associated with ingestion of unsafe water, lack of access to water (linked to inadequate hygiene), lack of access to sanitation, contact with unsafe water, and inadequate management of water resources and systems, including in agriculture. Infectious diarrhoea makes the largest single contribution to the burden of disease associated with unsafe water, sanitation and hygiene.

Six broad scenarios were characterized; these included populations with no access to improved water sources or no basic sanitation; those with access to fully regulated water supply and sanitation services; and an ideal scenario in which no disease transmission is associated with this risk factor. In addition, schistosomiasis, trachoma, ascariasis, trichuriasis and hookworm disease were fully attributed to unsafe water, sanitation and hygiene.

Exposure prevalence was determined from the WHO/UNICEF Global Water Supply and Sanitation Assessment 2000. This provides a synthesis of major international surveys and national census reports, which provide data for 89% of the global population. In 2000, the percentage of people served with some form of improved water supply worldwide reached 82% (4.9 billion), while 60% (3.6 billion) had access to basic sanitation facilities. The vast majority of diarrhoeal disease in the world (88%) was attributable to unsafe water, sanitation and hygiene.

Approximately 3.1% of deaths (1.7 million) and 3.7% of DALYs (54.2 million) worldwide are attributable to unsafe water, sanitation and hygiene. Of this burden, about one-third occurred in Africa and one-third in SEAR-D. In these areas, as well as in EMR-D and AMR-D, 4–8% of all disease burden is attributable to unsafe water, sanitation and hygiene. Overall, 99.8% of deaths associated with this risk factor are in developing countries, and 90% are deaths of children.

URBAN AIR POLLUTION

The serious consequences of exposure to high levels of urban ambient air pollution were made clear in the mid-20th century when cities in Europe and the United States experienced air pollution episodes, such as the infamous 1952 London fog, that resulted in many deaths and hospital admissions. Subsequent clean air legislation and actions reduced ambient air pollution in many regions. However, recent epidemiological studies, using sensitive designs and analyses, have identified serious health effects of combustion-derived air pollution even at the low ambient concentrations typical of Western European and North American cities (45). At the same time, the populations of the rapidly expanding megacities of Asia, Africa and Latin America are increasingly exposed to levels of ambient air pollution that rival and often exceed those experienced in industrialized countries in the first half of the 20th century (46).

Urban air pollution is largely and increasingly the result of the combustion of fossil fuels for transport, power generation and other human activities. Combustion processes produce a complex mixture of pollutants that comprises both primary emissions, such as diesel soot particles and lead, and the products of atmospheric transformation, such as ozone and sulfate particles formed from the burning of sulfur-containing fuel.

Air pollution from combustion sources is associated with a broad spectrum of acute and chronic health effects (47, 48), that may vary with the pollutant constituents. Particulate air pollution (i.e. particles small enough to be inhaled into the lung,) is consistently and independently related to the most serious effects, including lung cancer and other cardiopulmonary mortality (44, 49, 50). Other constituents, such as lead and ozone, are also associated with serious health effects, and contribute to the burden of disease attributable to urban air pollution. The analyses based on particulate matter estimate that ambient air pollution causes about 5% of trachea, bronchus and lung cancer, 2% of cardiorespiratory mortality and about 1% of respiratory infections mortality globally. This amounts to about 0.8 million (1.4%) deaths and 7.9 million (0.8%) DALYs. This burden predominantly occurs in developing countries, with 42% of attributable DALYs occurring in WPR-B and 19% in SEAR-D. Within subregions, the highest proportions of total burden occur in WPR-A, WPR-B, EUR-B and EUR-C, where ambient air pollution causes 0.6–1.4% of disease burden. These estimates consider only the impact of air pollution on mortality, and not morbidity, due to limitations in the epidemiologic database. If air pollution multiplies both incidence and mortality to the same extent, the burden of disease would be higher.

INDOOR SMOKE FROM SOLID FUELS

Although air pollutant emissions are dominated by outdoor sources, human exposures are a function of the level of pollution in places where people spend most of their time (51–53). Human exposure to air pollution is thus dominated by the indoor environment. Cooking and heating with solid fuels such as dung, wood, agricultural residues or coal is likely to be the largest source of indoor air pollution globally. When used in simple cooking stoves, these fuels emit substantial amounts of pollutants, including respirable particles, carbon monoxide, nitrogen and sulfur oxides, and benzene.

Nearly half the world continues to cook with solid fuels. This includes more than 75% of people in India, China and nearby countries, and

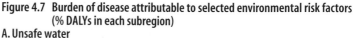

Figure 4.7 Burden of disease attributable to selected environmental risk factors (% DALYs in each subregion)

A. Unsafe water

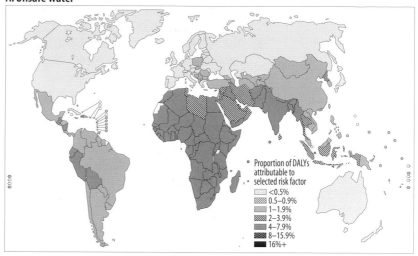

B. Indoor smoke from solid fuels

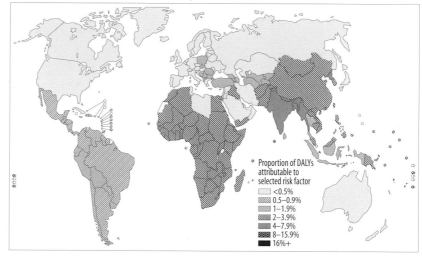

C. Urban air pollution

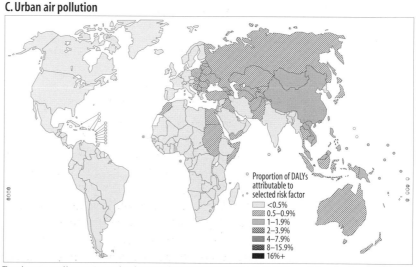

The values presented here are averages by subregion; variations occur within these subregions but are not shown here. For an explanation of subregions see the List of Member States by WHO Region and mortality stratum.

50–75% of people in parts of South America and Africa. Limited ventilation is common in many developing countries and increases exposure, particularly for women and young children who spend much of their time indoors. Exposures have been measured at many times higher than WHO guidelines and national standards, and thus can be substantially greater than outdoors in cities with the most severe air pollution.

Studies have shown reasonably consistent and strong relationships between the indoor use of solid fuel and a number of diseases. These analyses estimate that indoor smoke from solid fuels causes about 35.7% of lower respiratory infections, 22.0% of chronic obstructive pulmonary disease and 1.5% of trachea, bronchus and lung cancer. Indoor air pollution may also be associated with tuberculosis, cataracts and asthma.

In total, 2.7% of DALYs worldwide are attributable to indoor smoke, 2.5% in males and 2.8% in females. Of this total attributable burden, about 32% occurs in Africa (AFR-D and AFR-E), 37% in SEAR-D and 16% in WPR-B. Among women, indoor air smoke causes approximately 3–4% of DALYs in AFR-D, AFR-E, EMR-D, SEAR-D and WPR-B. The most important interventions to reduce this impact are better ventilation, more efficient vented stoves, and cleaner fuels.

Many other risks to health accumulate in the indoor environment, and housing has a key role in determining their development and impact (see Box 4.2).

LEAD EXPOSURE

Lead, because of its multiplicity of uses, is present in air, dust, soil and water. Lead enters the body mainly by ingestion or inhalation. Contamination of the environment has in-

---

Box 4.2 Housing and health

The primary purpose of buildings worldwide is to protect humans from the hazards and discomforts of outdoor environments and to offer a safe and convenient setting for living and human activity. Furthermore, people – especially in temperate and cold climates and in industrialized societies – spend most of their time indoors in buildings such as homes, offices, schools and day-care centres. This means that, from the perspective of exposure to environmental conditions and hazards, housing and indoor environments have important public health consequences for both physical and mental health.

The most extreme health impact of housing is found among the poorest sectors of societies in the form of a complete lack of housing, which affects millions of people worldwide. Lack of affordable housing for low-income households may mean diverting family resources from expenditure on food, education or health towards housing needs. Beyond this, both the physical structure of houses and their location can involve health risks.

Important parameters in indoor environments include the thermal climate, noise and light, and exposure to a large number of chemi-

cal, physical and biological pollutants and risk factors. While these parameters are also affected by human-related activities and outdoor sources (such as vehicle and industrial pollutants or local vegetation and insect ecology), human exposure is modified by housing characteristics such as building materials, number and size of rooms and windows, ventilation and energy technology. For example, a "leaky" house can lead to dampness and mould which may result in various forms of respiratory illness and allergic reactions; the use of building materials such asbestos or lead-based paint can increase exposure to these toxic substances; the use of inflammable or weak material such as wood, plastic or cardboard – particularly common in urban slums – poses increased risks of injuries; building design will influence exposure to disease vectors such as mosquitoes; inadequate ventilation or overcrowding will cause exposure to different pollutants and pathogens; poor lighting or heating will influence both physical and mental health as well as participation in activities such as education; and so on.

The location of housing and the organization of neighbourhoods also have public health impli-

cations, in particular in rapidly urbanizing developing countries, where a growing proportion of the population live in informal settlements or slums, often on the periphery of major cities. If housing is located on floodplains or steep hillsides, near sources of traffic, industrial activity, solid waste dumps or vector breeding sites, and away from services such as sanitation, transportation, schools or health facilities, public health will be affected directly (for example, through sanitation) or indirectly through access to food and education. In addition, organization of neighbourhoods has been shown to have an effect on mental and physical health, school attendance and performance, or prevalence of violence and crime.

Referring to housing as a "risk factor" would mask the important role that it plays in providing a setting for daily household and community activities. At the same time, it is important to acknowledge the important and complex roles that housing and neighbourhood design play in public health and to promote systematic inclusion of health in the design of housing, housing technology and the urban and regional planning processes.

Sources: *(54–56)*.

creased with industrial development and particularly the use of leaded petrol. Currently about 60 countries have phased out leaded petrol and approximately 85% of petrol sold worldwide is lead-free. Other important lead sources are more difficult to control, such as leaded kitchenware ceramics, water pipes and house paints.

Following control measures, lead levels have been steadily declining in industrialized countries but at least 5% of children still have elevated blood lead levels, with even higher rates in children of poorer households *(57)*. In many developing countries, where leaded gasoline is still used, lead can present a threat to more than half of children *(58)*. Rapidly increasing traffic loads have the potential to further increase blood lead levels. Worldwide, 120 million people are estimated to have lead levels of 5–10 µg/dl, with similar numbers above 10 µg/dl, and 40% of children have blood lead levels above 5 µg/dl. Overall, 97% of affected children live in developing regions. Industrial or cottage exposure to lead, such as from smelters or battery recycling, could only partly be assessed here, but can represent a large additional burden in certain regions.

Lead affects practically all body systems. Most toxic exposures occur at chronic low levels and can result in reductions in intelligence quotient (IQ) *(59)*, increased blood pressure, and a range of behavioural and developmental effects. The range and extent of adverse health effects has been appreciated only relatively recently. Furthermore, lead is now understood to be toxic, especially to children, at levels previously thought to be safe *(60)*. In more severe cases of poisoning, adverse health effects include gastrointestinal symptoms, anaemia, neurological damage and renal impairment *(61)*. Other adverse effects, such as reduction in IQ levels, behavioural disorders or renal function, can be discerned only through special examinations. These analyses estimate that lead results in about 234 000 (0.4%) deaths and 12.9 million (0.9%) DALYs. About one-fifth of this entire burden occurs in SEAR-D, and a further one-fifth in WPR-B.

CLIMATE CHANGE

Humans are accustomed to climatic conditions varying daily, seasonally and yearly. The recent concern over global climate change arises from accumulating evidence that, in addition to this natural climate variability, average climatic conditions measured over extended periods (conventionally 30 years or longer) are now also changing *(62)*. The most recent report (2001) from the United Nations Intergovernmental Panel on Climate Change (IPCC) estimates that the global average land and sea surface temperature has increased by 0.6 ±0.2 °C since the mid-19th century, with most change occurring since 1976 *(63)*. The 1990s was the warmest decade on record. Warming has been observed in all continents, with the greatest temperature changes occurring at middle and high latitudes in the northern hemisphere. Patterns of precipitation have also changed: arid and semiarid regions are apparently becoming drier, while other areas, especially mid-to-high latitudes, are becoming wetter. There is also evidence that where precipitation has increased, there has been a disproportionate increase in the frequency of the heaviest precipitation events. The causes of this climate change are increasingly well understood. The IPCC concluded that "most of the warming observed over the last 50 years is likely to be attributable to human activities", most importantly the release of greenhouse gases from fossil fuels.

Climate model simulations have been used to estimate the effects of past, present and future greenhouse gas emissions on future climate. Based on a range of alternative development scenarios and model parameters, the IPCC concluded that if no specific actions are taken to reduce greenhouse gas emissions, global temperatures are likely to rise between 1.4 °C and 5.8 °C from 1990 to 2100. Such a rise would be faster than any rise encountered since the inception of agriculture around 10 000 years ago. Predictions for precipitation and wind speed are less consistent, but also suggest significant changes.

Potential risks to human health from climate change would arise from increased exposures to thermal extremes (cardiovascular and respiratory mortality) and from increases in weather disasters (including deaths and injuries associated with floods). Other risks may arise because of the changing dynamics of disease vectors (such as malaria and dengue fever), the seasonality and incidence of various food-related and waterborne infections, the yields of agricultural crops, the range of plant and livestock pests and pathogens, the salination of coastal lands and freshwater supplies resulting from rising sea-levels, the climatically related production of photochemical air pollutants, spores and pollens, and the risk of conflict over depleted natural resources. Effects of climate change on human health can be expected to be mediated through complex interactions of physical, ecological, and social factors. These effects will undoubtedly have a greater impact on societies or individuals with scarce resources, where technologies are lacking, and where infrastructure and institutions (such as the health sector) are least able to adapt. For this reason, a better understanding of the role of socioeconomic and technological factors in shaping and mitigating these impacts is essential. Because of this complexity, current estimates of the potential health impacts of climate change are based on models with considerable uncertainty.

Climate change was estimated to be responsible in 2000 for approximately 2.4% of worldwide diarrhoea, 6% of malaria in some middle income countries and 7% of dengue fever in some industrialized countries. In total, the attributable mortality was 154 000 (0.3%) deaths and the attributable burden was 5.5 million (0.4%) DALYs. About 46% this burden occurred in SEAR-D, 23% in AFR-E and a further 14% in EMR-D.

OTHER ENVIRONMENTAL RISKS TO HEALTH

Traffic and transport form another component of environmental hazard in society. Traffic-related burden includes not only injury, but also the consequences of pollution with lead and the effects on urban air quality. Furthermore, as with many exposures assessed

---

Box 4.3 Road traffic injuries

Road traffic injuries were estimated to account for over 1.2 million deaths worldwide in 2000, amounting to 2.3% of all deaths. Many such deaths occur in young adults, with significant loss of life, so the proportion of disease burden measured in disability-adjusted life years (DALYs) is greater – about 2.8% of the total. Over 90% of these deaths occur in the middle and low income countries, where death rates (21 and 24 deaths per 100 000 population, respectively) are approximately double the rates in high income countries (12 per 100 000 population).

Differences in road use between industrialized and developing countries have implications for intervention policies. Driver or occupant deaths accounted for approximately 50–60% of national road traffic fatalities in industrialized countries in 1999, with the vast majority occurring on rural roads. Pedestrian involvement was higher in urban areas, with evidence for increased risk among children and over-60-year-olds. In developing countries, a far higher proportion of road deaths occurs among vulnerable users (pedestrians, bicyclists, other non-motorized traffic, and motor cyclists and moped riders) and among passengers of buses and trucks.

Road traffic crashes are largely preventable. Approaches to improving road safety fall into three broad groups: engineering measures (e.g. road design and traffic management), vehicle design and equipment (e.g. helmets, seat belts and day-time running lights) and road user measures (e.g. speed limits, and restrictions on drinking and driving).

The prospects for prevention can be estimated from some interventions. For example, in Thailand the introduction of a new motor cycle helmet law was followed by a reduction in fatalities of 56%; in Denmark, improved traffic management and provision of cycle tracks was followed by a 35% drop in cyclist fatalities; and in Western Europe it was estimated that lowering average vehicle speeds by 5km/hour could yield a 25% reduction in fatalities. Based on a model developed in the United Kingdom, which takes into account the numbers of cars per capita, it is estimated that, if the countries with the higher road traffic injury rates were to lower these rates to those of other countries in each region, death rates would fall by between 8% and 80%. The scope for improvement is highest in the poorest countries. Worldwide, it is estimated that 44% of road traffic fatalities – or 20 million DALYs – per year could be avoided by this method.

Sources: *(64–70)*.

here, there are complex interactions with other exposures – for example, the lost opportunity for physical activity and the economic effects of transport and traffic. Considerations related to road traffic injuries are outlined in Box 4.3.

SELECTED OCCUPATIONAL RISKS

Throughout the world many adults, and some children, spend most waking hours at work. While at work, people face a variety of hazards almost as numerous as the different types of work, including chemicals, biological agents, physical factors, adverse ergonomic conditions, allergens, a complex causal network of safety risks, and many and varied psychosocial factors. These may produce a wide range of health outcomes, including injuries, cancer, hearing loss, and respiratory, musculoskeletal, cardiovascular, reproductive, neurotoxic, skin and psychological disorders. Because of lack of adequate global data, only selected risk factors were evaluated in this report (see Table 4.7). The disease burden from these selected occupational risks amounts to 1.5% of the global burden in terms of DALYs.

Examples of other important work-related risk factors include pesticides, heavy metals, infectious organisms, and agents causing occupational asthma and chronic obstructive lung disease. Analyses at the global level may not show the magnitude of occupational risk factors, because only the workers employed in the jobs with those risks are affected. It is important to note that not only are the affected workers at high risk, but also that workplace risks are almost entirely preventable. For example, because health care workers constitute only 0.6% of the global population, hepatitis B in this group contributes negligibly to the global burden. These workers are, however, at high risk of hepatitis B, of which 40% is produced by sharps injuries (see Box 4.4). Policies to standardize needle usage and to increase immunization coverage will prevent these infections, which represent a heavy burden in the health personnel.

Stress at work has been shown in recent studies in industrialized nations to be associated with cardiovascular disease, but the risks will also exist in similar types of work in developing and industrializing nations. Policy-makers and decision-makers may wish to be guided by findings such as those illustrated in Box 4.5.

Table 4.7 Selected major risks to health: occupational hazards

Risk factor	Theoretical minimum exposure	Measured adverse outcomes of exposure
Work-related risk factors for injuries	Exposure corresponding to lowest rate of work-related fatalities observed: 1 per million per year for 16–17-year-olds employed as service workers in the United States	Injury
Work-related carcinogens	No work-related exposure above background to chemical or physical agents that cause cancer	Leukaemia, lung cancer
Selected airborne particulates	No work-related exposure	Chronic respiratory disease
Work-related ergonomic stressors	Physical workload at the level of that of managers and professionals	Lower back pain
Work-related noise	Less than 85 dB over eight working hours	Hearing loss

WORK-RELATED RISK FACTORS FOR INJURIES

Risk factors leading to injuries are present in every workplace. Industrial and agricultural workers have the highest risks, but even workers in offices, retail stores and schools are at risk *(73–75)*. Work-related falls, motor vehicle injuries, and contact with machinery result in nearly a thousand occupational deaths every day throughout the world. Disability is another consequence of work-related injury, sometimes requiring time lost from work, and sometimes resulting in a permanent inability to return to work. Reliable data about injuries are difficult to obtain, even in industrialized countries, because of variability in insurance coverage and in accuracy of the reporting systems. Nevertheless, occupational fatality rates reported in industrializing countries are at least two to five times higher than rates reported in industrialized countries *(76)*.

For this report, the numbers of workers at risk of injury were estimated by employment in broad occupational categories for each region, sex, and age. The corresponding fatal

Box 4.4 Sharps injuries among health care workers

Health care workers are at risk of infection with bloodborne pathogens because of occupational exposure to blood and body fluids. Most exposures are caused by "sharps" – contaminated sharp objects, such as syringe needles, scalpels and broken glass. The three infections most commonly transmitted to health care workers are hepatitis B virus (HBV), hepatitis C virus (HCV) and human immunodeficiency virus (HIV).

Among the 35 million health care workers worldwide, about three million receive percutaneous exposures to bloodborne pathogens each year; 2 million of those to HBV, 0.9 million to HCV and 170 000 to HIV. These injuries may result in 15 000 HCV, 70 000 HBV and 500 HIV infections. More than 90% of these infections occur in developing countries. Worldwide, about 40% of HBV and HCV infections and 2.5% of HIV infections in health care workers are attributable to occupational sharps exposures.

These infections are for the major part preventable, as shown by the low rates achieved in certain countries that have engaged in serious prevention efforts, including training of health care workers, HBV immunization, post-exposure prophylaxis and improved waste management. In addition to the disease burden caused to health care workers, the functioning of the health care system may be reduced because of impaired working capacity, in particular in developing countries where the proportion of health care workers in the population is already small compared with that in developed countries.

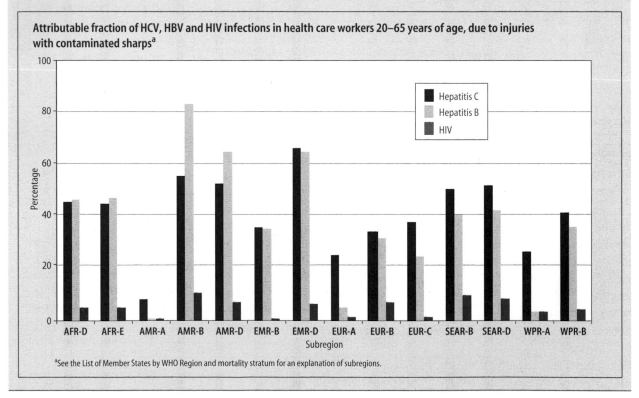

Attributable fraction of HCV, HBV and HIV infections in health care workers 20–65 years of age, due to injuries with contaminated sharps[a]

[a]See the List of Member States by WHO Region and mortality stratum for an explanation of subregions.

injury rates were obtained from an extensive literature survey. The analysis showed that overall approximately 310 000 workers lose their lives each year as a result of occupational injuries that are unintentional (from machines, motor vehicles, falls, poisonings, falling objects, fires and drowning) and intentional (homicide). Most of these deaths are preventable *(77)*. Occupational injuries represent 0.9% of world DALYs (13.1 million) and 16% of DALYs attributable to unintentional injuries in the working population aged 15–69 years. This burden, with its heavy toll in human suffering and monetary costs, affects mainly the developing regions such as SEAR-D and WPR-B. These two regions represent almost half of the workforce of the world.

WORK-RELATED CARCINOGENS

Many of the 150 chemical or biological agents classified as carcinogens are encountered in occupational settings *(78)*. The risk of developing cancer is influenced by the dose received, the potency of the carcinogen, the presence of other exposures (notably tobacco smoking), and individual susceptibility. Occupational cancers are entirely preventable through elimination of exposure, using proven occupational hygiene measures such as substitution of safer materials, enclosure of processes, and ventilation.

These analyses estimated the effects of occupational exposures to numerous known carcinogens on the occurrence of respiratory and bladder cancers, leukaemia, and mesothelioma.

Globally about 20–30% of the male and 5–20% of the female working-age population (people aged 15–64 years) may have been exposed during their working lives to lung carcinogens, including asbestos, arsenic, beryllium, cadmium, chromium, diesel exhaust, nickel and silica. Worldwide, these occupational exposures account for about 10.3% of cancer of the lung, trachea and bronchus, which is the most frequent occupational cancer. About 2.4% of leukaemia is attributable to occupational exposures worldwide. In total, the attributable mortality was 146 000 (0.3%) deaths and the attributable burden was 1.4 million (0.1%) DALYs.

WORK-RELATED AIRBORNE PARTICULATES

Millions of workers in a variety of occupations, such as mining, construction and abrasive blasting, are exposed to microscopic airborne particles of silica, asbestos and coal dust *(79–81)*. Inhalation of these particles may not only cause cancer of the lung, trachea and

---

Box 4.5 Coronary heart disease and work-related stress

Increasing evidence from industrialized countries links coronary heart disease with work-related stress, such as high psychological demands and low decision-making latitude among white-collar occupations including managers, administrators, supervisors and proprietors. Blue-collar workers are also at risk from high work pressure and cumulative workload, in combination with low-status control.

Low job control is associated with an increase in the risk of heart disease. Shiftwork, which tends to involve heavier work, more stress, less control, and less educated workers than regular day work, also increases risk. Mechanisms of action include disturbances to the circadian rhythm, fatigue, elevated levels of serum triglycerides, and the fact that shiftwork accentuates other risk factors for heart disease.

Overall, stress-related coronary heart disease is likely to be higher in blue-collar workers when the following factors are present: restricted discretion, shiftwork (particularly at night), imbalance between efforts and rewards, high demands, a poor psychosocial work environment, social isolation, physical inactivity, or occupational violence. These risk factors may be interactive. Recent estimates for Finland indicated that a substantial proportion of ischaemic heart disease results from the combined occupational risk factors of shift work, noise, exposure to engine exhausts, and environmental tobacco smoke.

Sources: *(71, 72)*.

bronchus, but also the non-malignant respiratory diseases silicosis, asbestos and coal and pneumoconiosis ("dusty lung").

Development of these diseases is influenced by the amount of exposure and the toxicity of the dust, and the diseases are characterized by long latency periods; therefore, even in countries in which exposures have been recognized and controlled, the disease rates are only gradually declining *(79)*. Rate trends in developing countries are mostly unknown but the magnitude of the problem is substantial *(81)*.

Studies estimate that 5–18% of asthma may be attributable to occupational exposure, with one review study suggesting a median value of 15% for the highest quality studies. One large population study estimates that 14% of chronic obstructive pulmonary disease is attributable to occupational causes. In total, the attributable mortality for chronic obstructive pulmonary disease was 243 000 (0.4%) deaths and the attributable burden was 3.0 million (0.2%) DALYs. Several tens of thousands of additional deaths are attributable to silica, asbestos and coal dust. At the global level, the burden appears low, but the risk to workers in mining, construction and other occupations is high. For example, most workers with long-term exposure to low-to-moderate silica concentrations will develop silicosis. These diseases are entirely preventable through efforts like those of the ILO/WHO global campaign to eliminate silicosis, including elimination of exposure through substitution of safer materials, wet methods, and ventilation.

WORK-RELATED ERGONOMIC STRESSORS

Low back pain is associated with many ergonomic stressors at work, including lifting and carrying of heavy loads, forceful movements, demanding physical work, whole-body vibration, frequent bending, twisting, and awkward postures *(82, 83)*. The factors leading to low back pain – physical, organizational and social factors at work, physical and social aspects of life outside the workplace, and physical and psychological characteristics of the individual – are complex and interrelated *(83)*. High rates of low back pain are reported for special groups of workers, such as farmers, nurses, heavy equipment operators, and construction workers *(84, 85)*. Although rarely life-threatening, low back pain causes much discomfort and can limit work, domestic and recreational activities.

Low back pain occurs frequently in industrialized countries; for example, half of all working Americans have back pain every year *(86)*. Although data from industrializing nations are limited, the rates reported in China are similar to those in industrialized countries (87). Much low back pain can be prevented, but successful intervention requires cooperation among partners, including management, labour, industrial engineers, ergonomists, medical practitioners and the scientific research community.

This analysis suggests that about 37% of back pain is attributable to occupational risk factors. Across regions, this varies comparatively little, from between 12% and 38% for women and between 31% and 45% for men. While not a cause of mortality, low back pain causes considerable morbidity, resulting in an estimated 0.8 million DALYs (0.1%) worldwide. It is a major cause of absence from work, and therefore induces a high economic loss *(84)*.

WORK-RELATED NOISE

Excess noise is one of the most common occupational hazards. Its most serious effect is irreversible hearing impairment. Noise-induced hearing loss typically begins in the frequency range of human voices, interfering with spoken communications. In the workplace, impaired communication sometimes leads to accidents. Exposure levels above 85 dB are considered to be hazardous for workers and are found especially among mining, manufacturing and construction workers, particularly in developing countries *(88, 89).*

These analyses used the WHO definition of hearing impairment, that establishes the threshold of hearing loss at 41 dB for 500, 1000, 2000 and 4000 Hz. A 25 dB threshold of hearing loss is more generally used in the occupational setting.

Based on the WHO definition, the analysis found that about 16% of hearing loss worldwide is attributable to occupational noise exposure. This amounted to about 415 000 (0.3%) DALYs. Overall, occupational noise was responsible for 4.2 million DALYs (0.3%). Noise-induced hearing loss is permanent and irreversible. It is also completely preventable. Fortunately, most occupational noise exposure can be minimized by the use of engineering controls to reduce noise at its source. A complete hearing loss prevention programme includes noise assessments, audiometric monitoring of workers' hearing, appropriate use of hearing protectors, worker education, record keeping, and programme evaluation *(90).*

OTHER RISKS TO HEALTH

Clearly, many thousands of other threats to health exist within and outside the categories outlined above. These include very large causes of disease burden, such as risk factors for tuberculosis (see Box 4.6) and malaria (which is currently responsible for 1.4% of global disease burden, with the vast majority of burden from this disease among children in sub-Saharan Africa). Genetics plays a substantial role in attributable burden (see Box 4.7). Technological developments could lead to considerable avoidable burden. In general, the approaches and methodology outlined in this report can be applied more widely, and as a

---

Box 4.6 Risk factors for tuberculosis

About 9 million new cases of tuberculosis (TB) occur each year. Including people who are also infected with HIV/AIDS, approximately 2 million patients die from TB annually. The global caseload is almost certainly rising, driven upwards in sub-Saharan Africa by the spread of HIV/AIDS and in Eastern Europe by the deterioration of health in general and of TB control in particular. There is a large reservoir of cases in Asia, and TB remains one of the most significant causes of ill-health and premature mortality.

One of the reasons for the persistent burden of tuberculosis is a failure to address the principal risk factors. The risks associated with TB can be put in three groups: the process of infection, progression to disease, and the outcome of a disease episode. Environmental factors that govern exposure to infecting bacilli include crowding, hospitalization, imprisonment, ventilation and the ambient prevalence of infectious (mostly sputum smear-positive) disease. Among factors that influence the progression to disease following infection, HIV co-infection is outstandingly important; others are age, sex, diabetes, to-

bacco, alcohol, TB strain virulence, and malnutrition. Factors that affect the outcome of a disease episode include where treatment is given (e.g. public or private sector), whether treatment is interrupted, and drug resistance. The adverse outcomes most commonly measured are treatment failure and death. Some other risk factors for TB are commonly invoked but ill defined, ethnicity and poverty among them. Ethnicity is often a marker for specific disadvantages, such as restricted access to health services.

While the study of risk factors is a necessary part of planning for TB control, it is not sufficient. Some major risk factors may not be amenable to change, at least as they are currently defined: there is nothing to be done about age per se, though one could investigate why, physiologically, adults are at greater risk of progressing to active disease than children. Further, the risk factor approach (based on observed variation) cannot be used to examine potentially effective interventions that do not yet exist. The absence of a new vaccine is not usually thought of as a risk factor for TB and yet common sense, backed by mathematical model-

ling, shows how effective immunization could be.

Despite some promising laboratory research, there is unlikely to be a new TB vaccine or drug before 2010. Meanwhile, the principal question for operational research is how to strengthen present curative services. With only 27% of new infectious cases being enrolled in DOTS therapeutic programmes, the main goal of TB control is to ensure broad national coverage rather than to target specific groups at risk. In this respect, it is important for patients to recognize the symptoms and know where to seek help, to receive the correct diagnosis and drug regimen, and to understand the importance of completing a course of treatment. There are some challenging questions here, whether or not they are framed in terms of risk factors: for a social intervention like DOTS, careful thought must be given to the design of case-control studies or randomized controlled trials, and still greater caution is needed when generalizing from the results.

Sources: *(91, 92).*

result the potential for prevention by focusing on causes of disease can be further refined. Two other groups of risk factors are described below (see Table 4.8).

UNSAFE HEALTH CARE PRACTICES

As well as their substantial benefits, health care practices may be a source of disease and death. In developing countries, nosocomial infections are increasingly recognized as a major problem in health care quality, although the burden of disease is difficult to estimate. Poor injection practices, including injection overuse and unsafe injection practices, constitute a subset that can be addressed because it is ubiquitous, has been studied in many countries and is associated with a particularly high toll of infection with bloodborne pathogens. Epidemiological studies have reported an association between injections and infection with bloodborne pathogens, including hepatitis B virus (HBV), hepatitis C virus (HCV) and human immunodeficiency virus (HIV) *(99–102)*. The causal nature of this association is supported by many criteria.

A safe injection is one that does not harm the recipient, the provider or the community. In reality, many injections in the world are unsafe. The risk to the community through unsafe sharps waste disposal has not been assessed, but is probably low. The risk to the provider (i.e. needlestick injuries, see Box 4.4) was studied among other occupational risks. The risk to the recipient is mainly secondary to the reuse of injection equipment.

Because injections are overused in many countries, unsafe injections have caused a substantial proportion of infection with bloodborne pathogens, accounting for an estimated 30% of hepatitis B virus infection, 31% of hepatitis C virus infection, 28% of liver cancer, 24% of cirrhosis and 5% of HIV infections. Overall, about 500 000 deaths (0.9%) are attributable to unsafe injection practices in medical settings worldwide, the attributable fractions are highest in South-East Asia, WPR-B and EMR-D. This results in about 10.5 million DALYs (0.7%), with 39% of this burden occurring in SEAR-D and 27% in WPR-B. In these areas,

---

Box 4.7 Genetics and attributable and avoidable burden

It is a common misconception that diseases are caused by *either* genetic·or environmental factors; almost all diseases are caused by both. Although it is not possible to estimate the attributable burden of disease from "genetic causes", it is potentially possible to estimate the burden attributable to certain gene mutations or alleles.

Diseases caused by mutations in single genes, such as phenylketonuria, tend to be rare, whereas the genetic influences on common causes of morbidity and mortality are more complex. In some cases single gene mutations which carry a high risk of disease can be identified but do not necessarily have a major impact on the incidence of disease in populations. For example, gene mutations which confer a high risk of breast cancer are important for carriers of those mutations but are present in only a small proportion of women who develop breast cancer.

Recent developments in genetics offer substantial potential for health gain through increasing the understanding of the biological basis of diseases, identification of high-risk individuals enabling targeted risk factor modification, and the potential for tailored treatment. The greatest possible gains lie in more direct applications. Pharmacogenetics promises to allow drug prescribing to be tailored to individuals likely to have most benefit or least susceptibility to adverse drug reaction. More important yet may be the discovery of disease susceptibility genes that allow identification of a protein in which altered function affects the disease process. This in turn could lead to interventions. While the avoidable burden of genetic disease cannot yet be quantified, especially for common chronic diseases that are influenced by multiple genes, it is likely to be substantial even if only a small fraction of the attributable burden is reversed.

The coming decades will see improved prevention and treatment through appropriate mixes of new genetic and traditional preventive strategies. Nonetheless, ambitious targets need not await these new interventions. Combinations of primary prevention, focusing on major risk factors, and secondary prevention have already achieved substantial reductions in major chronic diseases in just a few decades, during which time gene pools did not essentially alter. For example, age-specific reductions of 25–75% have been achieved in breast cancer mortality in the United Kingdom and United States, coronary disease in the United States and Scandinavia, stroke in Japan, and lung cancer in the United Kingdom. The potential to repeat such successes will clearly be greater if preventive efforts can be augmented by appropriate genetic-based interventions.

Sources: *(93–98)*.

Table 4.8 Selected other major risks to health

Risk factor	Theoretical minimum exposure	Measured adverse outcomes of exposure
Unsafe health care injections	No contaminated injections	Acute infection with hepatitis B, hepatitis C and HIV; liver cirrhosis, liver cancer
Childhood sexual abuse	No abuse	Depression, panic disorder, alcohol abuse/dependence, post-traumatic stress disorder and suicide in adulthood

unsafe injections result in about 0.7–1.5% of all disease burden. These estimates are based upon a mathematical model that was validated by epidemiological studies in most regions in the case of HBV and HCV infection. In the case of HIV infection, there is more uncertainty about the region-specific estimates, due to a lack of epidemiological studies. However, studies have been conducted in sub-Saharan Africa, where most HIV infection occurs, providing more confidence in the overall magnitude of attributable burden, and pointing to the importance of this particular mode of HIV transmission.

Unsafe injections are one form of risk in medical settings; some of the other risks are illustrated in Box 4.8.

ABUSE AND VIOLENCE

Abuse and violence are major causes of disease burden worldwide and there are many types: violence between individuals, including intimate partner violence, and collective violence orchestrated as part of wars and genocide. These are further outlined in Box 4.9. Child sexual abuse is another major component of burden resulting from abuse and violence in society.

Child sexual abuse (CSA) encompasses a range of sexual behaviours perpetrated by adults upon children. Abuse can be non-contact (including behaviours such as unwanted and inappropriate sexual solicitation or indecent exposure), contact (such as sexualized kissing, hugging, touching or fondling) or intercourse (including any penetrative act such as oral, anal or vaginal intercourse or attempted intercourse).

Box 4.8 Risks in the health care system

The complex combination of processes, technologies and human interactions that constitutes the modern health care delivery system not only brings significant benefits, but also an inevitable risk in the form of adverse events. This derives from the inherent risk of measurable harm in practice (human shortcomings), products (substandard or faulty products, side-effects of drugs or drug combinations, and hazards posed by medical devices), and procedures and systems (the possibility of failures at every point in the process of care giving). These risks are associated with different health care settings – hospitals, physicians' offices, nursing homes, pharmacies, and patients' homes.

Studies estimate the probability of patients suffering measurable harm in acute care hospitals at an alarming 16.6% in Australia, 3.8% in the United States, and around 10% in Denmark, the United Kingdom and a number of other European countries. Adverse events exact a high toll in disability and death, as well as in financial loss. Medical errors cause several tens of thousands of deaths annually in the United States alone. Although some deaths occur among people at high risk of death from their initial conditions, the loss of life years is still likely to be substantial. Estimates from the United Kingdom place the cost of additional hospital stays resulting from adverse events at approximately US$ 3 billion a year. The erosion of trust, confidence and satisfaction among the pub-

lic and health care providers must be added to these costs.

The situation in developing and transitional countries is not well known, but could be worse than that in industrialized nations because of counterfeit and substandard drugs and inappropriate or poor equipment and infrastructure.

The systems view is that risk is shaped and provoked by "upstream" systemic factors that include an organization's strategy, its culture, its approach towards quality management and risk prevention, and its capacity for learning from failures. System change as a means to reduce risk is therefore more potentially effective than targeting individual practices or products.

Sources: *(103–115).*

The prevalence of CSA is estimated from retrospective report and is higher than many find comfortable or plausible. In the review carried out as the basis for this report, prevalence estimates were available from 39 countries in 12 of the 14 country groupings, although data quality varied considerably between countries. After controlling for differences between studies, the prevalence of non-contact, contact and intercourse types of CSA in females was about 6%, 11% and 4%, respectively. In males it was about 2% for all categories. Thus over 800 million people worldwide may have experienced CSA, with over 500 million having experienced contact or intercourse types of abuse.

Not only is CSA common, it is also damaging. Research conducted in economically industrialized countries has shown that CSA increases the risk of a range mental disorders in later life, including depression, panic disorder, alcohol and drug abuse and dependence, post-traumatic stress disorder and suicide. Risks increase with the intrusiveness of the abuse.

Box 4.9 Violence

In 2000, violence caused 700 000 deaths in the world: about 50% by suicide, 30% by interpersonal violence, and 20% by collective violence.

Interpersonal violence

Interpersonal violence is defined as "the intentional use of physical force or power, threatened or actual, against another person that results in or has a high likelihood of resulting in injury, death, psychological harm, 'maldevelopment' or deprivation". As well as violence by strangers and acquaintances, it includes child maltreatment, spouse abuse, elder abuse and sexual violence. The true number of deaths is probably underestimated.

Worldwide, adolescents and young adults are the primary victims and perpetrators: interpersonal violence was the sixth leading cause of death among people aged 15–44 years in 2000. The highest estimated regional homicide rates per 100 000 population occurred in Africa (22.2) and the Americas (19.2), compared with Europe (8.4), the Eastern Mediterranean (7.1), South-East Asia (5.8) and the Western Pacific (3.4).

Many more people survive acts of interpersonal violence than die from them. Around 40 million children are maltreated each year. Rape and domestic violence account for 5% to 16% of healthy years of life lost by women of reproductive age. Between 10% and 50% of women experience physical violence at the hands of an intimate partner during their lifetime. Beyond the deaths and injuries, there are many profound health and psychological implications for victims, perpetrators and witnesses of interpersonal violence.

For individuals, risk factors include being a victim of child abuse and neglect, substance abuse, and being young and male. In families, marital discord, parental conflict, and low household socioeconomic status are important risks. In the community, low social capital and high crime levels contribute. In society generally, rapid social change, poverty and economic inequality, poor rule of law and high corruption, sex inequalities, high firearm availability, and collective violence are risk factors. In combination, these factors underlie the close relationship that exists between indicators of interpersonal violence and the socioeconomic context. Correlational studies show higher homicide rates among countries with lower per capita GDP. Findings consistently demonstrate that high levels of inequality coincide with high homicide rates and high rates of non-fatal violence among the poorest sectors of the population;

Interpersonal violence can be prevented and its destructive consequences lessened by focusing on these risk factors, ideally in combination and at different levels simultaneously. Home visits by nurses have shown effectiveness, as have various programmes on parent training, improving urban physical and socioeconomic structure, increasing protective knowledge in schools about sexual abuse, targeting the interaction between firearms and alcohol, and multimedia interventions aimed at reducing the social acceptability of violence. Almost all evaluations of such programmes have been conducted in industrialized countries. In the developing world it is projected that the burden of disease resulting from interpersonal violence will nearly double by 2020 unless preventive action is taken.

Collective violence

Collective violence is a broader term than war or conflict. It encompasses events such as genocide and applies when one group makes instrumental use of violence against another to achieve an objective. It is associated with major threats to health in what tend to be the world's poorer countries. In 2000, an estimated 310 000 deaths resulted directly from collective violence – mostly in Africa and South-East Asia.

Although a prominent feature of human history, collective violence has not received much systematic study. Today it is often characterized by varying degrees of state collapse or dysfunctional governance and a multiplicity of armed actors, often including child soldiers. Economic motivations or ethnic divisions have become more prominent causes of violence than political ideology. The results have often been indiscriminate attacks on civilians and degradation of social capital. Sometimes health infrastructure is specifically targeted, damaging access to water supplies and basic sanitation, and jeopardizing delivery of health interventions such as disease eradication programmes.

Indirect effects of collective violence arise from infectious disease, malnutrition, population displacement, psychosocial sequelae, and exacerbation of chronic disease. Mortality rates 80-fold higher than the baseline have been recorded in populations fleeing collective violence in Rwanda.

Risk factors for collective violence include the generalized availability of small arms, inequalities in access to educational, economic and political opportunities, and abuse of human rights. There is a need to combine efforts of the public health and social science sectors to guide progress in this area and to identify priority areas for intervention.

Sources: *(116, 117)*.

Uncertainty remains because of the lack of knowledge about the impact of cultural differences on CSA prevalence and its relationship with mental disorders. It is, however, certain that CSA causes a considerable burden of disease. It is estimated that about 33% of post-traumatic stress disorder in females and 21% in males is attributable to CSA. The attributable fraction for panic disorders is 11% worldwide, and CSA is estimated to cause about 5–8% of self-inflicted injuries, unipolar depression, and alcohol and drug use disorders. Overall, 0.1% of deaths worldwide (79 000) are attributable to CSA. Much of the burden is disabling rather than fatal, and occurs in the young. Thus CSA causes 8.2 million DALYS (0.6%); 0.4% in males and 0.8% in females. The highest proportion of burden (1–1.5% of total) occurs in females in AMR-A, SEAR-D, WPR-A and WPR-B.

GLOBAL PATTERNS OF RISKS TO HEALTH

Three major groupings of countries can be defined by geography, state of economic and demographic development, and mortality patterns. As can be seen from Figure 4.8, these

Figure 4.8 Amount and patterns of burden of disease in developing and developed countries

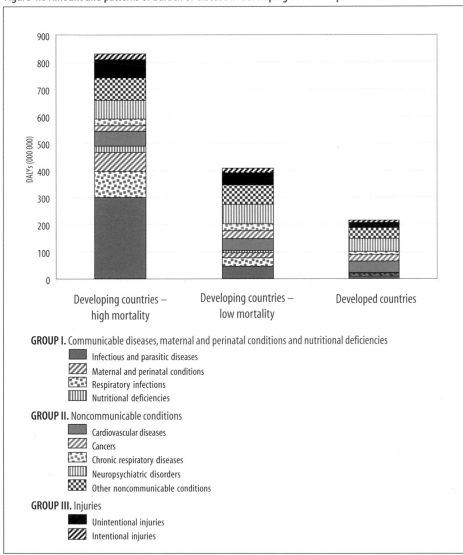

GROUP I. Communicable diseases, maternal and perinatal conditions and nutritional deficiencies
- Infectious and parasitic diseases
- Maternal and perinatal conditions
- Respiratory infections
- Nutritional deficiencies

GROUP II. Noncommunicable conditions
- Cardiovascular diseases
- Cancers
- Chronic respiratory diseases
- Neuropsychiatric disorders
- Other noncommunicable conditions

GROUP III. Injuries
- Unintentional injuries
- Intentional injuries

regions differ substantially in their disease patterns. This phenomenon reflects what is known as the "epidemiological transition" – as life expectancy increases, the major causes of death and disability in general shift from communicable, maternal and perinatal causes to chronic, noncommunicable ones. At present, about one-tenth of disease burden is caused by injury in all three regions.

The risk factors analysed in this report are responsible for a substantial proportion of the leading causes of death and disability in these regions, as shown by the mapping of risk factors to diseases and the range of population attributable fractions in Annex Tables 14, 15, and 16. Their ranking globally, and their distribution by broad region, is shown in Figure 4.9.

Additionally, the ranking of risks within major world regions, by level of development and affected disease or injury outcomes, is shown in Figure 4.10.

Perhaps the most striking finding is the extraordinary concentration of risks in the high mortality developing countries. Among these countries with just over two-fifths of the world's population, not only are the rates of disease and injury particularly high, but the contribution made by relatively few risk factors is particularly great. About one-sixth of the entire

Figure 4.9 Global distribution of burden of disease attributable to 20 leading selected risk factors

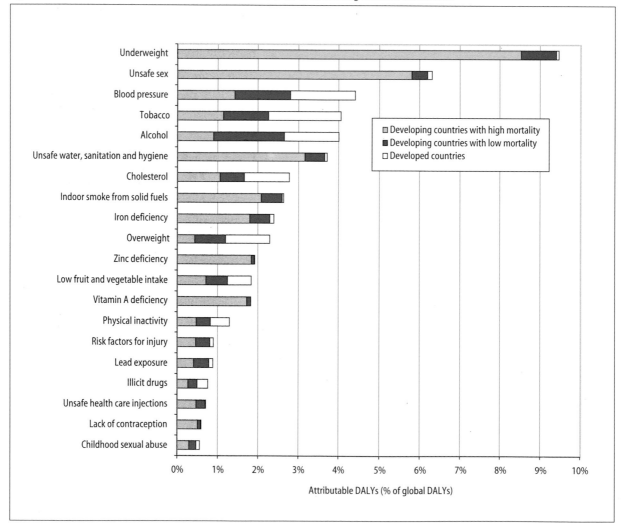

disease burden in these countries is attributed to underweight, with a substantial additional proportion attributable to micronutrient deficiencies. The burden resulting from these risks alone approaches that of the entire disease and injury burden in industrialized countries. Just over one-tenth of all disease burden in high mortality developing countries is

Figure 4.10 Burden of disease attributable to 10 selected leading risk factors, by level of development and type of affected outcome

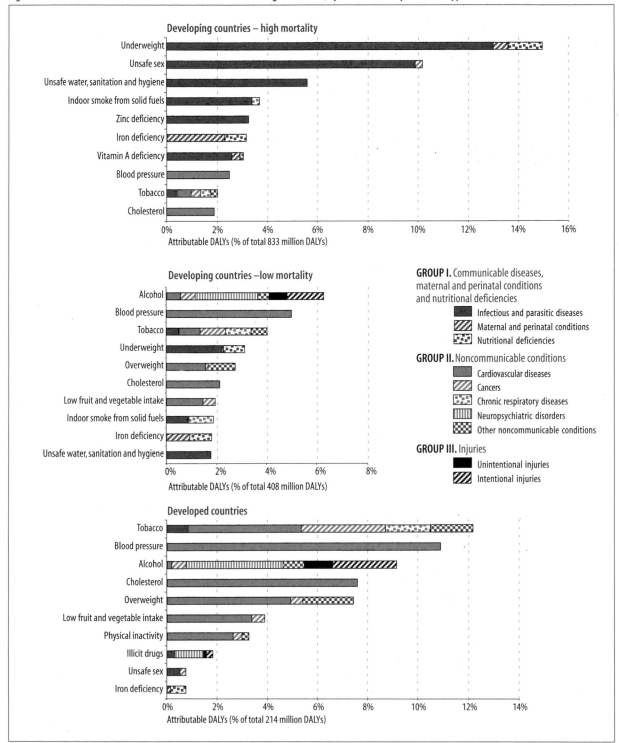

attributable to unsafe sex, with unsafe water accounting for about 4–5% of the burden. In all the high mortality developing regions, underweight, unsafe water, sanitation and hygiene, and indoor smoke from solid fuels feature in the leading six of these selected risks. In addition, unsafe sex is the leading risk in AFR-E and second leading risk in AFR-D. Virtually all of the substantial burden attributable to these risks is borne by developing countries.

For industrialized countries, with just over one-fifth of the world's population , tobacco is the leading risk factor, accounting for about 12% of all disease and injury burden. For both sexes, alcohol and blood pressure account for 9–10% of DALYs, and cholesterol and body mass for 6–7% of DALYs. Alcohol, blood pressure, overweight, cholesterol and tobacco are the leading five risks for each subregion in the industrialized group, varying only in their rank order.

An intermediate picture is seen for the low mortality, developing regions, with alcohol, tobacco and high blood pressure each accounting for about 4–6% of disease burden. Alcohol is the leading cause, alone accounting for about 6.2%. Indoor smoke from solid fuels and unsafe water and hygiene also feature in the ten leading risk factors for these areas. This double burden is seen most clearly for body weight – underweight and overweight are each responsible for about 3% of disease burden. Overall, however, the pattern of leading risks already most closely resembles that in industrialized countries.

These results provide a cross-sectional indication of an epidemiological transition for risk factors. The epidemiological transition that accompanies economic development has traditionally been understood in terms of outcomes, that is, patterns of disease and injury. This report shows some key drivers of this transition – risk factors that shape the development of disease and injury patterns.

The gradient of burden attributable to leading risks and diseases has a bearing on the appropriate degree of focus of public heath initiatives. In all three broad regions the leading disease or injury outcomes account for about three or four times more burden than the tenth ranked outcomes. However, the leading risk factor accounts for about 16 times more burden than the tenth ranked risk factor from this selected group in the industrialized countries. The ratio is less extreme but still considerable for high mortality developing countries, where the leading risk (underweight) accounts for about eight times more burden than the tenth ranked risk (cholesterol). For the low mortality developing countries, the ratio is even less marked, being about four-fold. Clearly, highly focused public health initiatives could be comparatively effective in the richest and the poorest countries, whereas in middle income countries the public health agenda of tackling major risks may have to be taken up on wider fronts.

Looking at the selected risk factors by proportion of attributable burden might obscure the vast absolute amount of burden caused by risk factors in the large developing regions. Because such a large proportion of the world's population live in developing countries, and background disease rates and risk factor levels are often high, the absolute number of DALYs attributable to each risk factor is greater than that in developed countries. Even for risks traditionally thought to be "Western", such as elevated body mass or cholesterol, more burden now occurs in developing than developed countries. The shift appears to have occurred for tobacco in the 1990s – about a decade ago more tobacco deaths occurred in the developed than the developing world. This report suggests the predominance of tobacco burden has now begun to shift to the developing world.

The distribution of attributable deaths and DALYs by age and sex is shown in Tables 4.9 and 4.10 and in Annex Table 8. Underweight and micronutrient deficiency-related burden clearly affect children almost exclusively, as do unsafe water and climate change. The burden in terms of DALYs due to other diet-related risks and occupational risks (except injury) is almost equally distributed among adults above and below the age of 60 years. The burden caused by addictive substances, unsafe sex, lack of contraception, risk factors for injury, unsafe health care injections and childhood sexual abuse mostly or almost all occurs in middle-aged adults. Diet-related and environmental risks and unsafe sex are about equally distributed among the sexes. However, about four-fifths of burden as a result of addictive substances, and about 60–90% of burden from separate occupational risks, occurs among men. Women suffer the majority of burden from childhood sexual abuse and all of the burden caused by a lack of contraception. Women are also affected more by those nutritional deficiencies that affect maternal conditions (iron and vitamin A deficiency).

One further major finding is the key role of nutrition in health worldwide. About one-fifth of the global disease burden can be attributed to the joint effects of protein–energy or micronutrient deficiency. In addition, almost as much burden again can be attributed to risk factors that have substantial dietary determinants – high blood pressure, cholesterol, overweight, and low fruit and vegetable intake. These patterns are not uniform within regions, however, and in some countries the transition has been much healthier than in others. The many and varied factors that determine national nutritional patterns are clearly a key determinant in achieving a healthier transition (see Box 4.10).

PUTTING IT ALL TOGETHER – WHAT IS POSSIBLE?

ESTIMATES OF THE JOINT EFFECTS OF SELECTED RISK FACTORS

The multicausal nature of disease often provides a choice among different preventive strategies and offers great potential benefit from simultaneous interventions. For example, modest reductions in blood pressure, obesity, cholesterol and tobacco use would more than halve cardiovascular disease incidence, if these reductions were population-wide and simultaneous. This section includes an assessment of gains in healthy life expectancy attributable to the leading 20 risk factors considered here.

As outlined previously, typically, population attributable fractions add up to less than the sum of components, because many diseases are caused by more than one risk factor. This is shown graphically in Figure 4.11, which shows the individual and joint contributions of three major risk factors to each major burden of disease outcome groups (group I: communicable, maternal, perinatal and nutritional conditions; group II: noncommunicable conditions; and group III: injuries) in three broad combinations of regions – demographically developed, developing low mortality, and developing high mortality. The size of each circle is proportional to the absolute disease burden.

This figure clearly shows how these selected major risks are responsible for a large fraction of current global disease burden, both across levels of development and type of outcome. It also shows how burden may be caused by more than one risk factor. The grouping by broad disease outcomes conceals some of the substantial population attributable fractions within the component clusters of disease. For example, of all childhood communicable diseases (including acute lower respiratory infection), 50% can be attributed to underweight, 23% to unsafe water, sanitation and hygiene, 13% to indoor smoke from solid fuels, and 63% to the joint effects of all three of these major risk factors. Similarly, 50% of cardiovascular diseases among those above the age of 30 years can be attributed to suboptimal blood pressure, 31% to high cholesterol and 14% to tobacco, yet the estimated joint effects of these three risks amount to about 65% of cardiovascular diseases in this group.

Using the assumptions outlined in Chapter 2, approximately 47% of global mortality can be attributed to the 20 leading risk factors and more than one-third attributed to the leading 10 risk factors. The likely impact of the 20 leading risks from the selected factors was estimated for 2000 in terms of potential gain in healthy life expectancy, as shown in Figure 4.12.

Had these risks not existed, then healthy life expectancy in 2000 might have been, on average, almost a decade greater globally. However, the gain varied considerably across regions, with the countries currently facing the world's largest risks to health having many times more healthy life years to gain than the richest countries. Thus the leading 20 risks were estimated to be responsible for 16 years lost in healthy life expectancy in AFR-E compared with slightly more than four years in WPR-A. Most of this was attributable to the leading few risks – for example, about 14 years lost in healthy life expectancy in AFR-E and 11 in AFR-D were attributable to the leading five risks in those regions. Notable also were the high mortality European regions of EUR-B and EUR-C, with particularly large attribut-

Table 4.9 Attributable mortality by risk factor, level of development and sex, 2000

	High mortality Developing countries AFR-D, AFR-E, AMR-D, EMR-D, SEAR-D		Low mortality Developing countries AMR-B, EMR-B, SEAR-B, WPR-B		Developed countries AMR-A, EUR-A, EUR-B, EUR-C, WPR-A	
	Males	Females	Males	Females	Males	Females
TOTAL DEATHS (000)	*13 758*	*12 654*	*8 584*	*7 373*	*6 890*	*6 601*
	(% total)	(% total)	(% total)	(% total)	(% total)	(% total)
Childhood and maternal undernutrition						
Underweight	12.6	13.4	1.8	1.9	0.1	0.1
Iron deficiency	2.2	3.0	0.8	1.0	0.1	0.2
Vitamin A deficiency	2.3	3.3	0.2	0.4	<0.1	<0.1
Zinc deficiency	2.8	3.0	0.2	0.2	<0.1	<0.1
Other diet-related risks and physical inactivity						
Blood pressure	7.4	7.5	12.7	15.1	20.1	23.9
Cholesterol	5.0	5.7	5.1	5.6	14.5	17.6
Overweight	1.1	2.0	4.2	5.6	9.6	11.5
Low fruit and vegetable intake	3.6	3.5	5.0	4.8	7.6	7.4
Physical inactivity	2.3	2.3	2.8	3.2	6.0	6.7
Sexual and reproductive health risks						
Unsafe sex	9.3	10.9	0.8	1.3	0.2	0.6
Lack of contraception	...	1.1	...	0.2	...	0.0
Addictive substances						
Tobacco	7.5	1.5	12.2	2.9	26.3	9.3
Alcohol	2.6	0.6	8.5	1.6	8.0	-0.3
Illicit drugs	0.5	0.1	0.6	0.1	0.6	0.3
Environmental risks						
Unsafe water, sanitation and hygiene	5.8	5.9	1.1	1.1	0.2	0.2
Urban air pollution	0.9	0.8	2.5	2.9	1.1	1.2
Indoor smoke from solid fuels	3.6	4.3	1.9	5.4	0.1	0.2
Lead exposure	0.4	0.3	0.5	0.3	0.7	0.4
Climate change	0.5	0.6	<0.1	<0.1	<0.1	<0.1
Occupational risks						
Risk factors for injury	1.0	0.1	1.4	0.1	0.4	0.0
Carcinogens	0.1	<0.1	0.5	0.2	0.8	0.2
Airborne particulates	0.3	<0.1	1.6	0.2	0.6	0.1
Ergonomic stressors	0.0	0.0	0.0	0.0	0.0	0.0
Noise	0.0	0.0	0.0	0.0	0.0	0.0
Other selected risks to health						
Unsafe health care injections	1.1	0.9	1.8	0.9	0.1	0.1
Childhood sexual abuse	0.1	0.2	0.1	0.2	0.1	0.1

able burden of healthy life expectancy, principally as a result of their large burden resulting from tobacco, alcohol, cholesterol and other major risks for noncommunicable diseases.

Such joint estimates have considerable uncertainty associated with them. As well as the technical assumptions necessary in making these estimates with limited data, the time-related issues should also be considered, with sequential rather than simultaneous changes occurring in real life. Thus there is the capacity of improved health to beget health. For example, improvements in nutritional status of children in developing countries might well lead to improved ability to avoid and reduce other risks in adulthood as well as the large, immediate threats of communicable diseases. For these reasons, it seems likely that these are conservative estimates of joint effects of major risks on healthy life expectancy.

The distribution of risks across levels of poverty as measured in this report, both within and between regions, suggests they are likely to explain a large proportion of current inequity in healthy life expectancy. The multicausal nature of many diseases means that tackling major risks at a population-wide level offers opportunities to lessen these differentials,

Table 4.10 Attributable DALYs by risk factor, level of development and sex, 2000

	High mortality Developing countries AFR-D, AFR-E, AMR-D, EMR-D, SEAR-D		Low mortality Developing countries AMR-B, EMR-B, SEAR-B, WPR-B		Developed countries AMR-A, EUR-A, EUR-B, EUR-C, WPR-A	
	Males	Females	Males	Females	Males	Females
TOTAL DALYs (000)	*420 711*	*412 052*	*223 181*	*185 316*	*117 670*	*96 543*
	(% total)	(% total)	(% total)	(% total)	(% total)	(% total)
Childhood and maternal undernutrition						
Underweight	14.9	15.0	3.0	3.3	0.4	0.4
Iron deficiency	2.8	3.5	1.5	2.2	0.5	1.0
Vitamin A deficiency	2.6	3.5	0.3	0.4	<0.1	<0.1
Zinc deficiency	3.2	3.2	0.3	0.3	0.1	0.1
Other diet-related risks and physical inactivity						
Blood pressure	2.6	2.4	4.9	5.1	11.2	10.6
Cholesterol	1.9	1.9	2.2	2.0	8.0	7.0
Overweight	0.6	1.0	2.3	3.2	6.9	8.1
Low fruit and vegetable intake	1.3	1.2	2.0	1.8	4.3	3.4
Physical inactivity	0.9	0.8	1.2	1.3	3.3	3.2
Sexual and reproductive health risks						
Unsafe sex	9.4	11.0	1.2	1.6	0.5	1.1
Lack of contraception	...	1.8	...	0.6	...	0.1
Addictive substances						
Tobacco	3.4	0.6	6.2	1.3	17.1	6.2
Alcohol	2.6	0.5	9.8	2.0	14.0	3.3
Illicit drugs	0.8	0.2	1.2	0.3	2.3	1.2
Environmental risks						
Unsafe water, sanitation and hygiene	5.5	5.6	1.7	1.8	0.4	0.4
Urban air pollution	0.4	0.3	1.0	0.9	0.6	0.5
Indoor smoke from solid fuels	3.7	3.6	1.5	2.3	0.2	0.3
Lead exposure	0.8	0.7	1.4	1.4	0.8	0.5
Climate change	0.6	0.7	0.1	0.1	<0.1	<0.1
Occupational risks						
Risk factors for injury	1.5	0.1	2.1	0.3	1.0	0.1
Carcinogens	0.1	<0.1	0.2	0.1	0.4	0.1
Airborne particulates	0.1	<0.1	0.8	0.1	0.4	0.1
Ergonomic stressors	<0.1	<0.1	0.1	0.1	0.1	0.1
Noise	0.3	0.1	0.5	0.3	0.4	0.3
Other selected risks to health						
Unsafe health care injections	0.9	0.8	1.1	0.5	0.1	0.1
Childhood sexual abuse	0.3	0.7	0.5	0.8	0.3	1.0

whatever their initial cause. The Commission on Macroeconomics and Health recently estimated that a 10% increase in life expectancy might increase GDP by 0.3% in the poorest countries of the world *(1)*. It is clear that many different combinations of reductions in these major risks could increase healthy life expectancy by at least 10% in these countries, especially if they were simultaneous and population-wide. Indeed, at least a quarter of all disease burden can be attributed to the leading three risks in high mortality developing areas and in developed regions, and at least one sixth in low mortality developing regions. Furthermore, these potential gains are averaged over a whole population, even though many people die from other causes. The average gain in healthy life expectancy would be much greater among those with averted events.

ESTIMATES OF AVOIDABLE BURDEN

Current action to focus on risks to health can change the future but not alter the past. It is possible to avoid future disease burden, but nothing can be done about attributable burden. The main policy use of attributable burden estimates should therefore be to help assess avoidable burden. In addition to the uncertainty involved in estimating attributable burden, making estimates of avoidable burden is particularly challenging because of uncertainty concerning predictions in risk factors and burden, and reversibility of risks. Despite these reservations, the policy relevance of avoidable burden information is considerable and justifies making estimates, given that appropriate caution will be exercised regarding their uncertainty. To maximize policy relevance, estimates can be made particularly for small-to-moderate risk factor reductions; that is, those that are likely to be achievable in the short term. A full range of estimates is essential, however, since, for example, a 5% distributional transition for one risk factor may be cost-effective in one region, whereas a 50% distributional transition may be cost-effective in another. Similarly, in one region, the same resources might be required to achieve a distributional transition of 1% for one risk factor as to achieve a 10% transition for another. Wide ranges of risk reductions have been assessed in the following chapter. As an example, the likely effects of a 25% distributional transition are estimated: that is, a 25% transition from current levels towards the theoretical

---

Box 4.10 Healthy risk factor transition

The "nutritional transition" encompasses changes in a range of risk factors and diseases. As a country develops and more people buy processed food rather than growing and buying raw ingredients, an increasing proportion of calories tends to be drawn from sugars added to manufactured food and from relatively cheap oils. Alongside the change in diet, changes in food production and the technology of work and leisure lead to decreases in physical exercise. The consequent epidemic of diet-related noncommunicable diseases (obesity, diabetes, hypertension and cardiovascular disease) coexists with residual undernutrition, and is projected to increase rapidly. For example, in India and China, a shift in diet towards higher fat and lower carbohydrate is resulting in rapid increases in overweight – among all adults in China and

mainly among urban residents and high income rural residents in India.

Countries which have completed the transition to overnutrition are experiencing a continual increase in levels of obesity, as high fat, high sugar and low exercise lifestyles permeate society. However, this transition may not be inevitable, and a key challenge for policy-makers is to generate a "healthier transition".

The Republic of Korea is an example of a country that has experienced rapid economic growth and the introduction of Western culture since the 1970s. There were large increases in the consumption of animal food products, and a fall in total cereal intake. Despite this, national efforts to retain elements of the traditional diet – very high in carbohydrates and vegetables – seem to have maintained low fat consumption and a low prevalence of obesity.

Civil society and government initiatives to retain the traditional diet and cooking methods in the Republic of Korea have been strong: mass media campaigns, such as television programmes, promote local foods, emphasizing their higher quality and the need to support local farmers. A unique training programme is offered by the Rural Development Administration. Since the 1980s, the Rural Living Science Institute has trained thousands of extension workers to provide monthly demonstrations of cooking methods for traditional Korean foods such as rice, kimchi (pickled and fermented Chinese cabbage) and fermented soybean food. These sessions are open to the general public in most districts in the country, and the programme appears to reach a large audience.

Sources: *(118–121)*.

minimum that occurs in 2000 and is maintained relative to "business as usual" exposure projections.

In this chapter, business as usual, or "drift", was first estimated to calculate what attributable burden would be in future years if there were no change in current trends in risk factor levels and distributions. For example, without further action it is predicted that in 2020 the disease burden attributable to tobacco will be nearly double its current levels. Similarly, there will be a one-third increase in the loss of healthy life as a result of overweight and obesity in 2020 compared with 2000. In contrast, 130 million DALYs per year are currently attributable to underweight, while it is estimated that 90 million will occur from this risk in 2010 even with all the benefits of economic development. Avoidable burden estimates the effects of changes in terms of deviations in risk levels from these predictions. Thus, avoidable burden is defined here as the fraction of total disease burden in a particular year that could be avoided with a specific reduction in current and future exposure compared to predicted current trends. The main estimates here are for a 25% distributional transition – roughly equated as a reduction of one quarter in current and future risk levels. The initial avoidable burden estimates are summarized in Tables 4.9 and 4.10 and Figure 4.13.

These estimates show, firstly, that underweight will remain one of the leading causes of avoidable burden in 2010 and 2020. This is despite the fact that the estimated global burdens attributable to childhood diseases, diarrhoea and other major causes of childhood mortality are expected to form a considerably lower proportion of the global disease burden in 2010 and 2020. For example, the business as usual trend for burden attributable to

Figure 4.11 Disease and risk factor burden

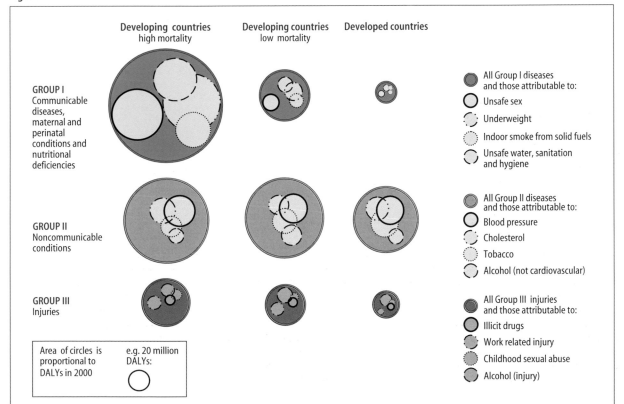

underweight suggests that it will be responsible for 90 million DALYs in 2010 and more than 60 million DALYs in 2020, with disease rates continuing to decline, but with increased population sizes. The risk factors of unsafe water, sanitation and hygiene, and indoor smoke from solid fuels assume lesser though still very substantial roles as causes of avoidable burden, as the exposure levels are predicted to decrease with economic development. The associated mortality and morbidity are also proportionally less important as a result of declining levels of related risk factors. Nonetheless, the avoidable burden remains substantial. Because these risks are high in the poor, both within and between countries, efforts to tackle them now are likely to reduce inequality significantly in the future.

The 10 leading risk factors in terms of avoidable burden in 2010 and 2020 are broadly similar to the 10 leading causes of attributable burden in 2000, although the ordering changes somewhat, reflecting expectations of demographic and social development. Most noticeably, the ranking of avoidable burden from reduction in unsafe sex is extremely high, making it the leading cause of avoidable burden and reflecting the benefits of preventing transmission and the continuing predicted epidemic of HIV/AIDS in some places where current effects are small but large increases may occur. If the benefits of reducing undernutrition and unsafe sex are additive, then a 25% reduction in these two risk factors alone would avoid an estimated 5% of global disease burden in 2010. These benefits would be substantially concentrated in sub-Saharan Africa, where the improvement in healthy life expectancy would be even greater.

The potential avoidable burden from decreases in the prevalence of unsafe sex are both substantial and rapid. For example, with a one-quarter reduction, a substantial number of deaths would be averted in 2010. These would mostly occur in young and middle-aged adults, and so the avoidable disease burden in terms of DALYs is even more substantial. Similarly, most of the benefits of reduction in alcohol consumption are rapidly achieved, since most of the attributable burden is to the result of injuries or neuropsychiatric diseases. One quarter reduction in alcohol use from its current trend could result in approximately

Figure 4.12 Estimated gain in healthy life expectancy with removal of 20 leading selected risk factors by subregion[a]

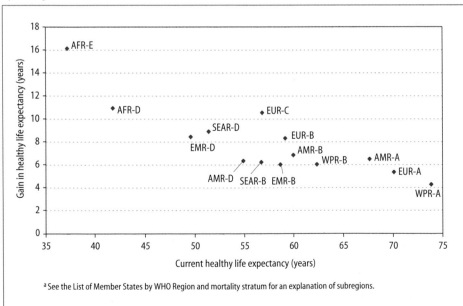

[a] See the List of Member States by WHO Region and mortality stratum for an explanation of subregions.

Table 4.11 Ranking of estimated attributable and avoidable burdens of 10 leading selected risk factors

Rank		Estimated attributable burden in 2000			Estimated avoidable burden after 25% distributional transition from 2001 in 2010			in 2020	
		DALYs (millions)	% total		DALYs (millions)	% total		DALYs (millions)	% total
1	Underweight	138	9.5	Unsafe sex	42	3.0	Unsafe sex	71	4.8
2	Unsafe sex	92	6.3	Blood pressure	25	1.7	Blood pressure	27	1.9
3	Blood pressure	64	4.4	Underweight	23	1.6	Tobacco	22	1.5
4	Tobacco	59	4.1	Tobacco	17	1.2	Cholesterol	17	1.2
5	Alcohol	58	4.0	Cholesterol	15	1.1	Underweight	16	1.1
6	Unsafe water, sanitation and hygiene	54	3.7	Alcohol	15	1.1	Alcohol	16	1.1
7	Cholesterol	40	2.8	Overweight	13	0.9	Overweight	15	1.0
8	Indoor smoke from solid fuels	39	2.6	Iron deficiency	9	0.6	Low fruit and vegetable intake	9	0.6
9	Iron deficiency	35	2.4	Low fruit and vegetable intake	9	0.6	Iron deficiency	7	0.5
10	Overweight	33	2.3	Unsafe water, sanitation and hygiene	8	0.6	Physical inactivity	6	0.4
Total DALYs		**1 455**			**1 417**			**1 459**	

15 million fewer DALYs in 2010. Shifting distributions of blood pressure and cholesterol by only a quarter of the distance towards the theoretical minimum from their current trends (on average by 5–10 mmHg systolic pressure or 0.3–0.6 mmol/l total cholesterol) could avert considerable disease burden. Such population-wide reductions could together avert a loss of tens of millions of years of healthy life, with most or all of the full potential reached before 2005 and the effects being approximately additive. Strategies to achieve this are outlined in the following chapter.

Another important feature of these estimates is the importance of reduction in tobacco use now. The benefits, although more delayed than those resulting from reduction of some other risks, are very large and long-lasting. This is seen in the estimated tens of millions of

Figure 4.13 Attributable DALYs in 2000 and avoidable DALYs in 2010 and 2020 following a 25% risk factor reduction from 2000, for 10 leading selected risk factors

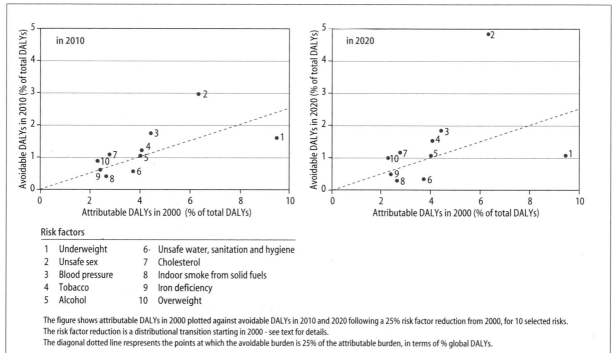

Risk factors

1	Underweight	6·	Unsafe water, sanitation and hygiene
2	Unsafe sex	7	Cholesterol
3	Blood pressure	8	Indoor smoke from solid fuels
4	Tobacco	9	Iron deficiency
5	Alcohol	10	Overweight

The figure shows attributable DALYs in 2000 plotted against avoidable DALYs in 2010 and 2020 following a 25% risk factor reduction from 2000, for 10 selected risks.
The risk factor reduction is a distributional transition starting in 2000 - see text for details.
The diagonal dotted line respresents the points at which the avoidable burden is 25% of the attributable burden, in terms of % global DALYs.

healthy life years to be saved in 2010 and 2020 as a result of preventing and reducing tobacco use. The potential avoidable burden from some other risks closely maps the attributable burden. For the risk factors that predominantly affect cardiovascular diseases (inadequate fruit and vegetable intake, physical inactivity, overweight, blood pressure and cholesterol) and for alcohol, the amount of disease burden avoidable in 2010 from a 25% reduction starting in 2000 is about one-third of the attributable burden in 2000. This "avoidability" is lower for underweight, micronutrient deficiencies, unsafe water, sanitation and hygiene, and indoor smoke from solid fuels – reflecting changing disease patterns as a result of the assumed demographic and social development – and for tobacco use, reflecting delayed benefits from cessation. In contrast, it is much higher for unsafe sex, reflecting the benefits of reduced communicable disease transmission and the predicted continuing HIV/AIDS epidemic.

However, these analyses only map out the potential for gain – what is required next are effective and cost-effective interventions to realize this potential.

THE NEED FOR COST-EFFECTIVENESS ANALYSES

Large gains in health are not possible without focusing on efforts to diminish large threats to health. These analyses have shown some major causes of disease and injury burden. While the risk factors were selected from a countless array of possible risks, there are, of course, many other distal factors (for example, lack of education) or proximal factors (for example, fat intake or osteoporosis) that lead to substantial disease burden and were not estimated in this work. However, there may be relatively few others that have population attributable fractions of more than 5% of all disease and injury burden in a particular region.

While many big challenges to health remain, there are also many different ways of meeting them – involving personal health interventions, non-personal health interventions, and intersectoral action. Not everything can be done in all settings, so some way of setting priorities needs to be found. The next chapter identifies costs and the impact on population health of a variety of interventions, as the basis on which to develop strategies to reduce risk.

REFERENCES

1. Commission on Macroeconomics and Health. *Macroeconomics and health: investing in health for economic development*. Geneva: World Health Organization; 2001.

2. *WHO global database on child growth and malnutrition*. Geneva: World Health Organization; 2002. Available from: URL: http://www.who.int/nutgrowthdb/

3. *Fourth report on the world nutrition situation: nutrition throughout the life cycle*. Geneva: United Nations Administrative Committee on Coordination Sub-Committee on Nutrition (ACC/SCN); 2000.

4. Rice AL, Sacco L, Hyder A, Black RE. Malnutrition as an underlying cause of childhood deaths associated with infectious diseases in developing countries. *Bulletin of the World Health Organization* 2000; 78:1207-21.

5. Grantham-McGregor SM, Ani CC. Undernutrition and mental development. In: Fernstrom JD, Uauy R, Arroyo P, editors. *Nutrition and brain*. Basel: Karger; 2001. Nestle Nutrition Workshop Series: Clinical and Performance Program Vol. 5. p. 1-18.

6. Pelletier DL. The relationship between child anthropometry and mortality in developing countries: implications for policy, programs and future research. *Journal of Nutrition* 1994; 124(Suppl.):2047S-81S.

7. Bleichrodt N. Developmental disorders associated with severe IDD. In: Hetzel BS, Dunn JT, Stansbury JB, editors. *The prevention and control of iodine deficiency disorders*. Amsterdam: Elsevier; 1987.

8. *Global prevalence of iodine deficiency disorders*. Geneva: World Health Organization; 1993. Micronutrient Deficiency Information System, Working Paper No.1.

9. Hetzel BS. Iodine deficiency disorders (IDD) and their eradication. *Lancet* 1983; 2: 1126-7.

10. Stoltzfus RJ, Dreyfuss ML. *Guidelines for the use of iron supplements to prevent and treat iron deficiency anemia*. Washington (DC): ILSI Press; 1998.

11. Sommer A, West KP, Jr. *Vitamin A deficiency: health, survival and vision*. New York: Oxford University Press; 1996.

12. Prasad AS. Discovery of human zinc deficiency and studies in an experimental human model. *American Journal of Clinical Nutrition* 1991; 53:403-12.

13. Sandstead HH. Zinc deficiency: a public health problem? *American Journal of Diseases of Children* 1991; 145:853-9.

14. *Infant and young child nutrition*. Geneva: World Health Organization; 2001. World Health Assembly Resolution WHA54.2.

15. Victora CG, Vaughan JP, Lombardi C, Fuchs SMC, Gigante LP, Smith PG, et al. Evidence for protection by breast-feeding against infant deaths from infectious diseases in Brazil. *Lancet* 1987; 2:319-22.

16. Prospective Studies Collaboration. Cholesterol, diastolic blood pressure, and stroke: 13 000 strokes in 45 000 people in 45 prospective cohorts. *Lancet* 1995; 346:1647-53.

17. Eastern Stroke and Coronary Heart Disease Collaborative Group. Blood pressure, cholesterol and stroke in eastern Asia. *Lancet* 1998; 352:1801-07.

18. Law MR, Wald NJ. Risk factor thresholds: their existence under scrutiny. *BMJ* 2002; 324:1570-6.

19. *Obesity: preventing and managing the global epidemic*. Geneva: World Health Organization; 2000. WHO Technical Report Series, No. 894.

20. Ness AR, Powles JW. Fruit and vegetables, and cardiovascular disease: a review. *International Journal of Epidemiology* 1997; 26:1-13.

21. World Cancer Research Fund and American Institute for Cancer Research. *Food, nutrition and the prevention of cancer: a global perspective*. Washington (DC): American Institute for Cancer Research; 1997.

22. *Physical activity and health: a report of the Surgeon General*. Altanta (GA): US Department of Health and Human Services, Centers for Disease Control and Prevention; 1996.

23. *Report on the global HIV/AIDS epidemic*. Geneva: Joint United Nations Programme on HIV/AIDS; 2002.

24. Corrao MA, Guindon GE, Sharma N, Shokoohi DF, editors. *Tobacco control: country profiles*. Atlanta (GA): American Cancer Society; 2000.

25. World Health Organization. *Tobacco or health: a global status report*. Geneva: World Health Organization; 1997.

26. Peto R, Lopez AD, Boreham J, Thun M, Heath CW. Mortality from tobacco in developed countries: indirect estimates from national vital statistics. *Lancet* 1992; 339:1268-78.

27. Liu BQ, Peto R, Chen ZM, Boreham J, Wu YP, Li JY, et al. Emerging tobacco hazards in China. 1. Retrospective proportional mortality study of one million deaths. *BMJ* 1998; 317:1411-22.

28. Niu SR, Yang GH, Chen ZM, Wang JL, Wang GH, He XZ, et al. Emerging tobacco hazards in China. 2. Early mortality results from a prospective study. *BMJ* 1998; 317:1423-4.

29. Dikshit RP, Kanhere S. Tobacco habits and risk of lung, oropharyngeal and oral cavity cancer: a population-based case-control study in Bhopal, India. *International Journal of Epidemiology* 2000; 29:609-14.

30. Gupta PC, Mehta HC. Cohort study of all-cause mortality among tobacco users in Mumbai, India. *Bulletin of the World Health Organization* 2000; 78:877-83.

31. *Health effects of exposure to environmental tobacco smoke:* Sacramento: California Environmental Protection Agency (Cal/EPA), Office of Environmental Health Hazard Assessment; 1997. Smoking and Tobacco Control Monograph 10.

32. Environmental Protection Agency (EPA). *Respiratory health effects of passive smoking: lung cancer and other disorders.* Washington (DC): US Environmental Protection Agency, Office of Health and Environmental Assessment; 1992.

33. Glantz SA, Parmley WW. Passive smoking and heart disease. Epidemiology, physiology, and biochemistry. *Circulation* 1991; 83:1-12.

34. Hackshaw AK, Law MR, Wald NJ. The accumulated evidence on lung cancer and environmental tobacco smoke. *BMJ* 1997; 315:980-8.

35. Jha P. *Curbing the epidemic: governments and the economics of tobacco control.* Washington (DC): The World Bank; 1999.

36. Law MR, Morris JK, Wald NJ. Environmental tobacco smoke exposure and ischaemic heart disease: an evaluation of the evidence. *BMJ* 1997; 315:973-80.

37. Strachan DP, Cook DG, editors. *Health effects of passive smoking in children.* A set of nine review articles appearing in *Thorax* 1997: 52 and 1998: 53.

38. Thun M, Henley J, Apicella L. Epidemiologic studies of fatal and nonfatal cardiovascular disease and ETS exposure from spousal smoking. *Environmental Health Perspectives* 1999; 107:841-6.

39. English DR, Holman CDJ, Milne E, Winter MJ, Hulse GK, Codde G, et al. *The quantification of drug-caused morbidity and mortality in Australia 1995.* Canberra: Commonwealth Department of Human Services and Health; 1995.

40. Rehm J, Gutjahr E, Gmel G. Alcohol and all-cause mortality: a pooled analysis. *Contemporary Drug Problems* 2001c; 28:337-61.

41. United Nations Office for Drug Control and Crime Prevention. *World drug report 2000.* Oxford: Oxford University Press; 2000.

42. *Global illicit drug trends 2000.* Vienna: United Nations Drug Control Programme; 2000.

43. Frischer M, Green ST, Goldberg D. *Substance abuse related mortality: a worldwide review.* Vienna: United Nations International Drug Control Programme; 1994.

44. Hulse G, English D, Milne E, Holman C. The quantification of mortality resulting from the regular use of illicit opiates. *Addiction* 1999; 94: 221-30.

45. Pope CA III, Dockery DW. Epidemiology of particle effects. In: Holgate ST, Koren HS, Samet JM, Maynard RL, editors. *Air pollution and health.* San Diego (CA): Academic Press; 1999.

46. Krzyzanowski M, Schwela D. Patterns of air pollution in developing countries. In: Holgate ST, Koren HS, Samet JM, Maynard RL, editors. *Air pollution and health.* San Diego (CA): Academic Press; 1999.

47. Committee of the Environmental and Occupational Health Assembly of the American Thoracic Society (ATS). Health effects of outdoor air pollution, Part 1. *American Journal of Respiratory and Critical Care Medicine* 1996; 153:3-50.

48. Committee of the Environmental and Occupational Health Assembly of the American Thoracic Society (ATS). Health effects of outdoor air pollution, Part 2. *American Journal of Respiratory and Critical Care Medicine* 1996; 153:477-98.

49. *Airborne particles and health: HEI epidemiologic evidence.* Boston (MA): Health Effects Institute; 2001. HEI Perspectives June 2001.

50. Samet JM, Cohen AJ. Air pollution and lung cancer. In: Holgate ST, Koren HS, Samet JM, Maynard RL, editors. *Air pollution and health.* San Diego (CA): Academic Press; 1999.

51. Bruce N, Perez-Padilla R, Albalak R. Indoor air pollution in developing countries: a major environmental and public health challenge. *Bulletin of the World Health Organization* 2000; 78:1078-92.

52. Smith KR, Samet JM, Romieu I, Bruce N. Indoor air pollution in developing countries and ALRI in children. *Thorax* 2000; 55:518-32.

53. Smith KR. Inaugural article: national burden of disease in India from indoor air pollution. *Proceedings of the National Academy of Sciences of the United States of America* 2000; 97:13286-93.

54. Spengler JD, Chen Q. Indoor air quality factors in designing a healthy building. *Annual Review of Energy and the Environment* 2000: 25:567-600.

55. Bornehag C-G, Blomquist G, Gyntelberg F, Järvholm B, Malmberg P, Nielsen A, et al. Dampness in buildings and health. Nordic interdisciplinary review of the scientific evidence on associations between exposure to "dampness" and health effects, NORDDAMP. *Indoor Air* 2001; 11:72-86.

56. Wargocki P, Bischof W, Brundrett G, Fanger O, Gyntelberg F, Hanssen SO, et al. Ventilation and health. *Indoor Air* 2002; in press.

57. Centers for Disease Control and Prevention. Blood lead levels in young children – United States and selected states, 1996–1999. *Morbidity and Mortality Weekly Report* 2000; 49:1133-7.

58. Kaiser R, Henderson AK, Daley WR, Naughton M, Khan MH, Rahman M, et al. Blood lead levels of primary school children in Dhaka, Bangladesh. *Environmental Health Perspectives* 2001; 109(6):563-6.

59. Schwartz J. Low-level lead exposure and children's IQ: a meta-analysis and search for a threshold. *Environmental Research* 1994; 65:42-55.

60. Lanphear BP, Dietrich P, Auinger P, Cox C. Subclinical lead toxicity in US children and adolescents. *Public Health Reports* 2000; 115:6.

61. Agency for Toxic Substances and Disease Registry (ATSDR). *Toxicological profile for lead (update)*. Atlanta (GA): US Department of Health and Human Services; 1999.

62. Parry MC, Rosenzweig C, Iglesis A, Fischer G, Livermore M. Climate change and world food security: a new assessment. *Global Environmental Change – Human and Policy Dimensions* 1999; 9: S51-S67.

63. Intergovernmental Panel on Climate Change. *Climate change 2001. Vol. 1: The scientific basis. Vol. II: Impacts, adaptation and vulnerability. Vol. III: Mitigation. Vol. IV: Synthesis report.* Cambridge: Cambridge University Press; 2001.

64. *The world health report 2001 – Mental health: new understanding, new hope.* Geneva: World Health Organization; 2001. Statistical annex.

65. *International Road Traffic and Accident Database (IRTAD)*. Paris: Organisation for Economic Co-operation and Development; 2001. Available from: URL: http://www.bast.de/htdocs/fachthemen/irtad/english/englisch.html (accessed November 2001).

66. Khon Kaen Accident Prevention Committee. Methodology and results of implementation of Khon Kaen Accident Prevention Committee responding to Anti-knock Helmet Act for Motorcyclists. *Trauma Center Bulletin* 1996; 1(2):1-3.

67. *Safety of pedestrians and cyclists in urban areas.* Brussels: European Transport Safety Council; 1999.

68. Dora C, Phillips M, editors. *Transport, environment and health.* Copenhagen: World Health Organization Regional Office for Europe; 2000. European Series, No. 89.

69. Jacobs GD. The potential for road accident reduction in developing countries. *Transport Reviews* 1982; 2(2):213-24.

70. *Review of road safety in Asia and the Pacific.* New York: United Nations Economic and Social Commission for Asia and the Pacific (ESCAP); 1998.

71. Bosma H, Peter R, Siegrist J, Marmot M. Two alternative job stress models and the risk of coronary heart disease. *American Journal of Public Health* 1988; 88(1):68-74.

72. Nurminen M, Karjalainen A. Epidemiologic estimate of the proportion of fatalities related to occupational factors in Finland. *Scandinavian Journal of Work, Environment & Health* 2001; 27(3):161-213.

73. National Institute for Occupational Safety and Health. *Worker health chartbook.* Cincinnati (OH): National Institute for Occupational Safety and Health (NIOSH); 2000.

74. Driscoll TR, Mitchell RJ, Mandryk JA, Healey S, Hendrie AL, Hull BP. Work-related fatalities in Australia, 1989 to 1992: an overview. *Journal of Occupational Health and Safety - Australia New Zealand* 2001; 17:45-66.

75. European Union (Eurostat). *Accidents at work in the European Union in 1993.* Available from: URL: http://europa.eu.int/comm/employment_social/h&s/figures/ accidents93_en.htm

76. Loewenson R. Assessment of the health impact of occupational risk in Africa: current situation and methodological issues. *Epidemiology* 1999; 10:632-9.

77. National Occupational Health & Safety Commission (NOHSC). *The causes of occupational accidents.* Available from: URL: http://www.nohsc.gov.au

78. International Agency for Research on Cancer. *IARC Monographs Programme on the Evaluation of Carcinogenic Risks to Humans.* Available from: URL: http://193.51.164.11

79. National Institute for Occupational Safety and Health. *Work-related lung disease surveillance report 1999.* Cincinnati (OH): Division of Respiratory Disease Studies, National Institute for Occupational Safety and Health (NIOSH); 1999.

80. Loewenson R. Globalization and occupational health: a perspective from southern Africa. *Bulletin of the World Health Organization* 2001; 79:863-8.

81. Chen W, Zhuang Z, Attfield MD, Chen BT, Gao P, Harrison JC, et al. Exposure to silica and silicosis among tin miners in China: exposure-response analyses and risk assessment. *Occupational and Environmental Medicine* 2001; 58:31-7.

82. Bernard BP, editor. *Musculoskeletal disorders and workplace factors.* Cincinnati (OH): National Institute for Occupational Safety and Health (NIOSH); 1997. DHHS (NIOSH) Publication No. 97-141.

83. Institute of Medicine. *Musculoskeletal disorders and the workplace: low back and upper extremities.* Washington (DC): National Academy Press; 2001.

84. Leigh JP, Sheetz RM. Prevalence of back pain among full-time United States workers. *British Journal of Industrial Medicine* 1989; 46:651-7.

85. Columbia University of Health Sciences (CUHS). *Counselling to prevent low back pain. Guide to clinical preventive services.* 2nd ed. Available from: URL: http://cpmcnet.columbia.edu/texts/gcps/gcps0070.html

86. Nachemson AL. Advances in low-back pain. *Clinical Orthopedics and Related Research* 1985; 200:266-78.

87. Jin K, Sorock G, Courtney T, Lian Y, Yao Z, Matz S, et al. Risk factors for work-related low back pain in the People's Republic of China. *International Journal of Occupational and Environmental Health* 2000; 6:26-33.

88. European Agency for Safety and Health at Work (EASHW). *Monitoring the state of occupational safety and health in the European Union - pilot study.* Luxembourg: EASHW. Available from: URL: http://agency.osha.eu.int/publications/ reports/stateofosh/

89. Goelzer B, Hansen CH, Sehrndt GA, editors. *Occupational exposure to noise: evaluation, prevention and control.* Berlin: Dortmund for the World Health Organization (WHO) and the Federal Institute for Occupational Safety and Health (FIOSH); 2001.

90. National Institute for Occupational Safety and Health (NIOSH). Work-related hearing loss. Available from: URL: http://www.cdc.gov/niosh/hpworkrel.html

91. *Global tuberculosis control: surveillance, planning, financing.* Geneva: World Health Organization; 2002. WHO document WHO/CDS/TB/2002.295.

92. Rieder HL. Epidemiologic basis of tuberculosis control. Paris: International Union Against Tuberculosis and Lung Disease (IUATLD); 1999.

93. Holtzman NA. Marteau TM. Will genetics revolutionize medicine? *New England Journal of Medicine* 2000; 343:141-4.

94. Peto R, Boreham J, Clarke M, Davies C, Beral V. UK and USA breast cancer deaths down 25% in year 2000 at ages 20-69 years. *Lancet* 2000; 355:1822.

95. Hunink MG, Goldman L, Tosteson AN. Mittleman MA, Goldman PA, Williams LW, et al. The recent decline in mortality from coronary heart disease, 1980-1990. The effect of secular trends in risk factors and treatment. *JAMA* 1997; 277:535-42.

96. Vartiainen E, Puska P, Jousilahti P, Korhonen HJ, Tuomilehto J, Nissinen A. Twenty-year trends in coronary risk factors in north Karelia and in other areas of Finland. *International Journal of Epidemiology* 1994; 23:495-504.

97. Shimamoto T, Komachi Y, Inada H, Doi M, Iso H, Sato S, et al. Trends for coronary heart disease and stroke and their risk factors in Japan. *Circulation* 1989; 9(3):503-15.

98. Peto R, Darby S, Deo H, Silcocks P, Whitley E, Doll R. Smoking, smoking cessation, and lung cancer in the UK since 1950: combination of national statistics with two case-control studies. *BMJ* 2000; 321:323-9.

99. Kane A, Lloyd J, Zaffran M, Simonsen L, Kane M. Transmission of hepatitis B, hepatitis C and human immunodeficiency viruses through unsafe injections in the developing world: model-based regional estimates. *Bulletin of the World Health Organization* 1999; 77:801-7.

100. Miller M, Pisani E. The cost of unsafe injections. *Bulletin of the World Health Organization* 1999; 77:808-11.

101. Reeler AV. Anthropological perspectives on injections: a review. *Bulletin of the World Health Organization* 2000; 78:135-43.

102. Simonsen L, Kane A, Lloyd J, Zaffran M, Kane M. Unsafe injections in the developing world and transmission of bloodborne pathogens. *Bulletin of the World Health Organization* 1999; 77:789-800.

103. Wilson RM, Runciman WB, Gibberd RW, Harrison BT, Newby L, Hamilton JD. The Quality in Australian Health Care Study. *Medical Journal of Australia* 1995;163(9):458-71.

104. Wilson RM, Harrison BT, Gibberd RW, Hamilton JD. An analysis of the causes of adverse events from the Quality in Australian Health Care Study, *Medical Journal of Australia* 1999; 170(9):411-5.

105. Leape LL, Brennan TA, Laird N, Lawthers AG, Localio AR, Barnes BA, et al. The nature of adverse events in hospitalized patients. Results of the Harvard Medical Practice Study II. *New England Journal of Medicine* 1991; 324:377-84.

106. Brennan TA, Leape LL, Laird NM, Hebert L, Localio AR, Lawthers AG, et al. Incidence of adverse events and negligence in hospitalized patients. Results of the Harvard Medical Practice Study I. *New England Journal of Medicine* 1991; 324:370-6.

107. Schioler T, Lipczak H, Pedersen BL, Mogensen TS, Bech KB, Stockmarr A, et al. Danish Adverse Event Study. Incidence of adverse events in hospitals. A retrospective study of medical records. *Ugeskr Laeger* 2001; 163: 5370-8. In Danish; abstract in English.

108. Vincent C, Neale G, Woloshynowych M. Adverse events in British hospitals: preliminary retrospective record review. *BMJ* 2001; 322:517-9.

109. The quality of health care/hospital activities: Report by the Working Party on Quality Care in Hospitals of the Sub-Committee on Coordination. Leuven: Standing Committee of the Hospitals of the European Union (HOPE); 2000.

110. Kohn LT, Corrigan JM, Donaldson MS, editors. To err is human: building a safer health system. Washington: National Academy Press for the Institute of Medicine; 2000.

111. Department of Health. An organisation with a memory. Report of an expert group on learning from adverse events in the NHS chaired by the Chief Medical Officer. London: The Stationery Office; 2000.

112. Progress in essential drugs and medicines policy 1998–1999. Geneva: World Health Organization; 2000. WHO document WHO/EDM/2000.2.

113. Leape LL, Bates DW, Cullen DJ, Cooper J, Demonaco HJ, Gallivan T, et al. Systems analysis of adverse drug events. *JAMA* 1995; 274:35-43.

114. Kovner C, Gergen PJ. Nurse staffing levels and adverse events following surgery. *Image – the Journal of Nursing Scholarship* 1998; 30:315-21.

115. Morris AH. Protocol management of adult respiratory distress. *New Horizons* 1993; 1:593-602.

116. Meddings DR. Civilians and war. A review and historical overview of the involvement of non-combatant populations in conflict situations. *Medicine, Conflict, and Survival* 2001; 17:6-16.

117. Krug EG, Dahlberg LL, Mercy JA, Zwi A, Lozano-Ascencio R, editors. *World report on violence and health*. Geneva: World Health Organization; 2002.

118. Popkin BM, Horton S, Kim S, Mahal A, Shuigao J. Trends in diet, nutritional status and diet-related noncommunicable diseases in China and India: The economic costs of the nutrition transition. *Nutrition Reviews* 2001; 59: 379-90.

119. Popkin BM. An overview on the nutrition transition and its health implications: the Bellagio meeting. *Public Health Nutrition* 2002; 5:93-103.

120. Kim S, Moon S, Popkin BM. The nutrition transition in South Korea. *American Journal of Clinical Nutrition* 2000; 71:44-53.

121. Lee M-J, Popkin BM, Kim S. The unique aspects of the nutrition transition in South Korea: the retention of healthful elements in their traditional diet. *Public Health Nutrition* 2000; 5:197-203.

CHAPTER FIVE

Some Strategies to Reduce Risk

This chapter puts forward the best available evidence on the cost and effectiveness of selected interventions to reduce some of the major risk factors discussed in Chapter Four. It looks at the extent to which these interventions are likely to improve population health, both singly and in combination. It illustrates how decision-makers can begin the policy debate about priorities with information about which interventions would yield the greatest possible improvements in population health for the available resources. The chapter examines a range of strategies to reduce different types of risk, and the possible impact of those strategies on costs and effectiveness. Many risk reduction strategies involve a component of behaviour change, and some types of behaviour change might require active government intervention to succeed. Different ways of attaining the same goal are discussed, for example, the population-wide versus the individual-based approach and prevention versus treatment. With regard to policy implications, the chapter concludes that very substantial health gains can be made for relatively modest expenditures on interventions. However, the maximum possible gains for the resources that are available will be attained only through careful consideration of the costs and effects of interventions.

5

Some Strategies to

Reduce Risk

From health risks to policy

*E*arlier chapters have quantified the burden of disease attributable to major risk factors, and shown the size of the potentially avoidable burden if the population distribution of risk is reduced across the board. This knowledge is important but it is only the first step required to decide how best to improve population health with the available resources. The second step involves assessing what types of intervention are available to decrease exposure to risks or to minimize the impact of exposure on health; to what extent they are likely to improve population health singly and in combination; and what resources are required to implement them. Chapter 4 quantified the importance of selected risk factors in different settings. This chapter evaluates selected interventions to reduce the impact on population health of some of those risk factors.[1]

Different types of evidence on intervention costs and effectiveness have been considered in the analysis detailed in this chapter. Some interventions have been widely implemented in many settings, and relatively good information on their costs and effects exists. The interventions for which it is easier to obtain this type of evidence are often those that focus on individuals rather than on populations as a whole, and the overall impact on population health of such interventions can be relatively small. Some types of population-based interventions with the potential to make very substantial improvements in population health have not been implemented very frequently or have not been evaluated very often. The evidence on the costs and effectiveness of these interventions is less certain, but it is important to consider them because they have the potential to make very substantial differences in health outcomes.

Cost-effectiveness analysis can be undertaken in many ways and there have been several attempts to standardize methods to make results comparable *(1–3)*. WHO has developed a standardized set of methods and tools that can be used to analyze the costs and population health impact of current and possible new interventions at the same time *(3)*. As part of WHO's CHOICE project, these tools and methods have been used to analyze a range of interventions that tackle some of the leading risks identified in Chapter 4.[2] The CHOICE project is intended to provide regularly updated databases on the costs and effects of a full range of promotive, preventive, curative and rehabilitative health interventions.

---

[1] This chapter represents a report on the first stage of a long-term work plan to evaluate the burden of all the major risks to health and the costs and effectiveness of all major interventions.

[2] CHOICE stands for CHoosing Interventions that are Cost-Effective – see www.who.int/evidence

To answer key policy questions on tackling risks to health, it is necessary to compare the costs and effectiveness of interventions to the situation that would exist if they were not done. This "counterfactual" scenario – what would happen in the absence of the interventions against a particular risk factor – is different from the counterfactual used in Chapter 4 to estimate the avoidable burden of disease. There the question was what would the burden have been if the distribution of risks could be lowered by 25%, 50% or even 100%. That is useful in showing the relative importance of different risk factors, but some of these risks can be reduced relatively easily, at low cost, and others cannot. Because health resources are always scarce in relation to need, choices must be made about how to allocate them between the substantial number of options available to reduce risks. The best way of doing this is to estimate, for each intervention, the gains in population health and the associated costs compared to the situation that would exist if the intervention were not undertaken.[3]

This chapter reports the best available evidence on the cost and effectiveness of selected interventions to reduce some of the major risk factors discussed in Chapter 4. The list of interventions is not exhaustive and the chapter does not include all the risk factors of Chapter 4. The ones for which interventions are considered here are highlighted in bold type in Table 5.1. A more comprehensive picture of interventions concerning diseases as well as additional risk factors (e.g. alcohol) will be presented in *The World Health Report 2003.*

The analysis is used to identify some interventions that are very cost-effective and some that are not cost-effective in different settings. It illustrates how decision-makers can begin the policy debate about priorities for allocating health resources with information about which interventions have the potential to yield substantial improvements in population health for the available resources.

This evidence will be only one input to the final decision about the best combination of interventions. Improving population health is the defining goal of health systems, but there are other social goals to which health systems contribute. Policy-makers will wish to consider the impact of different combinations of interventions on health inequalities and poverty and on the responsiveness of their systems, for example *(4).* Communities in different settings might differ in their ability and willingness to participate in specific risk-reduction activities, and particular activities might be more difficult to incorporate into existing health system infrastructure in some settings than in others. The information from this chapter is, therefore, one input – a key one, but not the only one – to the policy debate.

The analysis does not apply simply to interventions funded by government. WHO argues that governments should be good stewards of their health systems *(5).* If the population uses interventions that are ineffective, dangerous, or are simply not good value for money,

Table 5.1 Leading 10 selected risk factors as percentage causes of disease burden measured in DALYs[a]

Developing countries	
High mortality countries	
Underweight	**14.9%**
Unsafe sex	**10.2%**
Unsafe water, sanitation and hygiene	**5.5%**
Indoor smoke from solid fuels	3.7%
Zinc deficiency	**3.2%**
Iron deficiency	**3.1%**
Vitamin A deficiency	**3.0%**
Blood pressure	**2.5%**
Tobacco	**2.0%**
Cholesterol	**1.9%**
Low mortality countries	
Alcohol	6.2%
Blood pressure	**5.0%**
Tobacco	**4.0%**
Underweight	**3.1%**
Overweight	2.7%
Cholesterol	**2.1%**
Indoor smoke from solid fuels	1.9%
Low fruit and vegetable intake	**1.9%**
Iron deficiency	**1.8%**
Unsafe water, sanitation and hygiene	**1.7%**

Developed countries	
Tobacco	**12.2%**
Blood pressure	**10.9%**
Alcohol	9.2%
Cholesterol	**7.6%**
Overweight	7.4%
Low fruit and vegetable intake	**3.9%**
Physical inactivity	3.3%
Illicit drugs	1.8%
Unsafe sex	**0.8%**
Iron deficiency	**0.7%**

[a] Risk factors discussed in this chapter are in bold type.

---

[3] The term "intervention" is used in this chapter in a very broad sense. It includes any health action – any promotive, preventive, curative or rehabilitative activity where the primary intent is to improve health. Interventions in the chapter range from the introduction of a tax on tobacco products to treating hypertension to prevent a heart attack.

governments should find ways to encourage people to use resources more appropriately even if the finance is not provided by government. The evidence presented in this chapter will facilitate this process.

WHAT STRATEGIES CAN REDUCE RISKS TO HEALTH?

WHO defines the health system to include all actions whose primary intent is to improve health *(5)* and some activities that improve health fall outside this definition. Examples include reductions in poverty, and improvements in housing and education, which may well reduce exposures to some types of risks but are not primarily designed to improve health. This chapter is concerned mainly with interventions that have the primary intent of improving health.

Some interventions, however, are difficult to categorize strictly using this definition. One set that has traditionally fallen within the remit of public health covers improvements to water and sanitation. Many water and sanitation programmes fall outside the health portfolio, and clearly such improvements do have considerable amenity value outside health. However, clean water and improved sanitation are considered in this chapter because their attributable burden of disease is so significant. It must be noted, however, that although they improve health, many of their benefits are not readily incorporated into a cost-effectiveness framework and should be considered when comparing them with other types of health interventions.

A number of strategies have been used to reduce health risks that are seen as modifiable. They can be categorized broadly as interventions that seek to reduce risks in the population as a whole, and those which target individuals within the population. The former include intervention by governments through legislation, tax or financial incentives; engineering solutions such as the introduction of safety belts in motor vehicles or the provision of piped water; and health promotion campaigns targeting the general public. The latter include strategies to change health behaviours of individuals, often through personal interaction with a health provider; and strategies to change the behaviours of health providers, particularly in the way they interact with their clients.

Genetic screening is a valuable tool for some diseases associated with the risk factors described in this report, but individual genes are not susceptible to manipulation at present. Genetic screening is not considered further in this chapter.

RISK REDUCTION AND BEHAVIOUR

Many risk reduction strategies involve a component of behaviour change. Even engineering solutions, such as the provision of piped drinking-water, will not result in health improvements unless people are willing to use the new source. Social scientists argue that behavioural change first requires understanding *(6, 7)*.[4] A number of individual preferences or characteristics influence how people translate understanding into health behaviours, including how averse to health risks individuals are and how they value possible future health decrements compared with other competing choices in their lives such as wealth and lifestyle. These preferences are influenced by information and the influence of advertising and marketing.

"Perceived risk" is the subjective assessment of personal disease risk, based on an individual's interpretation of epidemiological and other types of data. There may be a difference

---

[4] In the case of addiction, individuals can struggle to change their behaviours despite recognition of the harmful effects to themselves and others *(8)*.

between risk perception as an individual and cultural concepts of risk acceptability by society. For example, although driving without a seat belt may be deemed so unacceptable by a society that legislation is enacted to enforce it, individuals within that society may perceive the risk to themselves as trivial and choose not to use a seat belt.

When it comes to risks to health, individuals and societies sometimes prefer to enjoy the benefits of an activity now without thinking about possible future health costs. High consumption of certain types of food, for instance, is perceived by some people to give current pleasure despite the risk of harmful health effects – to which they give less weight because they will occur in the future.

There is considerable variation in the rate at which people value and assess adverse events that might happen in the future. Some research has indicated that smokers "discount the future" more highly than non-smokers – for example, a given probability of developing lung cancer in 20 years is given less weight by smokers than by non-smokers (9). People who discount the future more highly value a given future health risk less highly than people who discount the future less highly, even if they have the same information. The question of how technically to incorporate this into the analysis is discussed later but the effectiveness of behavioural modification interventions is clearly influenced by variations in how people perceive the future.

A set of additional factors also influences the way people respond to risk-reduction interventions. Even when people have heard and understood the message that insecticide-treated nets prevent mosquito bites, and wish to use them to avoid both the nuisance value of mosquitoes and the risk of malaria, a number of factors may prevent them from doing so (10). These include the availability and affordability of nets in their locale and their sleeping arrangements (in a house, or on the street). These in turn will be affected by many factors including personal, community and health system characteristics.

One determinant is culture and the social support networks available, sometimes called social capital. Health system and provider characteristics, such as the way the health system is financed (for example, through social health insurance or user charges) or organized (for example, through managed care or a publicly funded system), also influence behaviours and, through them, the costs and effectiveness of interventions.

INDIVIDUAL-BASED VERSUS POPULATION APPROACHES TO RISK REDUCTION

Two broad approaches to reducing risk were defined earlier. The first is to focus the intervention on the people likely to benefit, or benefit most, from it. The second is to seek to reduce risks in the entire population regardless of each individual's level of risk and potential benefits. In some cases, both approaches could be used at the same time. Focusing on high-risk individuals can reduce costs at the population level because an intervention is provided to fewer people, but on the other hand it might also increase the costs of identifying the group of people most likely to benefit.

Focusing on people who are more likely to benefit has a significant impact on the health of a nation only when there are large numbers of them. For example, lowering cholesterol with drugs is effective in reducing overall mortality in a group of people at high risk of death from heart disease; targeting interventions to reduce cholesterol to the needs of these people focuses the interventions on a group of people likely to benefit.

However, only a small percentage of the population is at high risk of death from heart disease at any given time, and only some of them can be identified purely on the basis of their cholesterol levels. Recent evidence suggests that the group most likely to benefit from cholesterol reduction consists of individuals with combinations of risk factors, such as being male, with ischaemic changes, who smoke, are obese, are not physically active and have high blood pressure and high cholesterol *(11)*. Designing interventions for people with a combination of those risk factors might well prove to be more effective than treating people only on the basis of their levels of cholesterol *(12)*. This form of targeted approach will subsequently be called the "absolute risk approach".

The high-risk approach can be viewed as targeting the right-hand tail of the risk factor curves in Figure 5.1 *(13)*. The alternative is to try to shift the entire population distribution of risk factors to the left – like shifting the distribution of blood pressure for London civil servants in the direction of that of Kenyan nomads. This has the potential to improve population health to a much greater extent than a high-risk approach, while at the same time reducing the costs of identifying high-risk people. On the other hand, the costs of providing an intervention to the entire population would, in this case, be higher than providing it only to people in the right-hand tail. Which approach is the most cost-effective in any setting will depend on the prevalence of high-risk people in the population and the costs of identifying them compared with the costs of the available blood pressure reduction strategies.

THE ROLE OF GOVERNMENT AND LEGISLATION

Some areas of behavioural change are likely to be adopted relatively easily once information becomes available, assuming that the technology is affordable. Other types of behavioural change will benefit from active government intervention, particularly those where people have high rates of time discount or low rates of risk aversion. Government action is required if the full potential to improve population health through the reduction of alcohol and tobacco consumption is to be achieved, partly because of the addictive nature of these substances. Such action could be through changes in the law or financial incentives and disincentives. Road safety is another area where a significant number of people might not

Figure 5.1 Distributions of systolic blood pressure in middle-aged men in two populations

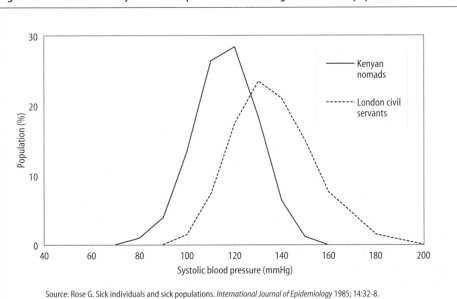

Source: Rose G. Sick individuals and sick populations. *International Journal of Epidemiology* 1985; 14:32-8.

choose to drive safely, or use seat belts or motorcycle helmets, but government action can encourage them to do so, thereby preventing injuries to themselves and to other people.

Increasing prices through taxation certainly reduces smoking *(14)* even if smuggling increases subsequently *(15)*. A particular focus of this chapter is to explore if this type of government action is cost-effective. In some countries there has been debate about whether governments should play this type of role, and information on the costs and impact on population health are important inputs to this debate.

DIFFERENT WAYS OF ATTAINING THE SAME GOAL

Different sets of interventions can be used to achieve the same goal and some interventions will reduce the burden associated with multiple risk factors and diseases. Interventions to reduce blood pressure, cigarette smoking and cholesterol all reduce cardiovascular disease, and each has been used separately and together with others at different times and in different settings. The effect of doing two at the same time might be more than would be expected by adding the benefits of doing the two interventions singly, or might be less. Much ischaemic heart disease mortality that has traditionally been attributed to particular risk factors is, in fact, caused by those factors in combination with other risk factors *(16)*. Partly as a result of these interactions, risk reduction strategies are generally based on a combination of interventions rather than just one.

The decision about which combination should be undertaken for the available resources is complex. It is necessary to determine the health gains, and the costs, of doing each possible intervention by itself and in combination with the other ways of reducing the burden for a given risk factor or disease. The analysis undertaken for this chapter followed that process by evaluating what would be achieved by each intervention alone and in combination with other interventions.

TECHNICAL CONSIDERATIONS FOR COST-EFFECTIVENESS ANALYSIS

The estimates, which provide the basis of the results reported in this chapter, were undertaken on a regional basis as part of the WHO CHOICE project. The six WHO regions were divided into mortality strata as described in earlier chapters, resulting in 14 epidemiological subregions. The total costs and total effects of each intervention were estimated separately for the 14 subregions. Eventually it is hoped that there will be sufficient data to make estimates at a country level, and even at the subnational level for large countries, but this is not currently possible.

Subregional analysis offers a valuable basis from which country analysts can work to calibrate the results to their settings. It is much more policy-relevant than a global analysis because the epidemiology, cost structures, and starting points (such as the availability of trained health staff and the history of health interventions) varies less within each subregion than across the world as a whole. The results are used here to identify interventions that are very cost-effective, cost-effective, and not cost-effective in each subregion.

Costs are reported in terms of international dollars rather than in US dollars, to account better for differences in cost structures between settings. Unit costs for most regions are higher using international dollars (I$) based on purchasing power parity exchange rates than they would be if official exchange rates had been used.[5] Effectiveness is measured in terms of disability-adjusted life years (DALYs) gained by the intervention. A brief description of the methods is found in Box 5.1, while full details of the methods and the calculations can be found on the WHO web site.[6]

It is not much value to provide decision-makers with information on the costs and effectiveness of interventions that are undertaken badly. Accordingly, the results reported here show what would be achieved if the interventions were undertaken in a relatively efficient manner. For example, we assume capacity utilization of 80% in most settings – for example, staff and capital equipment are fully occupied for 80% of the normal working day – except when estimating the effect of expanding coverage to very high levels. To reach 95% of the population it might be necessary to provide facilities in isolated areas where population numbers are insufficient to support such high rates of capacity utilization. The results, therefore, provide guidance on selected interventions that should be given high priority in the policy debate about resource allocation, but only if they are undertaken in an efficient manner.

Sets of interventions that interact in terms of effectiveness or costs are considered together, as stated earlier. For example, interventions to reduce risks associated with hypertension and high cholesterol interact. The analysis is based on estimates of the effects on population health of reducing blood pressure alone, reducing cholesterol levels alone, and doing both together.

In addition, many of the interventions are evaluated at different levels of coverage. For most, three levels were used (50%, 80% and 95%) and the impact on costs and effects of expanding coverage was incorporated.

The standard practice in this type of analysis is to discount both the health effects and the costs of the different programmes under consideration. There is no controversy about

---

Box 5.1 Methods for cost-effectiveness analysis

The cost-effectiveness analysis on which this report is based considered what would have happened if a set of interventions had not been implemented and compared the result with what happens on their implementation. Through a four-state population model, the number of healthy life years lived over a period of a hundred years by a population in the absence of that set of interventions is estimated by inputting parameters of incidence, remission, cause-specific and background mortality, and health state valuations reflecting the natural history of the disease. The parameters reflecting the natural history of the disease were mostly estimated by back-adjusting current rates using coverage and known effectiveness of interventions. The same four-state population model can then be rerun, reflecting changes in the parameters due to in-

terventions or combinations of interventions. For example, based on data from earlier chapters, vitamin A deficiency increases the risk of dying from diarrhoea. The impact of vitamin A supplementation is then mediated in the model by a decrease in case fatality rate for diarrhoea. Effectiveness data came from systematic reviews where available. The difference in the healthy life years gained by the population with and without the intervention is the impact of the intervention and is entered as the denominator of the cost-effectiveness ratio.

Costs covered in this analysis include expenses associated with running the intervention, such as administration, training and contact with the media. They also include costs incurred at the individual level such as counselling. Considerable effort was exerted to try to standardize the methodology used in collecting and classifying costs. The

quantities of inputs required to run each intervention were estimated by experts in 17 regions of the world and validated against the literature. Some individual-level costs were obtained by multiplying unit costs of inputs by the expected utilization of those inputs by the people covered by the programme. Unit costs for outpatient visits and laboratory tests were obtained from a review of literature and supplemented by primary data from several countries. The total costs for implementing a programme for 10 years constitutes the denominator of the cost-effectiveness ratio.

Stochastic uncertainty analysis was carried out for key parameters in both the numerator and denominator.

Sources: (3, 17–19).

---

[5] This is important to keep in mind when benchmarking the estimates in this chapter against those reported elsewhere, usually in US dollars. International dollars are derived by dividing local currency units by an estimate of their purchasing power parity (PPP) compared to a US$. PPPs are the rates of currency conversion that equalize the purchasing power of different currencies by eliminating the differences in price levels between countries.

[6] www.who.int/evidence

the appropriate discount rate to use for costs: the opportunity cost of capital. The discount rate for benefits is often thought to comprise two parts. One is a "pure" time preference for immediate over postponed consumption. The second relates to the fact that, as the prosperity of a society increases, the utility or benefit to it of a defined unit of consumption is less – that is, there is declining marginal utility of a unit of consumption as income rises. Many cost-effectiveness studies have assumed that this applies to health benefits as well and have discounted future health at a rate between 3% and 5% per year. This practice has long been debated, and some people have argued that the discount rate for health benefits should be close to zero and certainly less than the discount rate for costs (20–22).

This question is important for the analysis in the following section as it can change the relative priority of interventions. Not all health care programmes achieve results at the same rate. Public health and health promotion programmes in particular may take many years to produce tangible results, and applying a discount rate to the benefits of such programmes will reduce their apparent attractiveness compared with programmes that produce rapid benefits of a similar magnitude.

Common practice remains to discount costs and benefits at the same rate, so we follow the same practice in our baseline calculations using a rate of 3%. To be consistent with the approach used in Chapter 4 for measuring the burden of disease, age weights are also included in the baseline calculations.

The recent report of the Commission on Macroeconomics and Health suggested that interventions costing less than three times GDP per capita for each DALY averted represent good value for money and that, if a country could not afford to undertake them all from its own resources, the international community should find ways of supporting them (23). This report's classification of interventions is based on this principle, and defines very cost-effective interventions as those which avert each additional DALY at a cost less than GDP per capita, and cost-effective interventions as those where each DALY averted costs between one and three times GDP per capita.

Finally, cost-effectiveness analyses can be found in the published literature for some of the interventions discussed in this chapter, which does not, however, simply report the published results. The methods used for estimating costs and effectiveness varies considerably across the published studies and their results cannot be compared. Moreover, most provide insufficient information on how they estimated costs to be sure that all possible costs were included and valued appropriately. This report, therefore, re-estimated costs and effects using a standard approach for all interventions, although each study that could be found was evaluated to determine if the parameters it used could be incorporated.

CHOOSING INTERVENTIONS TO REDUCE SPECIFIC RISKS

The results reported in this chapter are important inputs to two types of policy questions. The first is how best to reduce the health burden associated with a specific risk factor, where information on the effectiveness and costs of the alternative interventions is one crucial input. The second is how best to reduce the health burden associated with risk factors in general, where information on the effectiveness and costs of interventions aimed as a variety of risk factors is critical. This section covers the first question, by reviewing the cost-effectiveness of selected interventions aimed at some of the main risk factors described in Chapter 4. The same organizing format followed in that chapter is followed here. The question of how to decide what combination of those risk factors should be given priority for any given level of resource availability is considered on page 139.

CHILDHOOD UNDERNUTRITION

The strategy of primary health care was adopted by the World Health Assembly in 1977 and outlined further in the 1978 Declaration of Alma-Ata on Health for All *(24)*. The Declaration encouraged governments to strive toward attaining Health for All by ensuring, at a minimum, the following activities: education concerning prevailing health problems, their prevention and control; promotion of food supply and good nutrition; safe water and basic sanitation; maternal and child health care which included family planning; immunization against major infectious diseases; prevention and treatment of locally endemic diseases; appropriate treatment of common diseases and injuries; and provision of essential drugs. Primary health care emphasized programmatic areas rather than diseases, and encouraged community and individual self-reliance and participation, an emphasis on prevention, and a multisectoral approach.

Subsequently, the concept of "selective primary health care" was proposed to allow for the scarcity of resources available to achieve health for all. It involved defining strategies focusing on priority health problems (including infant and child mortality), using interventions that were feasible to implement, of low cost, and with proven efficacy *(25, 26)*. UNICEF's GOBI strategy of 1982 emerged from this. At its foundation were four child health interventions which met the above criteria and which were considered to be synergistic – growth monitoring (G), oral rehydration therapy for diarrhoea (O), the promotion of breastfeeding (B) and childhood immunizations (I). Birth spacing/family planning (F), food supplementation (F) and the promotion of female literacy (F) were added subsequently (GOBI-FFF) *(27)*.

There has been subsequent analysis and discussion of the extent to which the specific interventions can be integrated into primary health care, and whether strategies should be modified in view of new knowledge and changing circumstances. However, concern with ensuring that child health strategies are based on feasible and affordable interventions – that are synergistic and of proven effectiveness – has remained. This chapter builds on that tradition by providing information on the costs and effects of selected interventions targeting key risk factors affecting the health of children. The results not only identify a group of interventions that are very cost-effective, but also illustrate how information on the costs and effectiveness of selected interventions can provide useful insights that can be used to re-assess, from time to time, the need to modify current approaches in view of changing knowledge and circumstances.

The focus is on interventions aimed primarily at the risk factors identified in Chapter 4 rather than all possible child health interventions. We have selected some interventions that can be delivered on a population-wide basis and some that focus on individuals, to illustrate how the two approaches interact. Childhood immunizations have not been included because they do not respond to one of the major risk factors of Chapter 4, and because it is already widely accepted that they are cost-effective *(28)*. The fact that interventions are not included here, therefore, should not be taken to imply that they are not cost-effective.

Childhood undernutrition (and breastfeeding)

Interventions

The childhood interventions were not evaluated in the A subregions where childhood undernutrition is not a major cause of burden.

Complementary feeding. One-time intensive counselling is provided to mothers on the appropriate complementary feeding practices and on the importance of continued breast-feeding. In addition, all infants aged 6 months to 1 year, regardless of nutritional status, are provided with ready-to-mix complementary food, which is collected every two months from a health centre by the carer. The intervention is estimated to shift positively the overall distribution of weight-for-age for children less than one year of age by 0.16 standard deviations (adapted from Caulfield & Huffman) *(29)*. It was then assumed that each cohort of children exposed to this intervention would continue to reap the benefits subsequently because of the knowledge and attitudes retained by the carer.

Complementary feeding with growth monitoring and promotion. All carers are given an initial intensive counselling session on appropriate complementary feeding prac-tices and the importance of continued breastfeeding. Carers are provided with growth charts and, during quarterly visits, the weight of the child is plotted and any deviations from ex-pected weight gain is discussed. Solutions are suggested and targets for weight gain are set. In addition, ready-to-mix complementary food is provided to all children from 6 months to 1 year of age who have been identified to have poor weight gain or are underweight.

Results

The impact of the two types of interventions is identical, but the costs of the more fo-cused approach of complementary feeding with growth monitoring and promotion are considerably lower than those for complementary feeding alone. Complementary feeding by itself is not cost-effective, while complementary feeding with growth monitoring is cost-effective in most regions. It is assumed that the benefits of the intervention in terms of carer's knowledge gained and attitudes changed will persist until the child is five years old. Interactions are considered below.

Iron deficiency

Interventions

Iron fortification. Iron, usually combined with folic acid, is added to the appropriate food vehicle made available to the population as a whole. Cereal flours are the most com-mon food vehicle and are the basis of the analysis, but there is also some experience with introducing iron to other vehicles such as noodles, rice, and various sauces *(30)*. The pro-portion of the population that consumes the food vehicle in sufficient quantities to absorb sufficient iron varies by region, from 65% to 95%, and this chapter explores the costs and effects in the event that fortification reaches 50%, 80% and 95% of the targeted population. Because of likely problems with absorption, fortification is considered only 50% as effica-cious as supplementation in the people who are covered, consistent with the assumptions of Chapter 4.

Iron supplementation. Iron is provided to pregnant women during antenatal visits. The assumed dose follows WHO guidelines, with daily supplementation of 60 mg elemen-tal iron, for six months during pregnancy and three months postpartum *(31)*. Three differ-ent levels of coverage are included – 50%, 80% and 95% – and it is assumed that only 67% of these women receive an effective dose because of less than perfect adherence *(32)*. For the women who currently attend antenatal clinics, only the costs of the iron and the additional time of the visit were included. However, expansion of coverage for iron supplementation purposes beyond current coverage of antenatal visits requires attributing the full cost of the necessary visits to the intervention.

Results

Even though many groups in the population are likely to benefit from iron fortification, only the impact on iron deficiency anaemia in pregnant women (with an impact on maternal health and prenatal mortality) has been included in the analysis. This understates the benefit, but these effects probably account for more than 95% of total deaths averted by fortification. Despite this, supplementation and fortification at 50% coverage are estimated to lead to increases in population health of almost 59 million and 29 million DALYs in turn globally when implemented over a 10-year period.

Supplementation yields greater improvements in population health than fortification, in all subregions with high child mortality (all D and E subregions), and at all levels of coverage. In the other subregions, supplementation has a larger impact on population health than fortification for equivalent levels of coverage. On a global basis, supplementation at 80% would gain just over 9 million DALYs per year compared to doing nothing.

On the other hand, fortification is always less costly than supplementation because it does not require a visit to a provider, and the unit cost of supplementation increases sharply with increasing coverage. This means that the cost-effectiveness of fortification is always lower than the cost-effectiveness of supplementation, regardless of the coverage of fortification. It, then, is the preferred option at low levels of resource availability.

However, in some settings iron fortification is hindered by the absence of ideal food vehicles that are eaten in sufficient quantities and it might be difficult to ensure coverage even as high as 50%. It is also hindered by the absence of ideal iron compounds that would be favorably absorbed, are stable and nonreactive, with little colour, and no taste of their own. Where people's diets are not based around cereal flours or another convenient food vehicle, supplementation is still a cost-effective option. Indeed, in areas with a high prevalence of iron-deficiency anaemia, it is still very cost-effective to spend the higher amounts on supplementation to achieve the greater population benefit. It is less cost-effective to take this option in areas where the burden from iron deficiency anaemia is relatively low, although the cost-effectiveness of switching from fortification to supplementation is between one and three times GDP per capita so does not fall into the band of cost-ineffective interventions.

VITAMIN A DEFICIENCY

Interventions

Vitamin A deficiency is negligible in the European region of WHO, while deaths due to pneumonia and diarrhoea are negligible in AMR-A and WPR-A. The following interventions are not evaluated in those areas.

Vitamin A supplementation. Oral vitamin A supplements are provided to all children under five years of age twice a year at a health centre. The dose is 200 000 i.u. for children from their first birthday. For those less than one year of age, the dose is 50 000–100 000 i.u. Effectiveness of the intervention is adjusted by adherence.

Vitamin A fortification. Fortification of a food staple with vitamin A (in this case assumed to be sugar), whether locally produced or imported or whether for industrial or domestic use, is assured through legislation. The amount of vitamin A required is calculated based on an estimation of the amount of recommended daily allowance anticipated to be taken in from other sources and the average per capita intake of sugar in different settings. A trend analysis of a number of different fortification programmes in central America shows a relative reduction of about 60% in the prevalence of vitamin A deficiency associated with the introduction of fortification *(33)*. Intervention includes provision of guidelines for quality control of sugar fortification in the mills, regular visits to mills by inspectors, and regular sampling and testing of sugar taken from mills, markets and homes for vitamin A content. Samples from homes are taken opportunistically during mass surveys carried out for other purposes.

Results

As with iron, vitamin A fortification is more cost-effective than supplementation in all regions, because of its lower costs. Supplementation will, however, have a substantially large benefit in terms of population health – approximately twice as high as fortification – although at a higher cost. It is also very cost-effective in its own right. Both remain either cost-effective or very cost-effective in all regions included in the analysis when coverage is increased to the maximum possible level.

ZINC DEFICIENCY

Interventions

Zinc supplementation. During one of the first immunization contacts in infancy, the health worker prescribes zinc gluconate or sulfate (10 mg in solution) as part of a routine. Thereafter, the zinc solution is administered by a carer at home daily to every child until the child reaches five years of age. Effectiveness of the intervention is adjusted by expected adherence for medications needing to be taken daily.

Zinc fortification. The intervention has the same characteristics as for Vitamin A fortification except the food vehicle is wheat, not sugar. Note that in the absence of effectiveness data, the assumption has been made that zinc fortification is half as efficacious as zinc supplementation, consistent with that made for iron fortification.

Results

As with iron and vitamin A, zinc supplementation and fortification both prove to be very cost-effective interventions in all subregions. Fortification is more cost-effective than supplementation and is also slightly more cost-effective than vitamin A supplementation in most regions evaluated. Even though zinc fortification is very cost-effective, the overall impact on population health of this intervention is lower than the gains associated with vitamin A fortification in regions where vitamin A deficiency is a problem. It should, of course, be remembered that no large-scale zinc fortification programme has yet been carried out, so the results are based on the effect on health of assumed increases in zinc intake.

OTHER INDIVIDUAL-BASED INTERVENTIONS FOCUSING ON CHILDREN UNDER FIVE YEARS OF AGE

Interventions

Although not strictly risk-reducing strategies, two ways of reducing the risk of death associated with the risk factors outlined above are considered here.

Oral rehydration therapy. Health workers are trained to use an algorithm for the assessment and management of dehydration caused by diarrhoea in children under five years of age. Children brought to a health facility with watery stools are assessed for signs of dehydration by a trained health worker. If severely dehydrated, the child is rehydrated in the health facility or referred to a higher-level facility if necessary. Children still able to take in fluids are provided with oral rehydration salts reconstituted in boiled then cooled water at a specified concentration. Advice is given on the frequency of the rehydration and also on danger signals for which the carer should watch. Programme implementation of this intervention has been estimated to achieve a relative reduction in case fatality rate of 36% *(34, 35)*.

Case management of pneumonia. Health workers are trained to assess and manage respiratory distress in children. A child brought to a health facility with a cough is assessed by a trained health worker for presence of rapid breathing and other signs of respiratory distress. Depending on which signs are present, the child is referred to a hospital for intravenous treatment with antibiotics, is prescribed a five-day course of antibiotics with instructions for follow-up, or the carer is provided advice on supportive management and on monitoring the respiratory status of the child. A metaanalysis of several large, community-based trials estimated that the intervention produced a relative reduction of 50% in case-fatality rate *(36)*. This effectiveness estimate was subsequently adjusted for adherence.

Results

The relative magnitude of the effect varies with epidemiology. For example, vitamin A supplementation achieves greater health effects than oral rehydration therapy in some areas (AMR-B, SEAR-B and WPR-B) but in the others the reverse is true. Both oral rehydration therapy and case management of pneumonia achieve substantially greater benefits than zinc fortification and supplementation, despite the zinc interventions being more cost-effective. Both forms of treatment are still very cost-effective in their own right in all subregions.

COMBINED INTERVENTIONS TO REDUCE RISKS IN CHILDREN UNDER FIVE YEARS OF AGE

Most of the childhood interventions considered above prove to be very efficient ways of improving population health. Zinc fortification, under the current assumption of effectiveness is, perhaps, the surprise, being more cost-effective than the other options in all regions. To the extent that the same food vehicles could be used to fortify zinc and iron, the cost-effectiveness of the combined intervention would be even more attractive, making it one of the most attractive options available of any type of intervention. However, zinc fortification by itself, despite its cost-effectiveness, would have a smaller impact on population health than the other interventions discussed in this section except for food supplementation. Moreover, it has yet to be used on the scale assumed for these calculations.

As yet there is little evidence from field studies about the impact of multiple interventions designed to improve the health of children under five years of age. An evaluation study to assess the impact of the integrated management of childhood illness strategy is currently under way (Box 5.2), which should provide evidence in the near future. In the meantime, we have modelled the interactions between the different combinations of interventions relating specifically to children described above (for example, not including iron) taking into account synergies in terms of costs and effects.

Except for the regions where Vitamin A deficiency is not a major cause of burden (EUR-B and EUR-C), the combination of zinc with Vitamin A fortification (or supplementation) with treatment of diarrhoea and pneumonia is the most cost-effective combination of preventive and curative actions, well under the cut-off point for very cost effective interventions.

This does not imply that other types of interventions are not cost-effective or should be excluded from consideration. It simply illustrates that addition of Vitamin A and zinc interventions to the curative care currently provided routinely in most settings would gain substantial improvements in child health at relatively low cost.

BLOOD PRESSURE AND CHOLESTEROL

Comprehensive approaches to the control of cardiovascular diseases take account of a variety of interrelated risk factors including blood pressure, cholesterol, smoking, body mass index, low levels of physical activity, diet and diabetes. They use a mix of population-wide and individual-based interventions, and countries that have developed comprehensive policies have seen cardiovascular disease mortality fall significantly. In Finland, for example, a comprehensive national strategy that combined prevention, community-based health promotion and access to treatment was associated with a 60% decline in mortality rates from cardiovascular diseases over a 25-year period (37–39).

Cardiovascular disease risk factors are associated with substantial health burdens in all countries, including the poorest countries, which makes it more important than ever to base strategies for their control on interventions that are affordable, feasible, effective and acceptable to communities. This section contributes to this process by reporting on the effectiveness and costs of selected interventions focusing on blood pressure and cholesterol. Box 5.3 reports on an intervention aimed at encouraging increased fruit and vegetable intake, while smoking is considered in a subsequent section.

Population-wide and individual-based interventions are evaluated, alone and in combination. All possible interventions or combinations could not be included here, nor is it possible to analyse all of the different ways of designing the interventions that are included. The information nevertheless shows that certain population-wide interventions that have not yet been widely implemented have the potential to be very cost-effective ways of improving population health and result in substantial health benefits. It also suggests that the combination of selected individual-based interventions with these population-wide interventions would also be cost-effective in most settings.

Box 5.2 Integrated Management of Childhood Illness: interventions that interact

Integrated Management of Childhood Illness (IMCI) is a broad strategy that encourages communities and health workers to see the child as a whole, not just as a single problem or disease. IMCI helps countries use their scarce health resources in efficient ways by combining prevention and treatment of the most common childhood illnesses into simple guidelines and messages. Countries adapt these guidelines to meet their needs and use them to train health workers at all levels, improve supervision, make sure essential drugs are available, and mobilize families and communities in support of child health.

Most of the 10.9 million child deaths in 2000 (99% of which occurred in developing countries) could have been prevented with available, inexpensive interventions that are already available to children in richer countries. These inequities could be reduced if IMCI is implemented at high levels of coverage. Over 80 developing countries have adopted IMCI as part of their national policy to improve child health. The challenge now is to scale up the strategy and to strengthen health systems so that they can deliver IMCI and other child and family services efficiently and effectively.

A multicountry evaluation of IMCI effectiveness, cost and impact is currently under way to obtain information about the barriers to IMCI implementation, the effects the strategy has on health services and communities, how much it costs, and how many lives it can save. The evaluation is being conducted in collaboration with Ministries of Health and technical assistance partners in Bangladesh, Brazil, Perú, Uganda, and the United Republic of Tanzania. The early results of the evaluation are already being used to improve the delivery of child health services in developing countries; for example, in the United Republic of Tanzania it has been shown that children in districts implementing IMCI are receiving better care than those in similar districts without IMCI.

Further information is available at: URL: http://www.who.int/child-adolescent-health and http://www.who.int/imci-mce

Blood pressure

Interventions

Population wide salt reductions. Two approaches were evaluated. The first involves cooperation between government and the food industry to include appropriate labelling about salt content on products and to ensure a stepwise reduction of salt in commonly consumed processed foods. This could be through multi-stakeholder initiatives such as the development of voluntary codes of conduct *(40)*. The estimated eventual effect would be a 15% reduction in sodium intake with corresponding reductions in regional age-specific and sex-specific mean systolic blood pressure levels *(41)*.

The second approach is based on legislative action to ensure a reduction of salt in processed food with appropriate labelling. It also requires collaboration between multiple stakeholders, with the addition of quality control and enforcement. As a result, costs are higher than the voluntary version, but effects on salt intake are also likely to be higher. An eventual 30% reduction in sodium intakes is assumed *(41)*.

Individual-based hypertension treatment and education. This strategy requires drug treatment; costing of treatment has been based on a standard regimen of 50 mg atenolol (beta-blocker) and 25 mg hydrochlorothiazide (diuretic) per day. Four visits to a health provider for medical check-ups and 1.5 outpatient visits for health education are required each year, with annual renal function, lipid profile, and blood sugar (only in A subregions) tests. Two variations of this intervention were evaluated – treatment for people with systolic blood pressures (SBP) of 160 mmHg and above, and for those with 140 mmHg and above. The intervention is expected to result in a one-third reduction of the difference between starting SBP and 115 mmHg. This reflects the observation that the lower the individual's SBP initially, the lower the typical reduction with treatment.

In subsequent sections, combined risk modification strategies that focus on the individual's absolute risk are analyzed. In addition, as with all the other interventions targeting major risks to ischaemic heart disease and stroke, the benefits of reducing blood pressure, cholesterol, and body mass index are modelled jointly, taking into account the interrelationships in these risks.

Results

In all subregions, population strategies to reduce blood pressure are very cost-effective. Legislation is potentially more cost-effective than voluntary agreements with industry – this effect is due to the assumption that legislation with enforcement will lead to a larger reduction in salt intake in the diet than voluntary agreements – but the trade-off between legislation and voluntary agreements is likely to depend on the national context.

Strategies to reduce blood pressure by treating individuals with a SBP greater than 160 mmHg fall into the most cost-effective category. Lowering the threshold to 140 mmHg implies many more individuals benefit from treatment but at a higher cost, and also increases the number of people suffering side-effects from treatment. The strategy would need to be considered carefully because whether it is cost-effective varies with such factors as epidemiology and costs. It is not cost-effective, for example, in AFR-D and AMR-D, and of borderline cost-effectiveness in AFR-E.

Combinations of individual treatment and population based approaches to reduce salt intake are cost-effective at the 160 mmHg SBP threshold in all settings. However, a focus on blood pressure alone is unlikely to be the most appropriate approach to reducing the risks associated with cardiovascular disease. To explore this, a strategy to act on multiple risk factors through population and individual treatment-based strategies at the same time is evaluated at the end of this section.

CHOLESTEROL

Interventions

Of the possible interventions, two are evaluated here.

Population-wide health education through mass media. Health education through broadcast and print media is expected to lead to a 2% reduction across the board in total cholesterol levels *(42)*.

Individual-based treatment and education. Two variations are evaluated. The first involves treatment for people with total cholesterol levels above the threshold of 6.2 mmol/l (240 mg/dl) and the second above 5.7 mmol/l (220 mg/dl). Treatment requires the daily intake of 30 mg of lovastatin, four annual visits to a health provider for evaluation, and 1.5 annual outpatient visits for health education sessions. Annual laboratory tests for total cholesterol levels are included in the costs in all regions and for hepatic function in low mortality, high-income areas (A subregions).

Results

In all subregions, population strategies to reduce cholesterol are very cost-effective. The total impact in terms of DALYs gained, however, is relatively small although this is based on evidence from studies with a relatively short period of follow-up. The long-term effect over generations is likely to be greater because overall cultural changes in dietary habits can be self-reinforcing.

Given that statins are now available at very low cost and are rather effective, using statins to reduce cholesterol is very cost-effective in all regions. Total population impacts in terms of DALYs averted are relatively large, though generally slightly smaller than the benefits gained from treating hypertension. The incremental cost-effectiveness of lowering the threshold from 6.2 to 5.7 mmol/l (240 to 220 mg/dl) is not in the very cost-effective category in AMR-D and SEAR-D, and is borderline in AFR-E.

COMBINING INTERVENTIONS TO REDUCE THE RISK OF CARDIOVASCULAR EVENTS

Interventions

Many different combinations are possible – for example, WHO recently convened a meeting to consider the integrated management of cardiovascular diseases by focusing on blood pressure, smoking cessation and diabetes *(43)*. This chapter evaluates different combinations of the interventions considered above for reducing blood pressure and cholesterol levels.

Individual-based treatment and education for systolic blood pressure and cholesterol. The combined costs and effects of individual management of treating systolic blood pressure over 140 mmHg and cholesterol over 6.2 mmol/l (240 mg/dl) have been evaluated for each region. In this intervention, some individuals receive treatment only for blood pressure, some only for cholesterol and some for both depending on measured tests.

Population-wide combination of interventions to reduce hypertension and cholesterol. This combination is based on the population-wide interventions described in the previous two sections – mass media for cholesterol and legislation for salt reduction.

Absolute risk approach. An alternative to focusing on cholesterol or blood pressure levels separately is to evaluate each individual's risk of a cardiovascular event in the next ten years. Several countries have already begun to implement this approach in practical clinical settings. All people with an estimated combined risk of a cardiovascular event over the next decade that exceeds a given threshold are treated for multiple risk factors as well as being provided with health education. Four different thresholds were evaluated – 5%, 15%, 25% and 35%.

Individual risks of a cardiovascular event for this analysis were based on age, sex, body mass index, serum total cholesterol, systolic blood pressure levels and smoking status. Lower cost and more practical implementation strategies for regions with less extensive infrastructure could result in risk assessment solely on the basis of age, sex, smoking status and body mass index, which would reduce the costs of implementing the approach.

People above the threshold level of risk are provided daily with 30 mg of lovastatin, 100 mg acetylsalicylic acid (aspirin), 25 mg thiazides, and 50 mg atenolol, regardless of levels of individual risk factors *(44)*. Annually they will make four visits to a provider for evaluation and 1.5 outpatient visits for health education sessions. In addition to the laboratory tests required to assess the initial level of risk, annual laboratory tests for renal function and lipid profiles are required in all regions with the addition of hepatic function and blood sugar tests in A subregions. The consequences of bleeding associated with the use of aspirin have been accounted for in the estimates of DALYs gained.

Combined population interventions and the absolute risk approach. As a final approach to reducing the burden associated with selected cardiovascular disease risk factors, the impact of a population strategy to reduce salt intake, lower cholesterol and reduce body mass index has been evaluated in combination with treatment based on an absolute risk threshold, for all of the cut-off points evaluated above. This combines most of the major known prevention strategies to reduce the burden of cardiovascular disease, except for smoking cessation which is discussed subsequently.

Results

The absolute risk approach for a theshold of 35% is very cost-effective in all subregions and is always more cost-effective than the alternative of treatment based on observed levels of blood pressure and cholesterol alone. As the threshold is lowered, the health benefits increase but so do the costs – in fact, it gets more and more expensive to obtain each additional unit of health benefit. The exact point at which policy-makers might choose to set the threshold will vary by setting and will take into account many factors in addition to cost-effectiveness, but it is always cost-effective (though not always very cost-effective) to reduce the threshold to 25%. In most subregions, moving to a 5% threshold would be cost-effective even taking into account the increase in side-effects. Overall, the potential to reduce the risk of cardiovascular events through this intervention is very impressive. Population-level effects exceeding a 50% reduction in events are possible.

The assumptions for the impact of the population interventions evaluated here are conservative and do not take into account long-term impacts such as permanent changes in dietary patterns. Combining population-based cholesterol reduction strategies with interventions to reduce salt intake at the population level is always very cost-effective. In addition, a strategy based on the combination of population-wide and individual-based interventions is also cost-effective in all settings. The most attractive strategy among all those evaluated appears to be the combination of salt reduction at a population level through legislation or voluntary agreements with health education through the mass media focusing on blood pressure, cholesterol and body mass, plus the implementation of an absolute risk approach to managing cardiovascular disease risks.

Where resources are very scarce, prime attention would be focused on prevention and promotion, combined with the less intense individual treatment options, for example, treating people whose overall risk of a cardiovascular event over 10 years exceeds 35%. Additional resources would allow consideration of whether the theshold for treatment should be lowered.

This section has focused only on blood pressure and cholesterol, and the addition of interventions to encourage increased physical activity, or to increase fruit and vegetable intake, should also be considered in the development of an overall strategy to deal with cardiovascular disease risks. A critical part of this would be a comprehensive approach to tobacco control. Interventions aimed at that end are discussed below because smoking affects not only cardiovascular diseases but also other important causes of burden.

LOW FRUIT AND VEGETABLE INTAKE

Interventions

Increasing the consumption of fruit and vegetables reduces the risks of ischaemic heart disease, stroke, and colorectal, gastric, lung and oesophageal cancers. A report of a population-based interventions designed specifically to encourage people to increase their consumption of fruit and vegetables is described in Box 5.3.

SEXUAL AND REPRODUCTIVE HEALTH

UNSAFE SEX AND HIV/AIDS

Interventions

Over the last two decades, international agencies, governmental organizations and representatives of civil society have collaborated to develop a range of approaches to respond to the AIDS epidemic. The cornerstone remains the combination of various preventive interventions, community action and participation, and appropriate care and treatment *(56)*. There has been continual reassessment of the role of particular types of interventions

---

Box 5.3 Cost-effectiveness of a national nutrition campaign

Although high consumption of fresh fruit and vegetables offers protection against many forms of cancer and coronary heart disease, dietary surveys in Australia indicate that many adults and children do not consume the recommended two servings of fruit and five servings of vegetables a day. The Australian and Victorian burden of disease studies reported that in 1996 approximately 10% of all cancers and 2.8% of the total burden of disease were attributable to insufficient intake of fruit and vegetables.

As part of a larger cost-effectiveness study of cancer control interventions, a national campaign to promote the intake of fruit and was analysed vegetables. The "2 Fruit 'n' 5 Veg" campaigns undertaken in Western Australia and Victoria used multiple strategies, including short, intensive mass media advertising and community-based consumer education through health facilities, food retailers and food service providers. Evaluation before and after the campaign showed that men improved their intake of fruits and vegetables by 11% and women by 6%. Full details of the methods are available from the authors on request.

The results of this analysis show that, while there is considerable uncertainty about the impact of a national campaign, it could avert between 6 and 230 deaths and save between 90 and 3700 DALYs. Campaign costs were estimated to be from just under US$ 1 million to US$ 1.8 million. The cost-effectiveness ratio for such a campaign lies between US$ 280 and US$ 9000 per DALY. If cost offsets (health service costs averted for prevented disease) are included – estimated at US$ 8.2 million – the intervention is "dominant", that is, health benefits are obtained at a net cost saving.

The favourable cost-effectiveness ratio of a fruit and vegetable campaign is similar to that estimated for national campaigns against tobacco use and skin cancer.

Sources: *(45–55)*.

in the overall strategy as new technologies and new information have become available and the epidemic has evolved. This process continues. The information presented in this section is designed to assist by providing information on the effectiveness and costs of selected preventive and curative interventions to reduce the health burden associated with unsafe sex. Although the consequences of unsafe sex can reduce population health in a number of ways, including through increased incidence of a range of sexually transmitted infections and unwanted pregnancies, this section focuses on HIV/AIDS as the leading cause of burden related to unsafe sex.

Many of the interventions that have been evaluated in the published literature, (for example, *(57)*, are really combinations of different types of health actions. For example, the effectiveness and cost data used to evaluate an intervention described as **voluntary counselling and testing (VCT)** were taken from a series of studies which described not only different mixtures of activities but also focused on different groups in the community. Some worked with female sex workers, and some also interacted with their clients. Some involved providing VCT to serodiscordant couples, others to pregnant women and yet others to people with other sexually transmitted infections. Many of these interventions also included health education and condom distribution. The estimates of effectiveness and costs for an intervention described as **outreach peer education programmes for commercial sex workers and their clients** were based on studies of activities that included many of the same components described for VCT above, to the extent that it is difficult to identify from the published literature what were the key components that made the intervention work.

Understanding the contribution of the different components would be very useful in deciding on the appropriate overall strategy. This analysis tries to contribute to this understanding by evaluating a set of individual interventions separately, and then considering their impact when undertaken together. The descriptions used below follow as closely as possible the way the interventions were undertaken in the studies from which effectiveness estimates can be derived.

At the same time, it is recognized that it is not possible to separate totally the impact of the different types of health actions which can be taken to reduce the burden associated with unsafe sexual practices. Encouraging sex workers to use condoms will have an effect on transmission only if clients can also be persuaded to use condoms. The interventions interact and the success of one requires the presence of the other. Similarly, the availability of condoms is a prerequisite for this and other preventive interventions. For this reason the report focuses less on the individual interventions in the discussion of the results, and more on the overall strategy which combines interventions.

In this regard, a separate intervention called **social marketing of condoms** is not evaluated, partly because no study was found which evaluated this activity for the prevention of HIV infections in isolation from other activities, and partly because the availability of condoms and people's willingness to use them are prerequisites for a number of other interventions. For that reason, condom distribution and the encouragement to use them have been incorporated into other interventions as appropriate. There may be various strategies for promoting access to and use of condoms, of which social marketing is only one.

A number of other interventions that are commonly undertaken or advocated have not been evaluated either. They include post-exposure prophylaxis, peer outreach for young people, and free-standing facilities for voluntary counselling and testing. In addition, the interventions that have been evaluated could be organized in various ways. The report has chosen one (or in some cases, several) specific options to enable the calculation of costs and outcomes, but the results could differ for other possible variations. The purpose of this exercise is not, therefore, to define rigidly the best combination of interventions in each setting. It is to provide valuable information on the effectiveness and costs of selected interventions and to show how this type of information can contribute to the continual reassessment of strategies to fight HIV/AIDS.

Interventions are not evaluated for the regions where injecting drug use plays an important role in transmission, limiting the analysis to the areas where unsafe sex is the dominant concern. EUR-B, EUR-C, WPR-B and the EMR subregions are not included in the discussion. The following interventions are evaluated singly and in combination.

Population-wide mass media using the combination of television, radio and print. This includes television and radio episodes as well as inserts in key newspapers during each year of intervention, with the intervention repeated every year. Development and administration costs to run the programme are included. Effectiveness depends on the coverage of the intervention, which is approximated by the proportion of the population reporting weekly access to any of the three types of media, based on national sample surveys from countries in each subregion *(58)*.

Voluntary counselling and testing (VTC) *(59)* in primary care clinics for anyone who wishes to use the services. Training of health workers is included. Testing is assumed to be based on a rapid test, to increase the proportion of individuals who receive their test results compared with standard assays. The proportion of the population using VCT where it has been made available has varied considerably across regions. In the Rakai study in Uganda *(60)*, approximately one-third of the population requested to be tested when VCT facilities were provided, and this proportion was similar in individuals positive and negative for HIV. Overall, this proportion was approximately twice the overall prevalence level in the population. In the United States, on the other hand, the proportion tested was nearly 45 times the prevalence level, with the probability of being tested among people with known HIV risk factors 2.3 times higher than in other people *(61)*.

Based on this, the assumed coverage of the intervention varied according to the average level of prevalence in each region. For A subregions, it was assumed that the total number tested over a five-year period would equal 45 times the average annual prevalence and that HIV-positive individuals would be 2.3 times as likely to be tested as HIV-negative individuals. For all other regions, the number tested over a five-year period equalled twice the average annual prevalence in each region.

School-based AIDS education targeted at youths aged 10–18 years. School-based education offers the opportunity to prime behaviour rather than seek to change it subsequently. The main effects would be to encourage a delayed age of sexual debut, a higher rate of condom use than in previous generations and a lower number of sex partners *(62)*. A scenario was evaluated where HIV education was provided during regular lessons to all enrolled students. Selected teachers are trained at each school and three different levels of geographical coverage were examined: 50%, 80% and 95% *(63)*.

Interventions for sex workers. Two versions were evaluated. The first involves initial training of selected sex workers so that they are then equipped to interact with their peers. Initial training is undertaken by social workers. In addition to outreach by peers, condoms are made available *(64)*. The second variation builds referral of sex workers for testing and possible treatment of sexually transmitted infections on top of the peer education and condom distribution *(65)*. Effectiveness estimates for the first version utilized results from Ngugi et al. *(64)* and Morisky et al. *(66)* among others; for the second, expanded version Njagi et al. *(67)* and Steen et al. *(68)* served as sources.

Peer outreach for men who have sex with men. Similar to the intervention for sex workers, this involves initial training of selected men to equip them to interact with their peers. This is only evaluated for A subregions, where men who have sex with men are an important cause of transmission and there is reasonable information on behaviours. Initial training is undertaken by social workers. In addition to outreach by peers, condoms are made available. Effectiveness estimates are based on Kahn et al. *(69)*, Mota et al. *(70)* and Haque et al. *(71)*.

Treatment of sexually transmitted infections (STI). The intervention evaluated here is provided in primary care facilities, available to anyone who requests it. Treatment involves not just the visits to a provider and drugs, but some counselling, advice on protection and condom distribution if requested. The mode of diagnosing these infections differs in developing and industrialized countries. Few tests are undertaken in C, D, and E subregions, and symptoms and signs are treated syndromically. In other regions, tests are usually conducted to identify the form of infection. This intervention was evaluated at two or three coverage levels depending on the region: current coverage levels, coverage at the level observed for antenatal care if antenatal care coverage exceeds current STI treatment coverage, and at 95% coverage. It is assumed that the current access to treatment is higher than the actual number treated (i.e., that not all patients with access will seek treatment), and that the same ratio of treatment-seeking to overall access would apply in the expanded coverage scenarios.

Maternal to Child Transmission (MTCT). Women seeking antenatal care are provided with information on the benefit and risks of using nevirapine for the prophylaxis of infection in their infant and are offered pre-test counselling. Women consenting for HIV-1 testing are also offered individual post-test counselling. HIV-positive women who accept prophylaxis are provided with a single dose of nevirapine for use at the onset of labour. If delivery is in a health care facility, a dose of nevirapine is given to the child, based on its weight. Where delivery does not take place in a health facility, the mother is requested to return to the antenatal clinic within 72 hours of delivery to be given a dose of nevirapine. Costs are based on each stage, and effectiveness takes into account not just the efficacy of the intervention but variations in likely acceptance and adherence across settings.[7] In A subregions, the costs include treatment with zidovudine, caesarean section delivery and infant food formulas.

Antiretroviral therapy (ARV) has also been evaluated. Although it is not an intervention designed to reduce the risks associated with unsafe sex behaviours, its role in poor countries is the source of much debate and discussion. Accurate estimates of potential coverage cannot be known at this early stage of scaling-up antiretroviral use, so it was assumed that health systems should be able to reach eventually the same proportion of the population with ARVs as they currently reach with antenatal care services.

Four different ARV interventions for people identified to have clinical AIDS are defined along two dimensions: (a) standard treatment vs standard treatment with more intensive monitoring of medication; (b) use of first-line drugs alone vs first- and second-line drugs where the latter are clinically necessary. The combinations range from standard treatment without second-line drugs to treatment with intensive monitoring and the option of second-line drugs. Standard treatment without second-line drugs may be undesirable for many reasons, but at the other extreme, the intensive monitoring option evaluated here incorporates more frequent monitoring than might be necessary or possible in some settings. The exact strategy chosen is likely to lie somewhere between the two extremes.

---

[7] Based on the information provided by the HIV/AIDS Department of WHO.

locations, high taxes on tobacco products, and health education and smoking cessation programmes have had considerable success *(76)*. Governments interested in choosing the best mix of interventions for their circumstances will focus on the cultural relevance of interventions, their resulting effects on population health, and costs.

Taxation. Tobacco taxes are generally established and collected by ministries other than the Ministry of Health, and in federal systems (such as the United States) they may be collected at more than one level of government (federal, state, county or city). The most common form of tobacco taxation is excise taxes on cigarettes.

Taxation increases the price to the consumer of tobacco products, leading to a decrease in consumption. At the same time, government tax revenues increase. Sometimes a portion of revenues from tobacco taxes is allocated to the health sector to promote health and discourage smoking behaviors. This in turn can help to make other types of tobacco control efforts both more effective and self-financing. This is particularly important to developing countries where resources to finance new public health initiatives are often very limited.

The effect of price changes on consumption is estimated from information about price elasticities of demand for tobacco products (the percentage change in consumption resulting from a 1% price increase). For every 10% real rise in price due to tobacco taxes, tobacco consumption generally falls by between 2% and 10% *(77)*. Studies suggest that the decrease is relatively larger for young smokers, for smokers with low incomes, and possibly for women. Regional price elasticities were estimated from a regression analysis of the relationship between the price elasticities observed in countries where studies had been undertaken and GDP per capita (in international dollars), with adjustments for differences in the age and sex structure of smokers.

Currently taxes on tobacco products account for approximately 44% of the final retail price of tobacco products, which translates to a 79% mark-up on the pre-tax price. This is a global average based on estimated regional data *(78)*. In the region with the highest rate of taxation, almost 75% of the final retail price consists of taxes (a mark-up on the pre-tax price of approximately 300%). Accordingly, this analysis evaluates three levels of taxation – the current average level (a 79% mark-up), the current maximum (a mark-up of 300%) and double the current maximum (a mark-up of 600% translating to a situation where taxes account for 89% of the final retail price).[8]

Since a majority of countries employ some combination of specific excise tax (based on quantity) and ad valorem taxes (based on value), a 50–50 split between the two forms is assumed; also, that the specific tax is not changed after the first year, so the real value of the price increase declines with inflation over time. In the last scenario (600% mark-up), it is not possible to know the price elasticity of demand because such rates of tax have been implemented in a few countries, so the elasticities observed at the current level of taxation are assumed to apply also at the higher rate.

Clean indoor air laws in public places, through legislation and enforcement. Laws banning smoking in indoor places were initially enacted as measures of fire prevention or as a means of ensuring food hygiene. Over time, legislation has increasingly acknowledged the strong evidence about the harmful effect of passive smoking, more commonly referred to as second-hand tobacco smoke.

---

[8] Because of the oligopolistic structure of the tobacco industry in most countries, price changes of tobacco products may at least match or most likely exceed the tax increase. To avoid the overestimation of the effectiveness of interventions, it is assumed that tax incidence is entirely borne by the consumers. It is also assumed that smuggling increases proportionally to the price changes.

Laws that control smoking in public places can protect non-smokers from the danger of passive smoking, but also encourage smokers to quit or reduce tobacco consumption *(79)*. Clean air laws that are strong and comprehensive can lead to a significant reduction in tobacco consumption. In addition, the posting of signs to indicate smoking and non-smoking areas tends to help prevent violations of the law.

Comprehensive bans on advertising of tobacco products through legislation. In countries where tobacco advertising is permitted, tobacco companies make advertising and promotion their single largest item of expenditure – often exceeding the amount spent on the purchase of the raw material, tobacco leaf. Large sums of money are also spent sponsoring sports and cultural events. This form of advertising generally associates tobacco with healthy and pleasurable activities and reaches wide audiences, many of them children and youth.

One of the principal arguments for enacting a ban on tobacco advertising is that it keeps young people free of pressures to commence smoking. Legislation to ban comprehensively tobacco advertising prohibits tobacco advertising in print, broadcasting, other mass media and billboards and at the point-of-purchase *(80)*. It also includes a ban on the tobacco industry's sponsorship of sports and other cultural events. A total ban on tobacco advertising also outlaws the distribution of free tobacco product samples as well as the distribution of items displaying tobacco company logos or trademarks such as T-shirts. This type of comprehensive intervention, evaluated here, can reduce tobacco consumption, while a more limited advertising ban has little or no effect *(81)*. Consequently, Australia, Canada, Finland, New Zealand, South Africa, Sweden and Thailand, to name a few, have enacted legal bans on tobacco advertising and promotion.

Information dissemination through health warning labels, counter-advertising, and various consumer information packages. Even in the most developed countries, the risks of tobacco use and the benefits of quitting are not fully appreciated by all segments of the population. Public health advocates argue that large numbers of individuals are not equipped to make fully informed decisions about their health particularly in relation to addictive substances. Accordingly, efforts are needed on the part of the government, media and the health sector to ensure that constant and continual anti-smoking messages are brought to the attention of the public, particularly young people in the regions where baseline levels of awareness are low.

The dissemination of health information often involves one or more of the following: (1) the provision of health education to the general public on the dangers of smoking and how to quit; (2) health education about the risks of tobacco use in schools; and (3) specific education for high-risk individuals. Information dissemination is also often referred to in the literature as health promotion or counter-advertising. Many different forms of information dissemination exist including: media advocacy, paid media advertising, community-based health promotion, school-based health education, and the issuance of noticeable health warning labels on tobacco products and tobacco advertisements. Experience with innovative graphic health warning labels such as those found in Brazil or Canada is as yet too limited to allow its inclusion, although early reports show that they are effective at discouraging smoking.

Here we evaluate an information dissemination package which has been shown to be effective to reduce tobacco consumption *(82)* and consists of: (1) special health information interventions (including issuance of health warning labels, mass media counter-advertising/anti-smoking campaigns, and public debates about anti-smoking legislation); and (2) health information shocks that capture various forms of anti-smoking publicity, including health reports published by large institutions (specifically, the 1964 US Surgeon General's Report and Reports from the American Cancer Society) as well as professional health publications that associate smoking with mortality.

Nicotine replacement therapy (NRT) targeted at all current smokers aged 20–60 years. Nicotine dependence is a critical barrier to successful smoking cessation. As a result, policy interventions to control smoking often aim to strengthen a smoker's motivation to quit (for example, increased health education, price policies and smoke-free policies) as well as reduce dependence-type barriers that stand in the way of quitting (for example, through pharmacological and behavioural treatments).

NRT includes pharmacological aids used to help smokers in their quest to stop smoking. NRT includes transdermal patches (commonly referred to as nicotine patches), nicotine chewing gum, nicotine nasal sprays, lozenges, aerosol inhalers and some classes of antidepressants, including biuproprion. Brief advice from a health provider coupled with NRT has been associated with sustained levels of smoking cessation in 6% of all smokers seeking to quit. This is sizably larger than the 1–2% per year who quit without any advice *(76)*.

To achieve successful and large-scale cessation rates, the introduction of NRT into a society is probably not sufficient by itself. When deciding to introduce NRT into a country's tobacco control policy, policy-makers need to ensure that health professionals (including doctors, nurses and pharmacists) have appropriate training so that they are confident and capable of providing advice and treatment to tobacco-dependent patients. Such costs were also included for the evaluation of the NRT intervention.

Results

The benefits of anti-smoking interventions for population health (in terms of DALYs) are estimated through the impact of reduced smoking on the incidence of cardiovascular disease, respiratory disease, and various forms of cancer. The interventions, not surprisingly, have a larger impact on population health in regions with a high prevalence of tobacco use, especially those in the second or third stage of the tobacco epidemic (for example, AMR-B, AMR-D, EUR-B, EUR-C, SEAR-B, SEAR-D and WPR-B).[9] Their cost-effectiveness also varies across regions, not only because of variations in exposure to tobacco but also differences in the efficiency of the tax collection system, the degree of anti-tobacco sentiment, and the amount of smuggling.

If only one intervention can be chosen, taxation is the intervention of choice in all regions. Not only does it have the greatest impact on population health, but it is also the most cost-effective option. Taxation also raises revenue for governments. For D and E subregions where price elasticities are generally high, taxation by itself could reduce tobacco consumption significantly. Higher rates of taxation achieve greater improvements in population health and are more cost-effective than lower rates. On purely health grounds, the higher the rate of taxation, the better.[10]

---

[9]   The second stage of the tobacco epidemic is characterized by rapidly increasing male smoking prevalence and gradually increasing female prevalence. In the third stage, male smoking prevalence reaches its peak and starts to decrease while female prevalence continues to increase *(76)*. The measure of tobacco exposure used here is the smoking impact ratio (SIR) defined in Chapter 4, and the effectiveness of each intervention was assessed by the changes of SIR as a function of the past tobacco consumption.

[10] It should be remembered that it is not possible to be certain how such levels would affect demand for and supply of tobacco products, although there are a few current examples of taxes involving a mark-up of around 600% on the pre-tax price. It should be also noted that the appropriate size of tax depends on various social factors.

To achieve even greater improvements in population health, the combination of taxation, comprehensive bans on advertising, and information dissemination activities would be affordable and cost-effective in the majority of subregions. Adding restrictions of smoking in public places increases the costs, but also gains even greater improvements in population health and is still very cost- effective in A, B and C subregions.

NRT by itself is not in the most cost-effective band of interventions, but does not fall outside the cut-off point of three times GDP per capita in many regions. When added to the other interventions as part of a comprehensive package, it certainly increases the costs of the package, but improves effectiveness as well. Although the additional cost of adding NRT to anti-smoking activities would be considerable, the additional expense would be justified on purely cost-effectiveness grounds in A, B and C subregions (with the exception of WPR-B).

ENVIRONMENTAL RISKS

UNSAFE WATER, SANITATION, AND HYGIENE

Interventions

Millennium development goals. The first intervention relates to the costs and effects of reaching the millennium development goal of halving the number of people with no access to safe water, giving preference to those who already have improved sanitation. To accomplish this, the choice of technology depends on a number of environmental factors and the cost, but the possibilities include public stand posts, bore holes, protected springs or wells, and collected rainwater. This does not mean that the new source of water is totally safe, but that some measures are taken to protect it from contamination.

A variation of this strategy is also considered: to halve the number of people without access to improved water *and* basic sanitation, using the same technologies for improving water described above. Low-cost technologies for provision of basic sanitation do not involve treatment of wastewater, and include septic tanks, simple pit latrines, and ventilated improved pit-latrines.

The cost-effectiveness of improving the current situation was evaluated. The current state of water and sanitation infrastructure in the different regions, determined largely by social and economic development in the past, was taken as the starting point from which interventions should be evaluated, just as the current state of education of the population helped to define the starting point for all interventions. For that reason it is not possible to evaluate interventions routinely at 50%, 80% and 95% coverage – coverage is already above that level in many settings. Accordingly, the costs and effectiveness of moving from the current level to 98% were routinely evaluated.

Disinfection at point of use. This involves using chlorine and safe storage vessels for people without current access to improved drinking sources. It also includes limited hygiene education. As opposed to the other interventions in this section, disinfection at point of use can be considered strictly as a health action – it is designed purely to improve health and is usually undertaken by the health sector.

Improved water supply and sanitation, low technologies. This provides the same type of water supply and basic sanitation improvements as described for the millennium development goals above but at a higher level of coverage.

Improved water supply and sanitation, with disinfection at point of use. This strategy adds disinfection at point of use to the low-technology strategy described above.

Improved water supply and sanitation, high technologies. The costs and effectiveness of using high technologies are also evaluated at the maximum possible level of coverage (98%). This involves provision of piped water to houses, with treatment to remove pathogens, quality monitoring and pollution control as well as sewage connection with partial treatment of wastewater.

Results

The interventions were not evaluated in EUR-A and AMR-A where virtually all people currently have access to safe water and basic sanitation. In the other areas, the main outcome evaluated was the reduction in the incidence and deaths from diarrhoeal disease. If improved water supply and basic sanitation were extended to everyone, 1.8 billion cases of diarrhoea (a 17% reduction of the current number of cases) would be prevented annually. If universal piped and regulated water supply was achieved, 7.6 billion cases of diarrhoea (69.5% reduction) would be prevented annually.

The millennium declaration goals specify access to safe drinking-water ("to halve, by the year 2015, the proportion of people who are unable to reach or to afford safe drinking-water"). This strategy would be the least costly to implement in each region, at a global cost of approximately I\$ 37.5 billion over 10 years. The gain is estimated to be approximately 30 million DALYs worldwide. Achieving universal access (evaluated at 98% coverage) of improved water supply and basic sanitation plus disinfection at point of use would result in an additional 553 million DALYs gained though at an additional cost of I\$ 449 billion. Each unit of additional health gains would cost of more than three times GDP per capita in some subregions.

The intervention which is consistently the most cost-effective across regions and would be classified as very cost-effective in all areas where it was evaluated was the provision of disinfection capacity at point of use. On purely cost-effectiveness grounds it would be the first choice where resources are scarce. Adding basic low technology water and sanitation to this option would also be either very cost-effective or cost-effective in most settings. It is likely that interventions targeting key behaviours such as improving hand washing practices would also provide considerable health benefits and prove to be cost-effective. As yet, moving to the ideal of piped water supply and sewage could not be considered a cost-effective means of improving health in poor areas of the world.

However, the principal driver for improvements to water supplies, apart from disinfection at point of use, is not health but economic development and convenience. These benefits may be tangible (time saved) or intangible (convenience, well-being). For example, Table 5.2 suggests that there would be a substantial benefits in terms of convenience involved in providing the interventions in this group in AFR-D and EMR-D. This might well be reflected in gains in economic output.

The great majority of costs also falls outside the health sector and is shared by diverse groups (gov-

Table 5.2 Time gains from improved access to water and sanitation in subregions AFR-D and EMR-D[a]

Potential outcomes achieved by:	Time gains by subregions (hours per year per capita)	
	AFR-D	EMR-D
halving the population without access to safe water	5.9	2.0
halving the population without access to safe water and by improving sanitation	44.1	19.4
disinfecting at point of use for water	88.2	38.8
improving sanitation (low technologies) + disinfection	88.2	38.8
increasing piped water systems and sewer connections	144.6	96.0

[a] See the List of Member States by WHO Region and mortality stratum for an explanation of subregions.

ernment, private sector, donors, nongovernmental organizations, communities and consumers). While it is possible to capture all the costs in a cost-effectiveness ratio, only health benefits have been included in these calculations. This certainly understates the benefits to society of improving water and sanitation. In addition, the cost-effectiveness ratios estimated for these interventions are based on conservative estimates of the health gains. Some possible longer-term benefits of preventing cases of diarrhoea, such as improved nutritional status, are not captured fully in an analysis focusing on the acute effects. Moreover, there will be benefits in different settings in terms of other health outcomes such as trachoma, schistosomiasis, and infectious hepatitis. The results for water and sanitation need to be interpreted in this light.

The burden of disease associated with unsafe water supply, sanitation and hygiene is concentrated in children in developing countries. Accordingly, emphasis should be placed on interventions likely to yield accelerated and affordable health gains in this group. Disinfection at point of use is an attractive option. The intervention has a large health impact in regions of high child mortality and the costs are relatively low. A policy shift to encourage better household water quality management using this technology (and probably better hygiene, although it was not analysed here), placing greater emphasis on achieving health gains associated with drinking-water access at the household level, would appear to be the most cost-effective water-related health intervention in many developing countries. This would complement the continuing expansion of coverage and upgrading of piped water and sewage services, which is naturally a long-term aim of most developing nations.

OCCUPATIONAL RISK FACTORS

Occupational risks have not been fully evaluated, but some information about intervention to reduce the burden associated with motor vehicle accidents is included in Box 5.4 and Box 5.5 summarizes the effectiveness and costs of various interventions to reduce the incidence of back pain associated with occupational ergonomic stressors. In that case, calculations are presented for three different types of settings, two with low mortality and one with high mortality (AMR-A, EUR-B, and SEAR-D).

Box 5.4 Reducing injuries from motor vehicle accidents

An estimated 1.2 million people died from road traffic injuries in 1998, raising such injuries to the rank of tenth leading cause of death worldwide. By 2020, they are expected to be the second leading cause of death. Interventions to reduce road traffic injuries are increasingly commonplace in industrialized countries, but little evidence is available from developing countries. WHO has recently commissioned a review of published and unpublished data sources and has critically examined the economic impact of interventions to prevent road traffic injuries and their potential applicability to developing countries.

The limited number of economic evaluations of interventions have used cost-benefit analysis where the outcome has been the assumed economic value of extending life and preventing accidents. One study of motorcycle helmet laws in the United States suggested that reduced costs of treating injuries exceeded the costs of introducing and policing the law by US$ 22.7 million. Motor vehicle inspection laws and the mandatory use of headlamps in daytime also reduced the subsequent costs of treating injuries, and the savings could also be substantially higher than the costs of introducing and administering the laws.

The installation of seat belts showed a net reduction in the costs of treatment by US$ 162 per vehicle, while seat belt regulations were found to be very cost-effective – costing just US$ 1406 per life saved. Although several economic evaluations of speed limits have been carried out, mostly in the United States, there is no clear consensus about the relative economic benefits of different speed limits. Speed bumps, deviations and other devices to calm traffic are used in many countries, but there have been very few comprehensive economic evaluations.

Only one of the studies reviewed focused on the developing world. As 90% of the world's population live in low and middle income countries, where the rates of road traffic injuries and fatalities are highest, it is essential for this major research gap in health information to be filled.

Sources: *(83–89)*.

HEALTH PRACTICES

UNSAFE HEALTH CARE INJECTIONS

Interventions

Decreased reuse of injection equipment without sterilization. This consists of the provision of new, single use injection equipment. This intervention included safe collection and management of sharps waste.

Decreased unnecessary use of injections. This consists of interactive, patient–provider group discussions.

The impact of these interventions singly and combined was assessed in terms of their potential impact on the incidence of HIV, hepatitis B and hepatitis C. Start-up activities

---

Box 5.5 Cost-effectiveness of interventions to reduce occupational back pain

The problem of back pain related to ergonomic stressors at work is widespread in highly industrialized and developing countries alike. Despite its prevalence and the toll it exacts from workers and their families with the concomitant economic losses, cost-effective interventions are available. Interventions for the prevention of back pain fall into three major categories: training of workers to raise their awareness of risks and improve their handling of hazardous jobs; engineering control, that is, physical measures that control exposure to the hazard, including equipment that assists with lifting, pushing and pulling; and a full ergonomics programme that includes both of these interventions together with further implementation procedures related to workplace organization and design.

Although there is considerable scientific uncertainty about the exact level of effectiveness of interventions on occupational ergonomic stressors, estimates obtained from several observational studies demonstrate that the largest improvement in population health – a 74% reduction in back-pain incidence – would be obtained from the full ergonomics programme. Lower benefits at the population level would be achieved by the other interventions: a 60% reduction by engineering control and training together, a 56% reduction by engineering control alone, and a 20% reduction by training alone.

The total costs of the worker training intervention are significantly lower than those of the full ergonomics programme. In the three subregions for which estimates are available (AMR-A, EUR-B

and SEAR-D), training is the most cost-effective option. It should be the first choice where resources are scarce. The costs of training are largely related to labour, the costs of engineering control are primarily capital expenditure, and the costs of a full ergonomics programme are equally related to both. As wage costs differ widely, the total costs of the interventions vary substantially across the subregions. Nevertheless, analysis suggests that full ergonomics programmes are cost-effective in the three subregions for their health effects alone, without allowing for the possible increase in productivity brought about by the interventions.

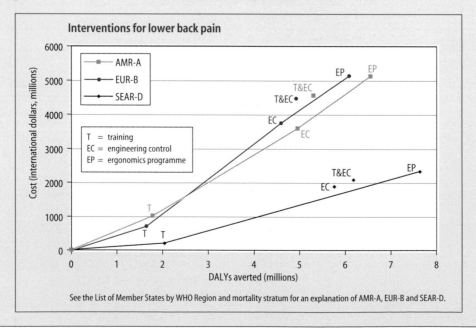

Interventions for lower back pain

T = training
EC = engineering control
EP = ergonomics programme

See the List of Member States by WHO Region and mortality stratum for an explanation of AMR-A, EUR-B and SEAR-D.

include a national planning workshop, the development and production of information, education and communication material, a workshop for the training of the trainers, the training of the procurement officer, and district planning workshops. The post-start-up activities included the supply of injection equipment, annual national follow-up work-shops, interactional group discussions between patients and health care providers, and annual monitoring surveys.

Results

These interventions were not evaluated in the low mortality subregions where the bur-den from unsafe injections is not significant (all A subregions). In the other mortality strata, reducing unnecessary use of injections will have a lower total impact on population health than reducing reuse of injection equipment without sterilization. The effect of doing both at the same time is less than additive, although doing both together does improve population health to a greater extent than doing simply one.

In approximately half the subregions (AMR-B, AMR-D, EUR-B and EUR-C), reducing reuse is also the most cost-effective option and it would be done as the first choice in the presence of severe resource constraints. However, in the other subregions (AFR-D, AFR-E, EMR-D, SEAR-B, SEAR-D and WPR-B), behavioural interventions to reduce overuse are more cost-effective than interventions to reduce reuse that require large quantities of injec-tion equipment. They would be done first if resources were scarce. In the event of additional resources being available, the combined intervention would be undertaken. In all cases, moving from the most cost-effective option to the combination has a cost-effectiveness ratio well below the cut-off point of three times GDP per capita.

COMBINING RISK REDUCTION STRATEGIES

The previous section reviewed the effectiveness, costs and cost-effectiveness of a series of interventions aimed at reducing specific risks to health. That analysis allows decision-makers with an interest in reducing the burden related to a specific cause – for example, cardiovascular disease or child undernutrition – to assess what types of interventions would be cost-effective in that area for the resources that are available. This section takes the broader perspective of a government as the steward of the entire health system. As argued earlier, one of the intrinsic goals of a health system is to improve population health, and information about how best to achieve this for the available resources is of vital importance. This requires not only deciding which combinations of interventions are cost-effective ways of reducing the risks associated with unsafe sex, for example, but also deciding which of the myriad of risks to health that could be targeted should be given priority.

The information considered in the previous section is used again to illustrate how cost-effectiveness analysis can make an important contribution to this debate. Figures 5.2 and 5.3 report the results for interventions considered in the previous section, for two of the 14 subregions, AFR-D and AMR-B.[11] Interventions that are both more costly and less effec-tive than alternative ways of achieving the same goal (for example, reducing the impact of unsafe sex) are not shown on the graphs so that the more cost-effective interventions can be identified more easily. That is why most of the interventions that are shown appear to be cost-effective. (The key to the interventions is found in Table 5.3.) The vertical axis depicts

---

[11] Full results for all interventions in all regions are found on the WHO web site: www.who.int/evidence

Figure 5.2. Cost and effects of selected interventions in subregion AFR-D

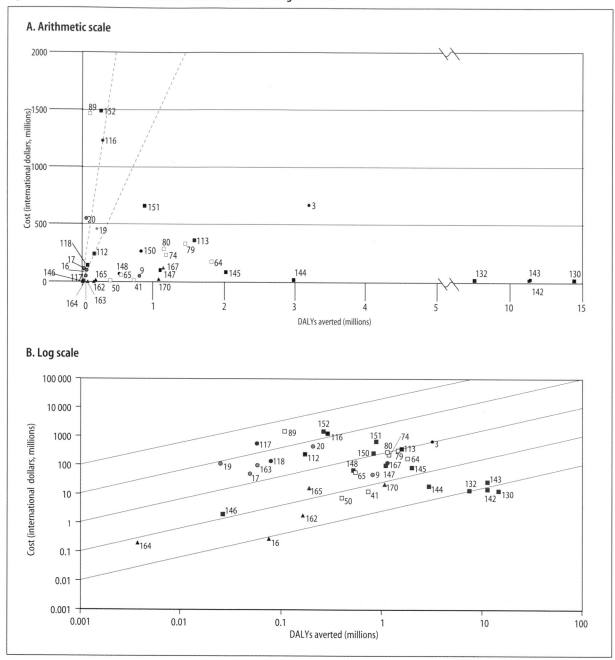

Figure 5.2. Cost and effects of selected interventions in subregion AFR-D

C. Legend

See the List of Member States by WHO Region and mortality stratum for an explanation of subregion AFR-D.
See Table 5.3 for a complete list of interventions.
For water and sanitation, only interventions considered to be purely health interventions are included.

Number	Legend	Description
		Unsafe water, sanitation and hygiene
3	●	Disinfection at point of use for population without improved water sources
		Addictive substances: Tobacco
9	◓	Doubling the maximum tax (2TAX)
16	◓	2TAX, Comprehensive ban (BAN) on advertising and Information dissemination (INF) through health warning labels, counter-advertising, and various consumer information packages
17	◓	2 TAX and BAN
19	◓	2TAX, Clean indoor air laws (LAW), BAN and INF
20	◓	2TAX, LAW, BAN, INF and Nicotine replacement therapy (NRT)
		Childhood undernutrition
41	□	Vitamin A fortification (VAF) of staple food, 95% coverage
50	□	VAF and Zinc fortification (ZF) of staple food, 95% coverage
64	□	VAF, ZF and Case management for childhood pneumonia (CM)), 80% coverage
65	□	VAF, ZF and Case management for childhood pneumonia (CM), 95% coverage
74	□	Vitamin A supplementation for all children aged 6 months to 5 years (VAS5), Zinc supplementation daily for all children 0–5 years of age (ZS5) and CM, 95% coverage
79	□	VAS5, ZS5, Oral rehydration therapy for diarrhoea (ORT) and CM, 80% coverage
80	□	VAS5, ZS5, ORT and CM, 95% coverage
89	□	VAS5, ZS5 , Improve complementary feeding through nutrition counselling and provision of nutrient-dense food for all underweight children aged 6–12 months identified through growth monitoring and promotion (CFGM), ORT and CM, 95% coverage
		Other nutrition-related risk factors and physical inactivity
112	■	Treatment with triple therapy (TRI) of hypertension-lowering drug (beta-blocker), statins and aspirin for individuals with absolute risk of cardiovascular event of 25% in 10 years
113	■	TRI with risk of 35% in 10 years
116	■	Legislation (LEG) to decrease salt content of processed foods, plus appropriate labelling and enforcement, Health education (HE) through mass media to reduce cholesterol and TRI with risk of 5% in 10 years
117	■	LEG, HE and TRI with risk of 15% in 10 years
118	■	LEG, HE and TRI with risk of 25% in 10 years
		Sexual and reproductive health
130	■	Mass media (MED), 100% coverage
132	■	Treatment of sexually transmitted infections (STI), enhanced coverage
142	■	Educating sex workers (EDS) and MED
143	■	EDS, MED and STI enhanced coverage
144	■	EDS, MED and STI, 95% coverage
145	■	EDS, MED, STI and School-based education (SBE) 50% coverage
146	■	EDS+STI, MED, STI 95% coverage and SBE 50% coverage
147	■	EDS+STI, MED, STI 95% coverage and SBE 80% coverage
148	■	EDS+STI, MED, STI 95% coverage and SBE 95% coverage
150	■	EDS+STI, MED, STI 95 % coverage, SBE 95% coverage, Voluntary counselling and testing (VCT) and Preventing mother-to-child transmission (MTCT)
151	■	Antiretroviral therapy: intensive monitoring, first-line drugs only (ARV2), EDS + STI, MED, STI 95% coverage, SBE 95% coverage, VCT and MTCT
152	■	Antiretroviral therapy: intensive monitoring, first- and second-line drugs (ARV4), EDS +STI, MED, STI 95% coverage, SBE 95% coverage, VCT and MTCT
		Unsafe injections
162	▲	Reduction in overuse of injections through interactive patient--provider group discussions (GD)
163	▲	Reduction in unsafe use of injections with single use injection equipment (SUI)
164	▲	GD and SUI
		Iron deficiency
165	▲	Iron supplementation (IS), 50% coverage
167	▲	IS, 95% coverage
170	▲	Iron fortification (IF), 95% coverage

Table 5.3 Cost-effective interventions

Number	Description	Number	Description
	Unsafe water, sanitation and hygiene	40	VAF, 80% coverage
1	Millennium development goal (MDG): to halve the proportion of people with no access to improved water sources	41	VAF, 95% coverage
		42	Zinc fortification (ZF) of staple food, 50% coverage
2	MDG and basic sanitation	43	ZF, 80% coverage
3	Disinfection at point of use for population without improved water sources	44	ZF, 95% coverage
		45	ORT and CM, 50% coverage
4	MDG, 98% coverage	46	ORT and CM, 80% coverage
5	Improved water supply, disinfection and basic sanitation (low technologies), 98% coverage	47	ORT and CM, 95% coverage
		48	VAF and ZF, 50% coverage
6	Piped water supply and sewer connection (high technologies), 98% coverage	49	VAF and ZF, 80% coverage
		50	VAF and ZF, 95% coverage
	Addictive substances: Tobacco	51	ZF and CM, 50% coverage
7	Global average tax rate (44% of the final retail price with a mark-up of 79%)	52	ZF and CM, 80% coverage
		53	ZF and CM, 95% coverage
8	Highest regional tax rate (75% of the final retail price with a mark-up of 300%)	54	VAS5 and ZS5, 50% coverage
		55	VAS5 and ZS5, 80% coverage
9	Doubling the maximum tax (2TAX) (89% of the final retail price with a mark-up of 600%)	56	VAS5 and ZS5, 95% coverage
		57	Zinc supplementation daily for all children aged 0--2 years (ZS2) and ZF, 50% coverage
10	Clean indoor air laws (LAW) in public places, through legislation and enforcement	58	ZS2 and ZF, 80% coverage
		59	ZS2 and ZF, 95% coverage
11	Comprehensive ban (BAN) on advertising of tobacco products through legislation and enforcement	60	VAF, ZF and ORT, 50% coverage
		61	VAF, ZF and ORT, 80% coverage
12	Information dissemination (INF) through health warning labels, counter-advertising, and various consumer information packages	62	VAF, ZF and ORT, 95% coverage
		63	VAF, ZF and CM, 50% coverage
13	Nicotine replacement therapy (NRT): 20 mg/day treatment with nicotine gum for three months, plus regular visits to a GP or health centre (1 per month) and a nurse counsellor (1.5 per month)	64	VAF, ZF and CM, 80% coverage
		65	VAF, ZF and CM, 95% coverage
		66	ZF, ORT and CM, 50% coverage
14	2TAX and INF	67	ZF, ORT and CM, 80% coverage
15	2TAX, LAW and INF	68	ZF, ORT and CM, 95% coverage
16	2TAX, BAN and INF	69	ZS5, ORT and CM, 50% coverage
17	2TAX and BAN	70	ZS5, ORT and CM, 80% coverage
18	2TAX, LAW and BAN	71	ZS5, ORT and CM, 95% coverage
19	2TAX, LAW, BAN and INF	72	VAS5, ZS5 and CM, 50% coverage
20	2TAX, LAW, BAN, INF and NRT	73	VAS5, ZS5 and CM, 80% coverage
		74	VAS5, ZS5 and CM, 95% coverage
	Childhood undernutrition	75	VAS5, ZS5 and ORT, 50% coverage
21	Oral rehydration therapy for diarrhoea (ORT), 50% coverage	76	VAS5, ZS5 and ORT, 80% coverage
22	ORT, 80% coverage	77	VAS5, ZS5 and ORT, 95% coverage
23	ORT, 95% coverage	78	VAS5, ZS5, ORT and CM, 50% coverage
24	Case management for childhood pneumonia (CM), 50% coverage	79	VAS5, ZS5, ORT and CM, 80% coverage
25	CM, 80% coverage	80	VAS5, ZS5, ORT and CM, 95% coverage
26	CM, 95% coverage	81	VAF, ZF, ORT and CM, 50% coverage
27	Vitamin A supplementation for all children aged 6 months to 5 years (VAS5), twice a year at the health centre, 50% coverage	82	VAF, ZF, ORT and CM, 80% coverage
		83	VAF, ZF, ORT and CM, 95% coverage
28	VAS5, 80% coverage	84	VAS2, VAF, ZS2, and ZF, 50% coverage
29	VAS5, 95% coverage	85	VAS2, VAF, ZS2, and ZF, 80% coverage
30	Zinc supplementation daily for all children aged 0--5 years (ZS5), 50% coverage	86	VAS2, VAF, ZS2, and ZF, 95% coverage
31	ZS5, 80% coverage	87	VAS5, ZS5, CFGM, ORT and CM, 50% coverage
32	ZS5, 95% coverage	88	VAS5, ZS5, CFGM, ORT and CM, 80% coverage
33	Improved complementary feeding (CF) through nutrition counselling and provision of nutrient-dense food for all children aged 6--12 months, 50% coverage	89	VAS5, ZS5, CFGM, ORT and CM, 95% coverage
		90	VAF, ZF, CFGM, ORT and CM, 50% coverage
34	CF, 80% coverage	91	VAF, ZF, CFGM, ORT and CM, 80% coverage
35	CF, 95% coverage		
36	Improved complementary feeding through nutrition counselling and provision of nutrient-dense food for all underweight children aged 6--12 months identified through growth monitoring and promotion (CFGM), 50% coverage		
37	CFGM, 80% coverage		
38	CFGM, 95% coverage		
39	Vitamin A fortification (VAF) of staple food, 50% coverage		

Number	Description	Number	Description
92	VAF, ZF, CFGM, ORT and CM, 95% coverage	135	SBE, 80% coverage
93	VAS2, VAF, ZS2, ZF and CM, 50% coverage	136	SBE, 95% coverage
94	VAS2, VAF, ZS2, ZF and CM, 80% coverage	137	Voluntary counselling and testing (VCT), 95% coverage
95	VAS2, VAF, ZS2, ZF and CM, 95% coverage	138	Preventing mother-to-child transmission (MTCT), antenatal care coverage
96	VAS2, VAF, ZS2, ZF, ORT and CM, 50% coverage	139	Educating men who have sex with men (EDM), 50% coverage
97	VAS2, VAF, ZS2, ZF, ORT and CM, 80% coverage	140	EDM, 80% coverage
98	VAS2, VAF, ZS2, ZF, ORT and CM, 95% coverage	141	EDM, 95% coverage
99	VAS2, VAF, ZS2, ZF, CFGM, ORT and CM, 50% coverage	142	EDS and MED
100	VAS2, VAF, ZS2, ZF, CFGM, ORT and CM, 80% coverage	143	EDS, MED and STI enhanced coverage
101	VAS2, VAF, ZS2, ZF, CFGM, ORT and CM, 95% coverage	144	EDS, MED and STI 95% coverage
		145	EDS, MED, STI 95% coverage and SBE 50% coverage
	Other nutrition-related risk factors and physical inactivity	146	EDS+STI, MED, STI 95% coverage and SBE 50% coverage
102	Voluntary cooperation of food manufacturers with government to decrease salt in processed foods, plus appropriate labelling	147	EDS+STI, MED, STI 95% coverage and SBE 80% coverage
103	Legislation (LEG) to decrease salt content of processed foods, plus appropriate labelling and enforcement	148	EDS+STI, MED, STI 95% coverage and SBE 95% coverage
		149	EDS+STI, MED, STI 95% coverage, SBE 95% coverage and VCT
104	Health education (HE) through mass media to reduce cholesterol	150	EDS+STI, MED, STI 95% coverage, SBE 95% coverage, VCT and MTCT
105	Hypertension-lowering drug treatment (DRG) and education (ED) on lifestyle modification including dietary advice, delivered by physicians to individuals with systolic blood pressure (SBP) >160 mmHg.	151	ARV2, EDS+STI, MED, STI 95% coverage, SBE 95% coverage, VCT and MTCT
		152	ARV4, EDS+STI, MED, STI 95% coverage, SBE 95% coverage, VCT and MTCT
106	DRG and ED with SBP >140 mmHg	153	EDS and MED
107	Cholesterol-lowering drug treatment (statins) and education (ED) on lifestyle modification including dietary advice, delivered by physicians to individuals whose serum cholesterol concentration (CHOL) exceeds 220 mg/dl (5.7 mmol/l)	154	EDS, MED and STI 95% coverage
		155	EDS+STI, MED and STI 95% coverage
		156	EDS+STI, MED, STI 95% coverage and SBE 80% coverage
108	Statins and ED with CHOL >240 mg/dl (>6.2 mmol/l)	157	EDS+STI, MED, STI 95% coverage and SBE 95% coverage
109	Nicotine replacement therapy (NRT) with medical advice and counselling, provided by physicians and outpatient carers to all smokers in the population	158	ARV1, EDS+STI, MED, STI 95% coverage and SBE 95% coverage
		159	ARV2, EDS+STI, MED, STI 95% coverage and SBE 95% coverage
110	Treatment with triple therapy (TRI) of hypertension-lowering drug (beta-blocker), statins and aspirin for individuals with absolute risk of cardiovascular event of 5% in 10 years	160	ARV2, EDS+STI, MED, STI 95% coverage, SBE 95% coverage and MTCT
		161	ARV4, EDS+STI, MED, STI 95% coverage, SBE 95% coverage and MTCT
111	TRI with risk of 15% in 10 years		**Unsafe injections**
112	TRI with risk of 25% in 10 years	162	Reduction in overuse of injections through interactive patient--provider group discussions (GD)
113	TRI with risk of 35% in 10 years		
114	LEG and HE	163	Reduction in unsafe use of injections with single use injection equipment (SUI)
115	DRG and statins and ED, with treatment of all individuals with SBP >140 mmHg and/or CHOL >240 mg/dl (>6.2 mmol/l)	164	GD and SUI
			Iron deficiency
116	LEG, HE and TRI with risk of 5% in 10 years	165	Iron supplementation (IS), 50% coverage
117	LEG, HE and TRI with risk of 15% in 10 years	166	IS, 80% coverage
118	LEG, HE and TRI with risk of 25% in 10 years	167	IS, 95% coverage
119	LEG, HE and TRI with risk of 35% in 10 years	168	Iron fortification (IF), 50% coverage
	Sexual and reproductive health	169	IF, 80% coverage
120	Antiretroviral therapy: standard monitoring, first-line drugs only (ARV1)	170	IF, 95% coverage
121	Antiretroviral therapy: intensive monitoring, first-line drugs only (ARV2)		
122	Antiretroviral therapy: standard monitoring, first- and second-line drugs (ARV3)		
123	Antiretroviral therapy: intensive monitoring, first- and second-line drugs (ARV4)		
124	Educating sex workers (EDS), 50% coverage		
125	Educating sex workers, 80% coverage		
126	Educating sex workers (EDS), 95% coverage		
127	EDS and treatment of sexually transmitted infections (EDS+STI), 50% coverage		
128	EDS+STI, 80% coverage		
129	EDS+STI, 95% coverage		
130	Mass media (MED), 100% coverage		
131	Treatment of sexually transmitted infections (STI), current coverage		
132	STI, enhanced coverage		
133	STI, 95% coverage		
134	School-based education (SBE), 50% coverage		

the annualized discounted costs of the intervention. All costs are included regardless of who pays.[12] The horizontal axis shows the yearly DALYs gained from this action.

The two rays drawn from the origin represent the cut-off points used to denote interventions as cost-effective and very cost-effective. All points on the lower ray (closer to the south-east corner) have a cost-effectiveness exactly equal to GDP per capita in the region. Interventions appearing to the right of it are defined as very cost-effective – most of the preventive interventions aimed at reducing unsafe sexual practices and improving child undernutrition fall in this category in both regions. All points on the upper ray (closer to the north-west corner) have a cost-effectiveness equal to three times GDP per capita, the cut point used to distinguish between cost-effective and cost-ineffective interventions. Points to the left of this ray would not be cost-effective in that region.

In AFR-D, preventive interventions to reduce the health effects of unsafe sex and the combined approach of population-wide and individual-based interventions for cardiovascular disease are among those in the most cost-effective category. On the other hand, treatment of people based purely on observed levels of blood pressure and cholesterol would not be cost-effective. In AMR-B, high rates of taxation to reduce smoking would be very cost-effective, but the combination of all the possible smoking-reduction interventions would not be in the most cost-effective category.

The figures show which interventions are in the the most cost-effective category. They also illustrate that it is possible for an intervention to be cost-effective but at the same time have a relatively small impact on population health. In AFR-D, for example, iron supplementation at 50% coverage (intervention 165) is cost-effective by itself. So is the combination of case management for pneumonia, ORT, vitamin A and zinc supplementation (intervention 80). The former would gain 1.28 million DALYs while the latter would gain 11.6 million. Despite the fact that both are very cost-effective, policy-makers need to have information about which one will have the greatest total impact on population health, and the total cost of achieving these health gains.[13]

In both figures, however, interventions cluster close to the origin and it is difficult to identify all of them clearly. Accordingly, the figures are redrawn with the axes on a logarithmic scale, enabling the individual interventions to be identified. In this case, the lines drawn obliquely across the figures represent lines of equal cost-effectiveness. All points on the line at the south-east extreme have a cost-effectiveness ratio (CER) of I\$ 1 per DALY gained. Because of the logarithmic scale, each subsequent line moving in a north-easterly direction represents a one order of magnitude increase in the CER, so all points on the next line have a CER of I\$ 10, and the subsequent line represents a CER of I\$ 100.

These figures illustrate more clearly that the variation in CERs across interventions within each region is substantial. In both subregions, some interventions (for example, preventive interventions aimed at reducing the incidence of HIV, and interventions to improve unsafe injection practices) gain each DALY at a cost of less than I\$ 10. On the other hand, adding nicotine replacement therapy to the cost-effective population-wide set of anti-smoking

---

[12] The points depict the total costs and total DALYs averted only for the most cost-effective interventions in any set (for example, interventions relating to unsafe sex). In other cases, the points show the additional costs and additional effects of moving from the most cost-effective option to that intervention. This is because decision-makers interested in maximizing population health for a given level of resources would first choose the most cost-effective intervention, then if additional resources were available, choose between alternative ways of using them based on the additional DALYs that would be gained from the additional expenditure.

[13] Iron supplementation at 50% coverage costs I\$ 38.2 million, while the combination of interventions would cost I\$ 1 billion at the regional level.

activities would cost more than I$ 10 000 per additional DALY gained (intervention 20). A similar range of cost-effectiveness ratios is observed in AMR-B.

The information on costs and effectiveness of a set of interventions targeting different risk factors can help to identify which interventions would be selected for given levels of resource availability in the different regions if the goal were to maximize population health.[14] In AFR-D, for example, a very severe restriction of resources would see most attention paid to preventive interventions to reduce the impact of unsafe sexual behaviours, unsafe injection use and micronutrient supplementation or fortification.

If the substantial increase in resources for health in Africa that is now becoming available allows all interventions costing less than three times GDP per capita to be funded, the optimal mix would include HIV prevention interventions combined with ARV treatment. It would include supplementation or fortification of vitamin A, iron and zinc in combination with treatment for diarrhoea and pneumonia in children. Disinfection at point of use would be combined with provision of improved sanitation facilities, and interventions designed to reduce the overuse of injections and unsafe injection practices would be introduced. Population-wide interventions to reduce the risks of cardiovascular disease would be combined with treatment of individuals with an absolute risk of an event in the next 10 years estimated to be above 25% (possibly even 15%), and high rates of taxation on cigarettes would be introduced and maintained.

These interventions are not exhaustive because not all risk factors were included, nor were all possible interventions analysed. However, they show that an annual expenditure of approximately I$ 6.8 billion would gain over 140 million DALYs in that region alone.

POLICY IMPLICATIONS

Very substantial health gains can be made for relatively modest expenditures on interventions to reduce risks. However, the maximum possible health gains will be attained only if careful consideration is given to the costs and effects of interventions. Risk reduction strategies need to be based on a thorough analysis of the best possible evidence on the health effects and the costs of technically feasible interventions, undertaken by themselves and in various combinations. The analysis of interactions between interventions is a critical but neglected question, which is the reason it has been given prominence in this chapter.

A selected number of interventions targeting some of the major risks to health have been discussed. Some that have not been considered are likely to also be cost-effective in different settings and will be included in *The World Health Report 2003*, but already a number of important messages emerge.

- A strategy to protect the child's environment is cost-effective in all settings. The components shown here to be very cost-effective include some form of micronutrient supplementation (depending on the prevalence of micronutrient deficiencies, either vitamin A, iron, or zinc) disinfection of water at point of use to reduce the incidence of diarrhoeal diseases; and treatment of diarrhoea and pneumonia.
- Preventive interventions to reduce incidence of HIV infections, including measures to encourage safer injection practices, are very cost-effective, although care needs to be taken when extrapolating the effectiveness of behaviour change interventions from one setting to another. The use of some types of antiretroviral therapy in conjunction with preventive activities is cost-effective in most settings. While directly

---

[14] As stated earlier, there are other goals of the health system as well and information on costs and effects will be only one of the inputs to the decision-making process.

Figure 5.3 Cost and effects of selected interventions in subregion AMR-B

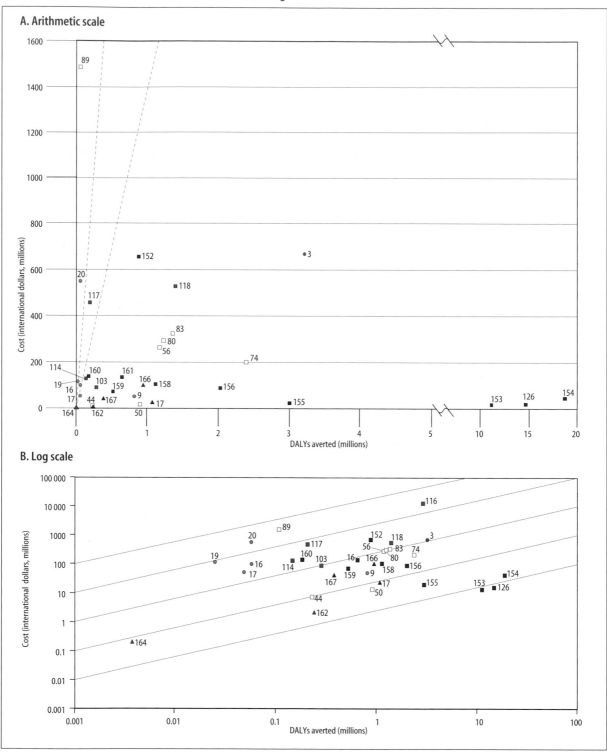

A. Arithmetic scale

B. Log scale

Figure 5.3 Cost and effects of selected interventions in subregion AMR-B

C. Legend

See the List of Member States by WHO Region and mortality stratum for an explanation of subregion AFR-D.
See Table 5.3 for a complete list of interventions.
For water and sanitation, only interventions considered to be purely health interventions are included.

Number	Legend	Description
		Unsafe water, sanitation and hygiene
3	●	Disinfection at point of use for population without improved water sources
		Addictive substances: Tobacco
9	●	Doubling the maximum tax (2TAX)
16	●	2TAX, Comprehensive ban (BAN) on advertising and Information dissemination (INF) through health warning labels, counter-advertising, and various consumer information packages
17	●	2TAX and BAN
19	●	2TAX, Clean indoor air laws (LAW), BAN and INF
20	●	2TAX, LAW, BAN, INF and Nicotine replacement therapy (NRT)
		Childhood undernutrition
44	□	Zinc fortification of food staple (ZF), 95%
50	□	Vitamin A fortification (VAF) of staple food and ZF, 95% coverage
56	□	Vitamin A supplementation for all children aged 6 months to 5 years (VAS5), twice a year at the health centre and Zinc supplementation daily for all children aged 0--5 years (ZS5), 95% coverage
74	□	VAS5, ZS5 and Case management for childhood pneumonia (CM), 95% coverage
80	□	VAS5, ZS5, Oral rehydration therapy for diarrhoea (ORT) and CM, 95% coverage
83	□	VAF, ZF, ORT and CM, 95% coverage
89	□	VAS5, ZS5, Improved complementary feeding through nutrition counselling and provision of nutrient-dense food for all underweight children aged 6–12 months identified through growth monitoring and promotion (CFGM), ORT and CM, 95% coverage
		Other nutrition-related risk factors and physical inactivity
103	■	Legislation (LEG) to decrease salt content of processed foods, plus appropriate labelling and enforcement
114	■	LEG and Health education (HE) through mass media to reduce cholesterol
116	■	Legislation (LEG) to decrease salt content of processed foods, plus appropriate labelling and enforcement, HE and TRI with risk of 5% in 10 years
117	■	LEG, HE and TRI with risk of 15% in 10 years
118	■	LEG, HE and TRI with risk of 25% in 10 years
		Sexual and reproductive health
126	■	Educating sex workers (EDS), 95% coverage
152	■	Antiretroviral therapy: intensive monitoring, first- and second-line drugs (ARV4), EDS+ Treatment of sexually transmitted infections (EDS+STI), Mass media (MED) 100% coverage, School-based education (SBE) 95% coverage, STI, 95% coverage, Voluntary counselling and testing (VCT) 95% coverage and Preventing mother-to-child transmission (MTCT)
153	■	EDS and MED
154	■	EDS, MED and STI 95% coverage
155	■	EDS+STI, MED and STI 95% coverage
156	■	EDS+STI, MED, STI 95% coverage and SBE 80% coverage
158	■	Antiretroviral therapy: standard monitoring, first-line drugs only (ARV1), EDS+STI, MED, STI 95% coverage and SBE 95% coverage
159	■	Antiretroviral therapy: intensive monitoring, first-line drugs only (ARV2), EDS+STI, MED, STI 95% coverage and SBE 95% coverage
160	■	ARV2, EDS+STI, MED, STI 95% coverage, SBE 95% coverage and MTCT
161	■	Antiretroviral therapy: intensive monitoring, first- and second-line drugs (ARV4), EDS+STI, MED, STI 95% coverage, SBE 95% coverage and MTCT
		Unsafe injections
162	▲	Reduction in overuse of injections through interactive patient--provider group discussions (GD)
164	▲	GD and Reduction in unsafe use of injections with single use injection equipment (SUI)
		Iron deficiency
166	▲	Iron supplementation (IS), 80% coverage
167	▲	IS, 95%
170	▲	Iron fortification (IF),95%

observed artiretroviral therapy combined with testing for resistance does not seem to be cost-effective in all settings, there might well be other reasons, that cannot be included in a standard cost-effectiveness framework, for pursuing it.

- Improved water supply based on disinfection at point of use is cost-effective in regions of high child mortality. While acknowledging that regulated piped water supplies will be the long-term aim of most countries, a policy shift towards household water management appears to be the most attractive short-term water-related health intervention in developing countries.

- In all settings at least one type of intervention to reduce the risks associated with cardiovascular disease was cost-effective. Population-wide salt and cholesterol lowering strategies are always very cost-effective singly and combined. Combining them with an individual risk reduction strategy is also cost-effective, particularly with interventions to reduce risk based on assessed levels of absolute risk. The cost-effectiveness of the absolute risk approach would improve further if it is possible to assess accurately individual risks without the need for laboratory tests, and further work towards testing this possibility is recommended. Additional interventions that were not evaluated here, such as those aimed at encouraging people to increase their physical activity levels, should also be considered when comprehensive strategies are being assessed in different settings.

- There is an important role for governments in encouraging risk reduction strategies. For example, taxes on cigarette products are very cost-effective globally and higher tax rates result in larger improvements in population health. In addition, governments would be well advised to consider taking steps to reduce the salt content of processed foods on a population-wide basis, either through legislation or through self-regulation. Both approaches would require consultation with a variety of stakeholders.

This report acknowledges that there are other goals of health policy in addition to improving population health. In choosing appropriate combinations of interventions, governments are also concerned with reducing poverty and other inequalities, and with questions of human rights, community acceptance and political needs. They must also consider how different types of interventions can be incorporated into the health infrastructure available in the country, or how the infrastructure could be expanded or adapted to accommodate the desired strategies. This is particularly important when considering if it is feasible to expand coverage to high levels. However, improving population health is the defining goal of a health system, the reason why it exists. The type of information reviewed in this chapter is one of the critical inputs required to inform the decision-making process about efficient ways to reduce risks to health.

REFERENCES

1. Mason J, Drummond M. Reporting guidelines for economic studies. *Health Economics* 1995; 4(2):85-94.

2. Gold MR, Siegel JE, Russel LB, Weinstein MC. *Cost-effectiveness in health and medicine*. New York: Oxford University Press; 1996.

3. Murray CJ, Evans DB, Acharya A, Baltussen RM. Development of WHO guidelines on generalized cost-effectiveness analysis. *Health Economics* 2000; 9(3):235-51.

4. Murray CJ, Frenk J. A framework for assessing the performance of health systems. *Bulletin of the World Health Organization* 2000; 78(6):717-31.

5. World Health Organization. *The World Health Report 2000: Health systems: Improving performance.* Geneva: World Health Organization; 2000.

6. Krummel DA, Humphries D, Tessaro I. Focus groups on cardiovascular health in rural women: implications for practice. *Journal of Nutrition Education and Behavior* 2002; 34(1):38-46.

7. Manne S, Markowitz A, Winawer S, Meropol NJ, Haller D, Rakowski W et al. Correlates of colorectal cancer screening compliance and stage of adoption among siblings of individuals with early onset colorectal cancer. *Health Psychology* 2002; 21(1):3-15.

8. West R. Theories of addiction. *Addiction* 2001; 96(1):3-13.

9. Torgerson DJ, Raftery J. Economic notes. Discounting. *British Medical Journal* 1999; 319(7214):914-5.

10. Okrah J, Traore C, Pale A, Sommerfeld J, Muller O. Community factors associated with malaria prevention by mosquito nets: an exploratory study in rural Burkina Faso. *Tropical Medicine & International Health* 2002; 7(3):240-8.

11. Collins R, Peto R, Armitage J. The MRC/BHF Heart Protection Study: preliminary results. *International Journal of Clinical Practice* 2002; 56(1):53-6.

12. Marshall T, Rouse A. Resource implications and health benefits of primary prevention strategies for cardiovascular disease in people aged 30 to 74: mathematical modelling study. *British Medical Journal* 2002; 325(7357):197.

13. Rose G. Sick individuals and sick populations. *International Journal of Epidemiology* 2001; 30(3):427-32.

14. Jha P, Chaloupka FJ. The economics of global tobacco control. *British Medical Journal* 2000; 321(7257):358-61.

15. Joossens L, Raw M. Smuggling and cross border shopping of tobacco in Europe. *British Medical Journal* 1995; 310(6991):1393-7.

16. Chang M, Hahn RA, Teutsch SM, Hutwagner LC. Multiple risk factors and population attributable risk for ischemic heart disease mortality in the United States, 1971-1992. *Journal of Clinical Epidemiology* 2001; 54(6):634-44.

17. Baltussen RMPM, Hutubessy RC, Evans DB, Murray CJL. Uncertainty in cost-effectiveness analysis. Probabilistic uncertainty analysis and stochastic league tables. *International Journal of Technology Assessment in Health Care* 2002; 18(1):112-9.

18. Baltussen RM, Adam T, Tan Torres T, Hutubessy RC, Acharya A, Evans DB, Murray CJL. *Generalized cost-effectiveness analysis: a guide.* Geneva: World Health Organization, Global Programme on Evidence for Health Policy; 2002.

19. Hutubessy RCW, Baltussen RMPM, Evans DB, Barendregt JJ, Murray CJL. Stochastic league tables: communicating cost-effectiveness results to decision makers. *Health Economics* 2002; 10(5):473-7.

20. Gravelle H, Smith D. Discounting for health effects in cost-benefit and cost-effectiveness analysis. *Health Economics* 2001; 10(7):587-99.

21. Tasset A, Nguyen VH, Wood S, Amazian K. Discounting: technical issues in economic evaluations of vaccination. *Vaccine* 1999; 17 Suppl 3:S75-S80.

22. Nissinen A, Berrios X, Puska P. Community-based noncommunicable disease interventions: lessons from developed countries for developing ones. *Bulletin of the World Health Organization* 2001; 79(10):963-70.

23. WHO Commission on Macroeconomics and Health. *Macroeconomics and health: investing in health for economic development. Report of the Commission on Macroeconomics and Health.* Geneva: World Health Organization; 2001.

24. World Health Organization. *Primary health care: report of the International Conference on Primary Health Care, Alma-Ata.* Geneva: World Health Organization; 1978. "Health for All" Series, No. 1.

25. Walsh JA, Warren KS. Selective primary health care: an interim strategy for disease control in developing countries. *New England Journal of Medicine* 1979; 301(18):967-74.

26. Warren KS. The evolution of selective primary health care. *Social Science and Medicine* 1988; 26(9):891-8.

27. Claeson M, Waldman RJ. The evolution of child health programmes in developing countries: from targeting diseases to targeting people. *Bulletin of the World Health Organization* 2000; 78(10):1234-45.

28. GAVI. *Immunize every child: GAVI strategy for sustainable immunization services. February 2000*. Working paper of the Global Alliance for Vaccines and Immunization, 2000 (unpublished document available on http://www.vaccinealliance.org).

29. Caulfield L, Huffman S, Piwoz E. Interventions to improve intake of complementary foods by infants 6 to 12 months of age in developing countries: impact on growth and on the prevalence of malnutrition and potential contribution to child survival. *Food and Nutrition Bulletin* 1999; 20:183-99.

30. UNICEF/UNU/WHO/MI. *Preventing Iron Deficiency in Women and Children. Technical Consensus on Key Issues*. Technical Workshop, UNICEF, New York, 7-9 October 1998. Boston: International Nutrition Foundation and Micronutrient Initiative; 1999.

31. Stoltzfus R, Dreyfuss M. *Guidelines for the use of iron supplements to prevent and treat iron deficiency anaemia*. Washington, D.C.: The International Nutritional Anaemia Consultative Group (INACG/WHO/UNICEF); 1998.

32. Galloway R, McGuire J. Determinants of compliance with iron supplementation: supplies, side effects, or psychology? *Social Science and Medicine* 1994; 39(3):381-90.

33. Mora JO, Dary O, Chinchilla D, Arroyave G. *Vitamin A sugar fortification in Central America. Experience and lessons learned*. Arlington, VA: MOST, The USAID Micronutrient Program; 2000.

34. Victora CG, Olinto MT, Barros FC, Nobre LC. Falling diarrhoea mortality in Northeastern Brazil: did ORT play a role? *Health Policy and Planning* 1996; 11(2):132-41.

35. Miller P, Hirschhorn N. The effect of a national control of diarrheal diseases program on mortality: the case of Egypt. *Social Science and Medicine* 1995; 40(10):S1-S30.

36. Sazawal S, Black RE. Meta-analysis of intervention trials on case-management of pneumonia in community settings. *Lancet* 1992; 340(8818):528-33.

37. World Health Organization. *Innovative care for chronic conditions: building bloks for action*. Geneva, World Health Organization, 2002 (unpublished document WHO/MNC/CCH/02.01).

38. Puska P. Development of public policy on the prevention and control of elevated blood cholesterol. *Cardiovascular Risk Factors* 1996; 6(4):203-10.

39. European Heart Network. *Food, nutrition and cardiovascular disease prevention in the European region: challenges for the new millenium*. Brussels: 2002.

40. Utting P. Regulating business via multistakeholder initiatives: a preliminary assessment. In: *Voluntary approaches to corporate responsibility*. Geneva: United Nations Non-Government Liaison Service; 2002. p. 61-130.

41. Lawes C, Feigin V, Rodgers A. *Estimating reductions in blood pressure following reductions in salt intake by age, sex and WHO region*. Auckland: Clinical Trials Research Unit, University of Auckland; 2002.

42. Tosteson AN, Weinstein MC, Hunink MG, Mittleman MA, Williams LW, Goldman PA et al. Cost-effectiveness of populationwide educational approaches to reduce serum cholesterol levels. *Circulation* 1997; 95(1):24-30.

43. World Health Organization. *Reduction of cardiovascular burden through cost-effective integrated management of cardiovascular risk: addressing hypertension, smoking cessation and diabetes*. Geneva, World Health Organization, 2002 (unpublished document NMH meeting report, 9-12 July 2002).

44. Law MR, Wald NJ. Risk factor thresholds: their existence under scrutiny. *British Medical Journal* 2002; 324(7353):1570-6.

45. Miller MR, Pollard CM, Coli T. Western Australian Health Department recommendations for fruit and vegetable consumption — how much is enough? *Australia and New Zealand Journal of Public Health* 1997; 21: 638-42.

46. *The health of New Zealanders 1996/7*. Wellington: New Zealand Ministry of Health; 1999.

47. *National nutrition survey*. Canberra: Australian Bureau of Statistics; 1996. Cat. No. 4801.0.

48. Mathers C, Vos T, Stevenson C. 1999. *The burden of disease and injury in Australia*. Canberra: Australian Institute of Health and Welfare; 1999. AIHW Cat. No. PHE 17.

49. Vos T, Begg S. *The Victorian Burden of Disease Study: mortality*. Melbourne: Public Health and Development Division, Victorian Government Department of Human Services; 1999.

50. Vos T, Begg S. *The Victorian Burden of Disease Study: morbidity*. Melbourne: Public Health and Development Division, Victorian Government Department of Human Services; 1999.

51. Carter R, Stone C, Vos T, Hocking J, Mihalopoulos C, Peacock S, et al. *Trial of Program Budgeting and Marginal Analysis (PBMA) to assist cancer control planning in Australia*. Canberra: Commonwealth Department of Health and Aged Care; 2000.

52. Dixon H, Borland R, Segan C, Stafford H, Sindall C. Public reaction to Victorian "2 fruit 'n' 5 veg every day" campaign and reported consumption of fruit and vegetables. *Preventive Medicine* 1998; 27: 572-82.

53. Mathers C, Stevenson C, Carter R, Penm R. *Disease costing methodology used in the Disease Costs and Impact Study 1993-94*. Canberra: Australian Institute of Health and Welfare; 1998. Health Expenditure Series No. 3, AIHW Cat. No. HWE 7.

54. Mathers C, Penm R, Sanson-Fisher R, Carter R, Campbell E. *Health system costs of cancer in Australia 1993-94*. Canberra: Australian Institute of Health and Welfare; 1998. Health Expenditure Series No. 4, AIHW Cat. No. HWE 4.

55. Mathers C, Penm R. *Health system costs of cardiovascular costs and diabetes in Australia 1993-94*. Canberra: Australian Institute of Health and Welfare; 1999. Health Expenditure Series No. 5, AIHW Cat. No. HWE 11.

56. UNAIDS. *Report on the global HIV/AIDS epidemic June 2000*. Geneva: UNAIDS; 2000.

57. Stover J, Walker N, Garnett GP, Salomon JA, Stanecki KA, Ghys PD et al. Can we reverse the HIV/AIDS pandemic with an expanded response? *Lancet* 2002; 360(9326):73-7.

58. Goldstein S, Scheepers E. *Soul City 4 impact evaluation: AIDS*. www.soulcity.org.za. 2000.

59. Sweat M, Gregorich S, Sangiwa G, Furlonge C, Balmer D, Kamenga C et al. Cost-effectiveness of voluntary HIV-1 counselling and testing in reducing sexual transmission of HIV-1 in Kenya and Tanzania. *Lancet* 2000; 356(9224):113-21.

60. Nyblade LC, Menken J, Wawer MJ, Sewankambo NK, Serwadda D, Makumbi F et al. Population-based HIV testing and counseling in rural Uganda: participation and risk characteristics. *Journal of Acquired Immune Deficiency Syndromes* 2001; 28(5):463-70.

61. Anderson JE, Carey JW, Taveras S. HIV testing among the general US population and persons at increased risk: information from national surveys, 1987-1996. *American Journal of Public Health* 2000; 90(7):1089-95.

62. Stanton BF, Li X, Kahihuata J, Fitzgerald AM, Neumbo S, Kanduuombe G et al. Increased protected sex and abstinence among Namibian youth following a HIV risk-reduction intervention: a randomized, longitudinal study. *AIDS* 1998; 12(18):2473-80.

63. Shuey DA, Babishangire BB, Omiat S, Bagarukayo H. Increased sexual abstinence among in-school adolescents as a result of school health education in Soroti district, Uganda. *Health Education Research* 1999; 14(3):411-9.

64. Ngugi EN, Wilson D, Sebstad J, Plummer FA, Moses S. Focused peer-mediated educational programs among female sex workers to reduce sexually transmitted disease and human immunodeficiency virus transmission in Kenya and Zimbabwe. *Journal of Infectious Diseases* 1996; 174 Suppl 2:S240-S247.

65. Levine WC, Revollo R, Kaune V, Vega J, Tinajeros F, Garnica M et al. Decline in sexually transmitted disease prevalence in female Bolivian sex workers: impact of an HIV prevention project. *AIDS* 1998; 12(14):1899-906.

66. Morisky D, Tiglao TV, Baltazar J, Detels R, Sneed C. *The effects of peer counseling on STD risk-behaviors among heterosexual males in the Philippines*. XIII International AIDS Conference, abstract WeOrD589, 2000 (unpublished document).

67. Njagi E, Kimani J, Plummer FA, Ndinya-Achola JO, Bwayo JJ, Ngugi EN. *Long-term impact of community peer interventions on condom use and STI incidence among sex workers in Nairobi*. Int Conf AIDS, 12:691 abstract no. 33515, 1998 (unpublished document).

68. Steen R, Vuylsteke B, DeCoito T, Ralepeli S, Fehler G, Conley J et al. Evidence of declining STD prevalence in a South African mining community following a core-group intervention. *Sexually Transmitted Diseases* 2000; 27(1):1-8.

69. Kahn JG, Kegeles SM, Hays R, Beltzer N. Cost-effectiveness of the Mpowerment Project, a community-level intervention for young gay men. *Journal of Acquired Immune Deficiency Syndromes* 2001; 27(5):482-91.

70. Mota M, Parker R, Lorenco L, Almeida V, Pimenta C, Fernandes MEL. *Sexual behavior and behavior change among men who have sex with men in Brazil, 1989-1994*. Third USAID HIV/AIDS Prevention Conference, abstract no.A-39, 1995 (unpublished document).

71. Haque A, Ahmed S. *Community based risks reduction approach among MSM: Bandhu Social Welfare Society : HIV/AIDS/STD prevention program*. XIII International AIDS Conference, abstract no. WePeD4745, 2000 (unpublished document).

72. Lee LM, Karon JM, Selik R, Neal JJ, Fleming PL. Survival after AIDS diagnosis in adolescents and adults during the treatment era, United States, 1984-1997. *JAMA : the Journal of the American Medical Association* 2001; 285(10):1308-15.

73. Pezzotti P, Napoli PA, Acciai S, Boros S, Urciuoli R, Lazzeri V et al. Increasing survival time after AIDS in Italy: the role of new combination antiretroviral therapies. Tuscany AIDS Study Group. *AIDS* 1999; 13(2):249-55.

74. McNaghten AD, Hanson DL, Jones JL, Dworkin MS, Ward JW. Effects of antiretroviral therapy and opportunistic illness primary chemoprophylaxis on survival after AIDS diagnosis. Adult/Adolescent Spectrum of Disease Group. *AIDS* 1999; 13(13):1687-95.

75. Stover J, Bollinger L, Cooper-Arnold K. *Goals model: for estimating the effects of resource allocation decisions on the achievement of goals of the HIV/AIDS strategic plan*. Glastonbury: The Futures Group International; 2001.

76. World Health Organization. *Guidelines for controlling and monitoring the tobacco epidemic.* Geneva: World Health Organization; 1998.

77. Chaloupka FJ, Hu TW, Warner KE, Jacobs R, Yurekli A. The taxation of tobacco products. In: Jha P, Chaloupka FJ, editors. *Tobacco control in developing countries.* Oxford: Oxford University Press; 2000. p. 237-72.

78. *Tobacco control country profiles.* Atlanta, GA: American Cancer Society; 2000. (also available at the World Bank web side: http://www1.worldbank.org/tobacco/countrybrief.asp).

79. Fichtenberg CM, Glantz SA. Effect of smoke-free workplaces on smoking behaviour: systematic review. *British Medical Journal* 2002; 325(7357):188.

80. World Health Organization. *Member states need to take action against tobacco advertising.* Press Release WHO/47. Geneva: World Health Organization; 2001. (http://www.who.int/inf-pr-2001/en/pr2001-47.html).

81. Saffer H, Chaloupka F. The effect of tobacco advertising bans on tobacco consumption. *Journal of Health Economics* 2000; 19(6):1117-37.

82. Kenkel D, Chen L. Consumer information and tobacco use. In: Jha P, Chaloupka FJ, editors. *Tobacco control in developing countries.* Oxford: Oxford University Press; 2000. p. 177-214.

83. *Global burden of injuries.* Geneva: World Health Organization; 1999.

84. Muller A. Evaluation of the costs and benefits of motorcycle helmet laws. *American Journal of Public Health* 1980; 70 (6): 586-92.

85. Fuchs VR. Motor accident mortality and compulsory inspection of vehicles. In: *The health economy.* Cambridge (MA): Harvard University Press; 1986. p. 169-80.

86. Rice DP, MacKenzie EJ, Jones AS, Kaufman SR, DeLissovoy GV, Max W, et al. *Cost of injury in the United States: a report to Congress.* San Francisco (CA): Institute for Health and Aging, University of California; and Injury Prevention Center, The Johns Hopkins University; 1989.

87. Graham JD, Thompson KM, Goldie SJ, Segui-Gomez M, Weinstein MC. Cost-effectiveness of air bags by seating position. *JAMA* 1997; 278(17): 1418-25.

88. Mannering F, Winston C. *Recent automobile occupant safety proposals in blind intersection: policy and the automobile industry.* Washington (DC): Brookings Institution; 1987. p. 68-88.

89. Kamerud DB. Benefits and costs of the 55 mph speed limit: new estimates and their implications. *Journal of Policy Analysis and Management* 1988; 7(2): 341-52.

CHAPTER SIX

Strengthening
Risk Prevention Policies

The two previous chapters have quantified the relative importance of various risk factors in different populations around the world and have proposed intervention strategies for some of them. Without doubt, information on the magnitude of disease and injury burden, and on the availability, effectiveness and cost-effectiveness of interventions is essential for prioritizing policy responses to reduce risks and improve overall levels of population health. Rapid health gains can only be achieved with focused interventions that reach large segments of the populations concerned. However, such strategies must take into account the broader framework of risk management considerations, some of which are highlighted in this chapter. It places the risks and intervention strategies outlined in Chapters Four and Five in the context of other considerations that need to be kept in mind when deciding on measures to reduce risk. A key issue is getting the right balance between efforts targeted on primary, secondary or subsequent prevention; another is the management of uncertain risks. The ethical implications of various programme strategies, including their impact on inequities in population health, must also be taken into account. This chapter argues that governments, in their stewardship role for better health, need to invest heavily in risk prevention, in order to contribute substantially to future avoidable mortality. It then shows how policy-relevant choices can be made and which risks should receive priority, particularly for middle and low income countries.

6

STRENGTHENING

RISK PREVENTION

POLICIES

CHOOSING PRIORITY STRATEGIES
FOR RISK PREVENTION

*I*n constructing health policies for the prevention of well-known risks, choices need to be made between different strategies. For instance, will preventing small risks in large populations avoid more adverse health outcomes than avoiding large risks in a smaller number of high-risk individuals? What priority should be given to cost-effective interventions for primary rather than secondary prevention, such as lowering blood pressure distribution by reducing dietary salt intake compared with treatment of people with high blood pressure? Should priority be given to preventing environmental and distal risks to health, such as tackling poor sanitation or inadequate nutritional intakes, rather than the more obvious proximal risks in a causal chain? What is the most appropriate and effective mix of these strategies?

In practice there is rarely an obvious and clear choice. These strategies are usually combined so as to complement each other *(1)*. In general, however, it is more effective to give priority to:
- population-based interventions rather than those aimed at high-risk individuals;
- primary over secondary prevention;
- controlling distal rather than proximal risks to health.

POPULATION-BASED INTERVENTIONS OR HIGH-RISK INDIVIDUAL TARGETS?

There is a "prevention paradox" which shows that interventions can achieve large overall health gains for whole populations but might offer only small advantages to each individual. This leads to a misperception of the benefits of preventive advice and services by people who are apparently in good health *(2, 3)*. In general, population-wide interventions have the greatest potential for prevention. For instance, in reducing risks from blood pressure and cholesterol, shifting the mean of whole populations will be more cost-effective in avoiding future heart attacks and strokes than screening programmes that aim to identify and treat all those people with defined hypertension or raised cholesterol levels, as shown in Figure 6.1 *(4–6)*. A similar approach can be used to modify behavioural risks and environmental exposures. For example, lowering the population mean for alcohol consumption will also predictably reduce the number of people suffering from alcohol abuse *(7)*. Often both approaches are used and successfully combined in one strategy.

Figure 6.1 Case studies of distribution shifting and cardiovascular disease in Finland and Japan

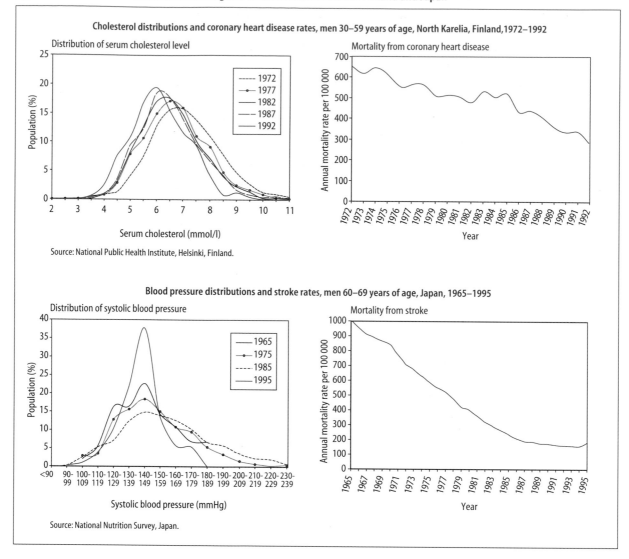

Cholesterol distributions and coronary heart disease rates, men 30–59 years of age, North Karelia, Finland,1972–1992

Distribution of serum cholesterol level

Source: National Public Health Institute, Helsinki, Finland.

Blood pressure distributions and stroke rates, men 60–69 years of age, Japan, 1965–1995

Distribution of systolic blood pressure

Source: National Nutrition Survey, Japan.

DISTAL OR PROXIMAL RISKS TO HEALTH?

Although most epidemiological research and intervention analysis has focused on the more immediate risks for major diseases, tackling distal risks to health such as education and poverty can yield fundamental and sustained improvements to future health status. Enough is known about the predominant role of distal factors on health and survival to justify vastly greater efforts to reduce poverty and improve access to education, especially for girls. There is huge potential for major health gains through sustained intersectoral action involving other ministries and agencies concerned with development.

PRIMARY OR SECONDARY PREVENTION?

Risk reduction through primary prevention, such as immunization, is clearly preferable as this actually lowers future exposures and hence the incidence of new disease episodes over time. For long-term health gains it is usually preferable to remove the underlying risk.

The choices may well be different, however, for different risks, depending to a large extent on how common and how widely distributed is the risk and the availability and costs of effective interventions. Large gains in health can be achieved through inexpensive treatments when primary prevention has failed. Secondary prevention is based on screening exposed populations for the early onset of subclinical illnesses and then treating them. This approach can be very effective if the disease processes are reversible, valid screening tests exist, and effective treatments are available.

MANAGING THE RISK PREVENTION PROCESS

As identifying and preventing risks to health is a political procedure, risk prevention requires its own decision-making processes if determined leaders from ministries of health and the public health community are to be successful (8). Other important factors which determine whether policies are adopted include public perceptions of the risks and benefits involved, perceived levels of dread and scientific uncertainty, how widely the risks are distributed and how inequitable or unfair are the health outcomes (9). Special interest groups and the media also have major roles in influencing these issues. Finally, there are important lessons for achieving success in risk communications that should be more widely disseminated, including the implications for more transparent government and greater openness by the scientific community (10). Successfully tackling risks to health involves many stakeholders from different sections in society, a combination of scientific and political processes, many qualitative and quantitative judgements, a range of intersectoral actions by different agencies and opportunities for open communication and dialogue (11).

Success in risk prevention will be largely determined by the strength of the political leadership from the ministry of health. Risk management is by no means a linear process and, although it typically involves an iterative decision-making process, action will be necessary in all four of the main components of assessment, management, communication and surveillance (see Figure 6.2).

Figure 6.2 Implementing risk prevention

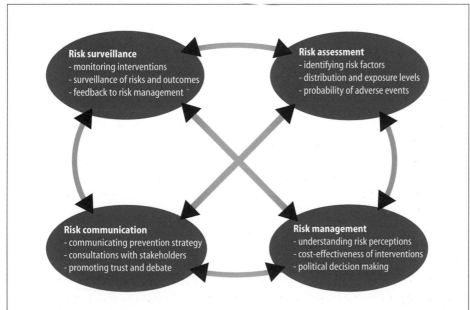

IDENTIFYING PRIORITY RISK FACTORS FOR PREVENTION

The scientific basis for the burden attributable to the main risk factors addressed in this report is reasonably well understood; for these risks, remaining data gaps should not diminish the importance of adopting control policies today if disease burden is to be lowered in the near future. Much of the scientific and economic information necessary for making health policy decisions is already available.

Many of these are also well known, common, substantial and widespread. They are also more likely to have cost-effective risk reduction strategies. Lack of uncertainty and availability of cost-effective interventions for large risks leads to agreement in society about the need for action. Examples would be increasing tobacco consumption, particularly in Asia and Eastern Europe, and the role of unsafe sex in the HIV/AIDS epidemic, particularly in Africa. Many of these risks are common to populations in both industrialized and developing countries, though the degree of exposure may vary.

Risk factors with smaller disease burdens should also not be neglected; although smaller than other factors, they still contribute to the total burden of disease in various regions. Large industrial activity involving coal, ambient air pollution and lead exposure, for example, has health effects comparable to other major risk factors. Some risks, such as occupational ones, are concentrated among certain sectors of society. This implies not only that these sectors are disproportionately affected, but also that the concentration makes targeting risk easier, as successful occupational safety interventions and policies in many regions have shown. For other risk factors, such as childhood sexual abuse, ethical considerations may outweigh direct contributions to disease burden. Even though the burden of disease attributable to a risk factor may be limited, highly effective or cost-effective interventions may be known. Reducing the number of unnecessary medical injections coupled with the use of sterile syringes are effective methods for controlling transmission of communicable diseases. Similarly, reductions in exposure to lead or ambient air pollution in industrialized countries in the second half of the 20th century were achieved by effective use of technology which often also led to energy saving and other benefits. In the case of these risk factors, therefore, the benefits to population health stemming from risk assessment, together with other considerations, provide the best possible policy guides for specific actions.

The management of risk factors or hazards that have uncertain or highly uncertain risk probabilities or adverse consequences, such as exposure to climate change or genetically modified foods, is considered in the next section, in the context of cautionary approaches and the use of the precautionary principle.

The national context is very important for assessing the options for risk prevention. For instance, in many middle and low income countries a lack of scientific expertise and equipment may mean that appropriate data for making local risk assessments are not available. In addition, many risks may also have low priority for any political action. In these situations, public awareness of risk factors may need to be enhanced and knowledge about the most dangerous risk factors brought openly to public attention, while interest groups and the mass media may need to be encouraged to debate publicly local risks to health. Any leadership for political action will have to come from the ministries of health. Collective actions at regional and international levels are also called for, as many risk factors and risks to health are not limited by national borders. This is where the World Health Organization can play an effective advisory and coordinating role.

ASSESSMENT AND MANAGEMENT OF HIGHLY UNCERTAIN RISKS

People who work in the public health arena regularly face surprises and controversies. While these are at times caused by special interest groups, they often reflect unmet challenges to health management capabilities and a lack of preparedness. In these situations prevention becomes a particularly politicized process, which leads to a need for better communications, trust, dialogue, information sharing and planning to contain panic *(11, 12)*. Planning for high uncertain risks should be an important component of the activities of the major organizations entrusted with public health management.

In recent years the public has requested much greater caution in the management of highly uncertain risks, leading to use of the term "precautionary principle". Considerable debate exists on what the precautionary principle actually means and there is no generally accepted definition. The most basic definition of the precautionary principle is that adopted at the United Nations Conference on the Environment and Development in 1992: "Where there are threats of serious or irreversible environmental damage, lack of full scientific certainty shall not be used as a reason for postponing cost-effective measures to prevent environmental degradation" *(13)*.

Although the principle is widely seen as a part of regulatory action, it is not actually embodied in any international legal agreement. If it has to be used to resolve difficult risks, how will it be interpreted by different group interests? A summary of the features of the "weak", "moderate" and "strong" positions for and against the possible use of the precautionary principle within regulatory frameworks are summarized in Box 6.1.

It is important to recognize that, because of a lack of scientific knowledge and scarce resources no public agency can prepare for the infinitely large number of eventualities. The risk assessment, risk management and risk communication tools that have been discussed for dealing with many health hazards that are now familiar can nonetheless be helpful, if appropriately employed, in tackling highly uncertain risks.

Box 6.1 Contrasting views of the role of the precautionary principle within different world views of regulation

Weak precaution	*Moderate precaution*	*Strong precaution*
Presumption of unfettered market-led development and technological innovation.	Underlying presumption of unfettered market-led development and technological innovation, but recognition that this can sometimes be overthrown by high levels of societal concern.	No presumption of either market-led or technologically driven development.
Regulators intervene only on positive scientific evidence of risk and only use interventions that are demonstrably cost-effective.	Presumption about interventions as under 'weak precaution', but with case by case flexibility to shift the need for proof towards the risk creator.	Risk creator has to demonstrate safety of activity. Little acceptance of cost-effectiveness arguments.
Presumption of risk management. Banning very rare.	Underlying presumption of risk management. Banning possible, but only as last resort.	Presumption of risk avoidance. Banning very likely.
Presumption of free trade based on objective scientific criteria. Individual preferences and societal concerns given no weight.	Underlying presumption of free trade on the basis of scientific criteria. Recognition that individual preferences and societal concerns do matter.	No automatic presumption of free trade. Individual preferences and societal concerns are dominant.

Adapted from: *(14)*.

Defining what is "highly uncertain" depends on context. Risks may be highly uncertain because they are:

- hidden risks, that are unstudied or insufficiently thought about. Risks may be hidden because they are unknown or rare phenomena; they are common phenomena that are statistically invisible (which might happen if data are gathered in categories that fail to reveal the risk); or they have been ignored because it was thought that nothing could be done about them;
- surprises;
- fresh controversies. There is inadequate and inconclusive information, but it can be reasonably expected that new information will be obtained which may well resolve outstanding key questions;
- persistent controversies, which endure even after a great deal of research to try to resolve them. Persistence of controversy is likely to be reinforced by differences in political or academic perspectives which inhibit communication between the parties and impede the establishment of common terms and agreement on approaches to information gathering. Special interest groups play a role in fostering controversy.

For any given risk, some or all of these categories can be a part of its development. For example, an unknown risk such as bovine spongiform encephalopathy (BSE) may emerge as a surprise, lead to serious controversies, and later on become familiar.

Assessment and management of highly uncertain risks can be adaptive, based on the following principles.

- Management should start with what is already known, acknowledge openly the major scientific uncertainties, and highlight uncertainties about human behaviour that affect the risk.
- Explicit analysis of what new information might become available on what time scales, and what it might show. A summary of this analysis should form a distinct section of the assessment.
- Development of a plan for acquiring and managing new information and presentation of the plan as a portion of the management options to be considered. Management goals should be defined broadly so that growing knowledge can be effectively utilized; the acquisition of new knowledge should be one of these goals.
- Improving assessment and performance is necessarily iterative; it is impossible to get everything right the first time, especially when uncertainties are large.

There may be threats that are irreversible, affect a large number of people, or rapidly expand the problem. Rapid diagnosis and response are therefore appropriate, and can often prevent major damage from occurring, especially in situations involving irreversible changes or rapid spread of the uncertain hazard. Characteristics of hazards such as persistence, irreversibility, and depth and breadth of impact are thus of particular concern.

Within the realm of highly uncertain risks, it is important to recognize that adaptive management should not be confined to particular, already specified, hazards. Rather, in order to use limited resources effectively, there should be investment in risk management efforts which do not focus on particular hazards but which will improve capabilities for identifying emerging hazards and for coping with them.

The management of highly uncertain risks involves infrastructure development in various international and national public agencies. The aims of such agencies are to search for hidden hazards, maintain a capability for responding to surprises and controversies, monitor the development of surprises and controversies and assess the effects of interventions, manage the development of new knowledge and access to it, and evaluate human behaviour as a contributor to hazards. Agencies that monitor and manage food safety or disposal of toxic waste are examples.

It is not necessarily the case that prioritization requires making the choice between managing known risks and focusing on uncertain risks. The two activities are complementary to a considerable extent. Improved capabilities in managing known risks will be a resource to draw upon when dealing with new risks, and capabilities at detecting risk possibilities, assessing uncertainty, and learning from experience will inform and improve the management of familiar risks. Furthermore, avoiding or reducing some uncertain risks, such as global climate change or toxic chemicals, can be achieved with interventions such as energy efficiency or use of alternative chemicals which may provide other economic benefits.

Risk management is by now an international task. Many risks cross boundaries, so that actions in one country or region have an impact in another. In the case of management of uncertain risks, an important aspect of strengthening capabilities will be partnerships between specialists – experts in dealing with particular hazards – from different countries. But the overall build-up of risk management capability will be fragmented unless there is active coordination involving generalists in the country and associated with international agencies.

ETHICAL CONSIDERATIONS IN RISK PREVENTION

Medical ethics is a well-developed subject but it is mainly concerned with individual patient–doctor relationships and there has been little application of its principles to public health and even less to risks to health (15, 16). However, there is a wide range of ethical issues concerning risk exposures and risk outcomes, mainly to do, firstly, with balancing the rights, freedoms and responsibilities of individuals against achieving greater risk prevention using population-wide approaches and, secondly, protecting those individuals at high-risk exposures. In addition, strong regulatory and legal mechanisms may be required, which can affect both individuals as consumers as well as those in high-risk groups.

There are four fundamental ethical principles that are widely used throughout the world in medical practice, commonly called autonomy, non-maleficence, beneficence and justice (17). Each is a complex ethical principle, but when applied to public health and risk factors they might each be paraphrased respectively as protecting the rights of the individual and informed choice, do no harm or injury, produce benefits that far outweigh risks, and achieve a more equitable and fair distribution of risks and benefits. The application of these principles requires that whole populations and exposed or affected individuals, together with a wide range of other concerned stakeholders, have free and open access to all the information. Freedom should exist for full representation and transparent decision-making. These are all frequently problematic issues in risk management.

When conflict exists between these principles in particular risk situations, one principle – for example distributive justice – may have to override another one. When this is necessary, which one is given priority should be declared and made explicit. If this is not done, the result can be even greater public and professional controversy and a loss of trust in political decision-makers. These principles are ethical guidelines and considerable judgement and negotiation is required for their use in many risk prevention situations. As there is little previous experience of applying these principles to risks to health, especially in developing countries, few accepted legal requirements or norms based on custom and practice are available. Thus each situation has often to be examined on a case-by-case basis *(15)*.

Conflicts of interest, both personal and corporate, represent an important ethical issue that is receiving increasing international attention. Few organizations have enforceable guidelines for disclosing and handling conflicts of interest, particularly between personal and professional medical roles and between public organizations, such as ministries of health, and private-for-profit companies. For instance, disclosure of personal interests, such as when experts have close links to the global alcohol, tobacco and food industries, is rarely even a voluntary requirement.

RISK COMMUNICATIONS AND THE ROLE OF GOVERNMENTS

The public, particularly poor people, believe that their governments have an important duty to reduce the extent to which they are exposed to hazards and that they should do all they reasonably can to reduce risks, such as making sure that environments, foods and medicines are safe. This is particularly important where individuals have little control over their exposure to risks, because these risks are either not readily apparent or exposure is not under voluntary control *(18–20)*. Although governments cannot set out to reduce risks to zero, they can aim to reduce them to a lower and more acceptable level. In addition, people are naturally anxious to understand how their governments make risk management decisions.

How can governments satisfy the public that they are actively pursuing this objective? How should the relevant risk information be communicated? Some important lessons have been learned on the role of dialogue in risk communication between the public and governments *(20, 21)*. These lessons cover the most effective ways to handle and communicate with the public about important risks and are well illustrated by the recent epidemic of BSE in the United Kingdom (see Box 6.2). Practical guidelines for better communication have also been published *(22, 23)*. The main points can be summarized as follows.

- Release a full account of the known facts. Governments and public agencies are often tempted to present simplified explanations and not to reveal the full facts. In addition, uncertainties included in decision-making are often glossed over and reassuring advice is frequently presented to the public. This is now recognized to be a major mistake. Political credibility and public trust are rapidly lost if the public believes it has not been given the full information on the risks that affect it.

Box 6.2 Important lessons for governments on developing better risk communications

- To establish credibility it is necessary to generate trust
- Trust can only be generated by openness
- Openness requires recognition of uncertainty, where it exists
- The public should be trusted to respond rationally to openness
- The importance of precautionary measures should not be played down on the grounds that the risk is unproven
- Scientific investigation of risk should be open and transparent

- The advice and reasoning of advisory committees should be made public
- The trust that the public has in scientists, experts and professionals, such as chief medical officers, is precious and should not be put at risk
- Any advice to the public from such experts and advisory committees should be, and should be seen to be, objective and independent of government and political influence.

Adapted from: *(10)*. p. 266.

- Information should be released by an independent and trusted professional agency. It is also very important who communicates the information. This should be done by recognized experts who are well qualified in the subject and who are seen to be fully trustworthy, politically independent and without conflicts of interest. For public health in many countries, this important function is often best performed by the chief medical officer. For controversial information, in general, the public does not trust any messages conveyed by politicians or politically appointed spokespersons.

- An atmosphere of trust is needed between government officials, health experts, the general public and the media. This trust has to be developed and fostered. Condescending attitudes and the withholding of information can rapidly lead to public cynicism and accusations of a cover-up or a hidden scandal. Trust is easily lost but very difficult to regain.

The importance of developing trust between all parties has considerable implications for greater open government and its role in civil society. For instance, regulatory agencies need to be seen to be independent from political pressures, scientific information needs to be in the public domain, meetings of scientific advisory committees and their records need to be accessible for public scrutiny, and the mass media need to be free to investigate risks and publish their findings *(10)*.

STRENGTHENING THE SCIENTIFIC EVIDENCE BASE

There have been many scientific advances in risk assessment since the subject was established in the 1960s. However, it started by focusing largely on new technologies and external environmental threats and has only latterly been extended to take into account major biological and behavioural risks to health, such as blood pressure, unsafe sex and tobacco consumption. In addition, the science of risk assessment developed mainly in North America and later in Europe, while to date there has been little application of this science in middle and low income countries. Research studies are needed to see if the lessons learned on risk perceptions and communications in industrialized countries also remain applicable in developing countries. In addition, while some reasonable global data exist, such as for risks leading to cardiovascular diseases *(6, 24)*, data sources for other important risk factors require substantial improvement, especially for most middle and low income countries. There is an urgent need, therefore, to establish new data sources for developing countries.

The most important aspects of strengthening the scientific evidence base in risk assessment and management include the following activities.

- Collection of new scientific data on risk factors and exposures. For the most common and important risks to health, collection of the essential new data needs to be replicated in many more countries. This will require international support for methodological developments in such areas as standardized protocols, data collection instruments, approaches to statistical analysis, data archiving and exchange, and dissemination and use of research findings. Both qualitative and quantitative approaches will be necessary. Ongoing, regular collection of surveillance data is needed, in order to monitor trends in existing risk factors and to detect changes in exposure to risks and health outcomes associated with them.

- Establishment and support of new risk intervention research. Substantial public funding is required to undertake relevant research studies, particularly in developing countries, and to establish and develop regional centres of excellence in risk intervention research, training and advice. New research is needed, firstly, to compare risk perceptions in cross-national studies; secondly, to gather data on the frequency of risk factors and their levels in middle and low income populations; and thirdly, to evaluate the effectiveness and costs of different combinations of interventions. Strong support from the multilateral agencies and international donor and scientific communities will be essential.

- Coordination of research activities in different sectors. Given the complex and interdisciplinary nature of risk intervention research, coordination of both support and funding will be necessary at national and international levels. In countries this may require the establishment of new initiatives, such as research funds, specialized research units, appointment of government scientific advisers, and creation of new and independent scientific advisory committees that are free from political controls.

Urgent need for international action

This report has documented the substantial gains in healthy life expectancy that populations everywhere can expect from even modest reductions in exposure to major risk factors such as underweight, unsafe sex, tobacco use and elevated blood pressure. Scientific uncertainty should not be allowed to delay the control of large and important risk factors, many of which are already causing a large amount of disease burden. This burden is expected to increase dramatically unless widespread action is taken by individuals, civil society, governments and international organizations. For example, the consumption of tobacco could be substantially reduced, particularly in developing countries.

Enough reliable information exists about the causes of disease and injury to act today to reduce drastically the disease burden and achieve the potential gains foreseen in this report. Moreover, substantial agreement on what needs to be done also exists between the international scientific community and those charged with improving the public health. Strategies to achieve these potential gains, particularly in developing countries, ought to involve a question of balance. It is a balance between the priority of sharply reducing the burden from exposures such as underweight and poor water and sanitation, which are largely confined to poorer populations, and the priority of reducing or preventing further population exposure to factors such as tobacco, elevated blood pressure and cholesterol.

To achieve a truly healthier future, risk management strategies will need to focus simultaneously on what are now global risks to health, and not just on the more immediate challenges to survival. The World Health Organization and other parties in international development have a clear role to ensure that scientific knowledge is translated into action and to guide and encourage the global health community (see Box 6.3). This may well require a readiness to overcome opposition from influential special interest groups and powerful corporations that have most to lose from policies aimed at improving risk prevention and strengthening regulatory practices.

As this report shows, much is already known about how to reduce effectively risks to health. That reduction will require sustained policy action and commitment by governments and other partners. Key elements of this commitment will be the creation or strengthening of national institutions to implement and evaluate risk reduction programmes, and more effective engagement of sectors such as transport, education and finance to capitalize on the potential for greatly reducing population exposures.

Clearly, the world is facing global risks to health. Yet it is equally clear that dramatic reductions in risk and a healthier future for all can be achieved. What is required now is a global response, with strong and committed leadership, supported by all sectors of society concerned with promoting health.

Box 6.3 Examples of successful international concerted action

Scientific uncertainty should not be allowed to delay the control of large and important risk factors, given the evidence that substantial future reductions could be achieved. International partnerships have proved to be a powerful way forward, as the following examples show.

Framework Convention for Tobacco Control (FCTC)

Unless prevention is given a high priority, tobacco will kill about 10 million people each year by 2030 and 70% of the deaths will be in developing countries. The Framework Convention is being developed by the World Health Organization, based on its Constitution, and is currently under negotiation between the great majority of Member States. It will be an international legal instrument to which countries can sign up, to reduce the harm caused by tobacco. It comprises aspects such as advertising, regulation, smuggling, taxation, smoke-free zones and treatment of addiction. As many of these issues transcend national borders, regional and international cooperation is called for. The Framework Convention facilitates a multisectoral approach but also recognizes that the health sector has a leading responsibility to combat the tobacco epidemic. The first full draft Convention was issued in July 2002 and it is expected to be adopted in May 2003. In the next phase individual protocols will be developed.

web site http://www.who.int/tobacco/

Stop-TB Partnership

Each year tuberculosis causes two million deaths, many in association with HIV/AIDS. It is a disease of poverty, for which a very cost-effective drug treatment (DOTS) is available. In 2000, ministers from 20 of the 22 countries which account for 80% of the global TB burden issued the Amsterdam Stop-TB Declaration, setting explicit objectives to reduce the disease. The Stop-TB Partnership, which has an open membership of governments, nongovernmental organizations, foundations, individuals and others, is hosted by the World Health Organization. It is an advocacy and advisory public–private partnership that aims to detect 70% of all new infectious TB cases and cure 85% of them by 2005 and to halve deaths from TB by 2010. This called for a global DOTS expansion plan, strengthening of national control programmes, ensuring universal access to TB drugs, and promoting research into new drugs and vaccines.

web site http://www.stoptb.org

Global Alliance for Vaccines and Immunization (GAVI)

Following a fall in immunization coverage in many poor developing countries, this new international public–private partnership was launched in January 2000, with an initial donation of US$ 750 million from the Bill and Melinda Gates Foundation. Other members are governments, UNICEF, the World Bank, nongovernmental organizations and the vaccine industry. It is hosted by the World Health Organization and has a board and specialized task forces. It aims to raise coverage in the 74 poorest countries and to introduce new vaccines, including hepatitis B and Haemophilus influenzae type B. GAVI is making a five-year commitment. By June 2002, over US$ 900 million had been committed to 60 countries, mainly in Africa and Asia. GAVI has also been seen as a potential model for the new Global Fund to Fight AIDS, Tuberculosis and Malaria.

web site http://www.vaccinealliance.org

REFERENCES

1. Rose G. *The strategy of preventive medicine.* Oxford: Oxford University Press; 1992.

2. Rose G. Strategy of prevention: lessons from cardiovascular disease. *British Medical Journal* 1981; 282:1847-51.

3. Rose G. Sick individuals and sick populations. *International Journal of Epidemiology* 1985; 14:32-8.

4. Kinlay S, O'Connell D, Evans D, Halliday J. The cost-effectiveness of different blood-cholesterol lowering strategies in the prevention of cardiovascular disease. *Australian Journal of Public Health* 1994; 18:105-10.

5. Rodgers A, Lawes C, MacMahon S. Reducing the global burden of blood pressure- related cardiovascular disease. *Journal of Hypertension* 2000; 18(Supplement):S3-6.

6. Magnus P, Beaglehole R. The real contribution of the major risk factors to coronary epidemics – time to end the "Only 50%" myth. *Archives of Internal Medicine* 2001; 161:2657-60.

7. Rose G, Day S. The population mean predicts the number of deviant individuals. *British Medical Journal* 1990; 301:1031-4.

8. Dowie J. *Towards value-based, science-informed public health policy: conceptual framework and practical guidelines*. Geneva: World Health Organization; 2001. Background paper for *The World Health Report 2002*.

9. Slovic P, Gregory R. Risk analysis, decision analysis, and the social context for risk decision making. In: Shanteau J, Mellers BA, Schum DA, editors. *Decision science and technology: reflections on the contributions of Warne Edwards*. Boston: Kluwer Academic; 1999. p. 353-65.

10. Phillips, Lord, Bridgeman J, Fergusan-Smith M. *The Bovine Spongiform Encephalopathy (BSE) Inquiry (The Phillips Inquiry). Findings and conclusions, Volume 1*. London: The Stationery Office; 2001.

11. Pidgeon N. Risk perception. In: *Risk analysis, perception and management*. London: Royal Society; 1992. p. 89-134.

12. Bickerstaff K, Pidgeon N. *World Health Organization and Department of Health Conference on Risks to Public Health, London 23–24 October 2001*. Geneva: World Health Organization; and London: Department of Health; 2001. Report commissioned for *The World Health Report 2002*.

13. UNCED. *United Nations Conference on the Environment and Development, Rio de Janeiro, Brazil, 3–14 June 1992*. New York: United Nations; 1992.

14. ILGRA. *The precautionary principle: policy and application*. London: Department of Health Inter-departmental Liaison Group on Risk Assessment; 2001.

15. Hall W, Carter L. *Ethical issues in risk management*. Geneva: World Health Organization; 2001. Background paper for *The World Health Report 2002*.

16. Roberts MJ, Reich MR. Ethical analysis in public health. *Lancet* 2002; 359:1055-9.

17. Beauchamp TL, Childress JF. *Principles of medical ethics*. 5th edition. New York: Oxford University Press; 2001.

18. Slovic P. Informing and educating the public about risk. *Risk Analysis* 1986; 6:403-15.

19. Covello V, McCallum D, Pavlova M. *Effective risk communication: the role and responsibility of government and nongovernment organizations.* New York: Plenum Press; 1989.

20. Renn O. The role of communication and public dialogue for improving risk management. *Risk Decision and Policy* 1998; 3:5-30.

21. Calman K. Communication of risk: choice, consent and trust. *Lancet* 2002; 360:166-8.

22. Lum MR, Tinker TL. *A primer on health risk communication: principles and practices*. Atlanta (GA): US Department for Health and Human Services, Agency for Toxic Substances and Disease Registry; 1994.

23. Department of Health. *Communicating about risks to health: pointers to good practice*. London: The Stationery Office; 1998.

24. Ibrahim S, Smith GD. Systematic review of randomised controlled trials of multiple risk factor interventions for preventing coronary heart disease. *British Medical Journal* 1997; 314:1666-71.

CHAPTER SEVEN

Preventing Risks and Taking Action

More emphasis on preventing the causes of important diseases is the key to improving world health. Tackling major risks effectively could lead to up to ten years more of healthy life expectancy globally. Although the world faces some common, large and certain risks to health, effective and affordable interventions are available. Very substantial gains can be made for relatively modest expenditures, but bold government policies will be required. They should prioritize the most important risks and shift the main focus to include preventive measures that can be applied to the whole population. For example, governments can decide to aim for increased taxes on tobacco; legislation to reduce the proportion of salt and other unhealthy components in foods; stricter environmental controls and ambitious energy policies; and stronger health promotion and health safety campaigns. Reducing major risks will in turn reduce inequities in society, and promote both healthy life and sustainable development.

7

PREVENTING RISKS

AND TAKING ACTION

FOCUSING ON PREVENTION MEANS FOCUSING ON RISKS

*I*n order to protect and improve health around the world, much more emphasis is needed on preventing the actual causes of important diseases – the underlying risks to health – as well as treating the established diseases themselves. Prevention can best be achieved through concerted efforts to identify and reduce common, major risks and by taking advantage of the prevention opportunities they present.

This report shows that about 47% of global mortality is attributable to the leading 20 risk factors that have been assessed in earlier chapters, and that more than one third of that burden is attributable to just 10 of those factors. Tackling these risks effectively could lead to almost a decade more of healthy life expectancy globally. The potential improvements in global health are much greater than generally realized – extra years of healthy life expectancy could be gained for populations in all countries within the next decade.

The greatest gains would be in some of the poorest nations – with perhaps ten more healthy life years achievable. The potential benefits extend across all countries and all levels of socioeconomic development. Even in the most developed countries of North America and Europe, another five or so years of healthy life expectancy for the population is within reach.

Looking towards the potential global burden of disease in the next two decades, Chapter 4 showed that reducing risk by 25% will result in large amounts of that burden being avoided. Translated into human terms, this offers the prospect of millions of premature deaths being averted, and of many more millions of people being spared years of disease, disability and ill-health. It might mean, for example, that in the year 2010 more than a million deaths from HIV/AIDS and the loss of 40 million healthy life years related to unsafe sex would be averted, as would more than a million deaths and over 35 million lost healthy life years from cardiovascular diseases related to blood pressure and cholesterol.

However, Chapter 4 also gave a measure of the cost of inaction. It predicted that by the year 2020 there will be nine million deaths caused by tobacco, compared to almost five million a year now; five million deaths attributable to overweight and obesity, compared to three million now; and that the number of healthy life years lost by underweight children will be 60 million, which although less than half the 130 million now, is still unacceptably high.

This report represents one of the largest research projects ever coordinated by the World Health Organization. It has quantified many of the important global risks and assessed the cost-effectiveness of measures to reduce them. The ultimate goal is to support governments in all countries to lower the impact of these risks.

The conclusions have already been described as a wake-up call to health leaders around the world. They are also the basis for building a healthier future for entire populations across the world.

THE WORLD FACES SOME COMMON, LARGE AND CERTAIN RISKS TO HEALTH

Leading 10 selected risk factors as percentage causes of disease burden measured in DALYs

Developing countries	
High mortality countries	
Underweight	14.9%
Unsafe sex	10.2%
Unsafe water, sanitation and hygiene	5.5%
Indoor smoke from solid fuels	3.6%
Zinc deficiency	3.2%
Iron deficiency	3.1%
Vitamin A deficiency	3.0%
Blood pressure	2.5%
Tobacco	2.0%
Cholesterol	1.9%
Low mortality countries	
Alcohol	6.2%
Blood pressure	5.0%
Tobacco	4.0%
Underweight	3.1%
Overweight	2.7%
Cholesterol	2.1%
Low fruit and vegetable intake	1.9%
Indoor smoke from solid fuels	1.9%
Iron deficiency	1.8%
Unsafe water, sanitation and hygiene	1.8%

Developed countries	
Tobacco	12.2%
Blood pressure	10.9%
Alcohol	9.2%
Cholesterol	7.6%
Overweight	7.4%
Low fruit and vegetable intake	3.9%
Physical inactivity	3.3%
Illicit drugs	1.8%
Unsafe sex	0.8%
Iron deficiency	0.7%

There are countless risks to health, but even among the selected major risks in this report, relatively few are responsible for large amounts of the global disease burden. Almost all of them are more common among the world's poor than the better-off. Until now, their true impact has been underestimated, particularly in developing countries.

The picture that has emerged from this research gives an intriguing – and alarming – insight into current and important causes of diseases and death and the factors underlying them. Human behaviour and societies are changing around the world and global changes are having a large impact on people's health.

The table, left, shows the top 10 selected risk factors as causes of disease burden in high and low mortality developing countries and in developed countries. While this table shows the burden attributable to the selected factors at a global level, it does not show the high risks faced by certain sections of the population (for example, the many people whose occupations place them at high risk of life-threatening injury or chronic disease), or the burden resulting from major diseases (such as malaria, tuberculosis and HIV/AIDS which in total cause more than 10% of global disease burden). Also, the combined effects of the risk factors in this table will be less than the sum of their separate effects.

- At least 30% % of all disease burden occurring in high mortality developing countries, such as those in sub-Saharan Africa and South-East Asia, is due to just five risk factors: underweight, unsafe sex, micronutrient deficiencies, unsafe water, and indoor smoke. Risks associated with food insecurity, hunger and malnutrition still dominate the health of the world's poorest nations. Most of the childhood deaths in developing countries each year are associated with malnutrition. In addition, the consequences of unsafe sex are fuelling the HIV/AIDS epidemics in Africa and Asia.

- In low mortality developing countries, such as the People's Republic of China and most countries in Central and South America, the top five risk factors cause at least one sixth of their total disease burden. These populations face a double burden of risks. Indeed, the analysis on which this report is based shows how these countries already face many of the same risks as industrialized countries – tobacco and high blood pressure, for example – while also having to contend with major remaining problems of undernutrition and communicable diseases.

- At the same time in the developed countries of North America, Europe and the Asian Pacific, at least one-third of all disease burden is attributable to these five risk factors: tobacco, alcohol, blood pressure, cholesterol and obesity. The tobacco epidemic alone kills about 2.4 million people every year in industrialized countries. In addition, suboptimal levels of blood pressure and cholesterol each cause millions of deaths annually, and increasing levels of overweight are leading to epidemics of obesity and diabetes.

The world is living dangerously – either because it has little choice, or because it is making the wrong choices. Today there are more than six billion people coexisting on this fragile planet. On one side are the many millions who are dangerously short of the food, water and security they need to live. Developing countries still face a high and highly concentrated burden from poverty, undernutrition, unsafe sex, unsafe water, poor sanitation and hygiene, iron deficiency and indoor smoke from solid fuels. On the other side lies unhealthy consumption, particularly of tobacco and alcohol. The risks from blood pressure and cholesterol, strongly linked to heart attacks and strokes, are also closely related to excessive consumption of fatty, sugary and salty foods. They become even more dangerous when combined with the deadly forces of tobacco and excessive alcohol consumption. Obesity, a result of unhealthy consumption coupled with lack of physical activity, is itself a serious health risk.

All of these risk factors – blood pressure, cholesterol, tobacco, alcohol and obesity – and the diseases linked to them are well known to wealthy societies. The real drama is that they now also increasingly dominate in low mortality developing countries where they create a double burden on top of the infectious diseases that always have afflicted poorer countries. They are even becoming more prevalent in high mortality developing countries.

EFFECTIVE AND AFFORDABLE PREVENTIVE INTERVENTIONS ARE AVAILABLE

Every country has major risks to health that are known, definite and increasing, sometimes largely unchecked; cost-effective interventions exist but are underutilized.

Very substantial health gains can be made for relatively modest expenditures. Chapter 4 examined in detail the cost-effectiveness of many interventions. Some of the most important findings are briefly described below.

- A strategy to protect the child's environment is cost-effective in all settings, with very cost-effective components including some form of micronutrient supplementation, such as vitamin A, iron, and zinc; disinfection of water at point of use to reduce the incidence of diarrhoeal diseases; and treatment of diarrhoea and pneumonia.
- Improved water supply based on disinfection at point of use is cost-effective in regions of high child mortality. While acknowledging that regulated piped water supplies will be the long-term aim of most countries, a policy shift towards household water management appears to be the most attractive short-term water-related health intervention in developing countries.
- Preventive interventions to reduce the incidence of HIV infections, including measures to encourage safer injection practices, are very cost-effective. The use of some

types of antiretroviral therapy in conjunction with preventive activities is cost-effective in most settings.

- At least one type of intervention to reduce the risks associated with cardiovascular disease is cost-effective in all settings. Population-wide salt and cholesterol lowering strategies are always very cost-effective singly and combined. The most attractive combined strategy to reduce the risks associated with cardiovascular disease appears to be the combination of salt reduction at a population level through legislation or voluntary agreements, health education through the mass media focusing on blood pressure, cholesterol and overweight; plus the implementation of an individual risk reduction approach.

> **Some of the affordable solutions described in this report are closely related to two priority actions that WHO has outlined for the coming years:**
>
> • promoting healthy environments for children;
>
> • reinvigorating WHO's work on diet, food safety and human nutrition, linking basic research with efforts to tackle specific nutrient deficiencies in populations and the promotion of good health through optimal diets – particularly in countries undergoing rapid nutritional transition.

- Tobacco, of course, is a major risk for cardiovascular disease. In terms of interventions, the greatest tobacco-related improvements in population health would be a combination of tobacco taxation, comprehensive bans on advertising, and information dissemination activities, all of which would be affordable and cost-effective in most parts of the world. Adding restrictions of smoking in public places increases the costs, but also gains even greater improvements in population health and is still very cost-effective in industrialized countries.

NARROWING THE GAP BETWEEN POTENTIAL AND ACTUAL BENEFIT: A KEY RESEARCH PRIORITY

Despite the availability of cost-effective interventions to reduce risks, this report says there is a large potential benefit that is not realizable with current strategies and technologies. Unacceptably large gaps remain in understanding the effects of exposures on populations at different stages of development. Similar uncertainties apply to how health systems might be better adapted to achieve substantial overall health gains through more affordable preparations and delivery methods. More fundamental research is needed in order to transfer effectively the scientific knowledge on hazards that will help change human behaviour and lower individual risks. If policy-makers are to be more effectively engaged in applying measures that have proven benefits in risk reduction, the political context of knowledge transfer and risk management needs to be better understood and utilized. A key research priority is the development of new interventions, particularly for leading diseases. Together with more efficient primary prevention, these interventions can be expected to reduce substantially the risk burden in all populations.

POPULATION-WIDE PREVENTION STRATEGIES: KEY TO RISK REDUCTION

"It makes little sense to expect individuals to behave differently from their peers; it is more appropriate to seek a general change in behavioural norms and in the circumstances which facilitate their adoption." (Rose, 1982)

The great potential of prevention strategies that aim to achieve moderate, but population-wide, reductions in risks is yet to be fully recognized. Only a fraction of the benefits forecast in this report would arise from strategies directed towards the minority of people at high risk above commonly used thresholds (such as severe underweight, hypertension or obesity). However, achieving this potential requires a change in "ownership" of responsibility for tackling these big risks – away from individuals at the extremes and towards governments and ministries of health tackling population-wide risk levels. Not only do governments need to increase non-personal health services, but they must also ensure much broader access to cost-effective personal health services.

GOVERNMENT RESPONSIBILITY FOR HEALTH

REDUCING MAJOR RISKS TO HEALTH WILL PROMOTE SUSTAINABLE DEVELOPMENT

The most important rationale for dealing with major risks is, of course, a humanitarian one. However, it is increasingly clear that investment in health is also a means of stimulating economic growth and reducing poverty. The development goals that challenge governments cannot be reached in the face of widespread ill-health, particularly among poor people. Alleviation of hunger and malnutrition is a fundamental prerequisite for poverty reduction and sustainable development. In many countries, particularly those in sub-Saharan Africa, the AIDS epidemic is a national emergency that undermines develop-

> **There are several other compelling reasons for governments to play a greater role in tackling major risks to health:**
>
> - **Reducing major risks to health will promote sustainable development**
>
> - **Reducing major risks can reduce inequities in society**
>
> - **Governments need to prioritize and focus on the most important risks**
>
> - **Exercising stewardship means fulfilling the government's responsibility to protect its citizens**

ment, compounding the impact of conflict, food shortages and other causes of poverty. It drives and perpetuates the poverty of individuals, families and societies. Promoting safe sex to reduce HIV/AIDS must be at the core of public policy, of poverty reduction strategies, of action for sustainable development, and of human security. It requires intensive and concerted action by many different agencies across different sectors, coordinated by government.

REDUCING MAJOR RISKS CAN REDUCE INEQUITIES IN SOCIETY

Almost all the risk factors assessed in this report occur more commonly in the poor, who typically also have less autonomy and fewer resources to reduce risks. While personal services are more likely to be adopted by the well-off, and hence may even increase inequalities, government-directed population-wide changes can benefit whole communities. The benefits of such changes are likely to be greatest in the poor among whom risks are greatest, and thus inequalities will be reduced. Tackling major risks has the potential to substantially reduce inequalities worldwide.

GOVERNMENTS NEED TO PRIORITIZE AND FOCUS ON THE MOST IMPORTANT RISKS

Many major risks require considerable resources to forge the essential social consensus required for tackling them. For example, a mixture of public and private sector agreements and legislation are required to create the social milieu for health gains resulting from tobacco taxation or gradual changes to food manufacturing. Achieving such changes in the social milieu are a substantial challenge for governments. Since all risks cannot be targeted simultaneously, there should be a focus on those with the greatest potential for short and long-term improvement.

Exercising stewardship means fulfilling the government's responsibility to protect its citizens

Although governments rarely can hope to reduce risks to zero, they can aim to lower them to a more acceptable level, and explain, through open communication with the public, why and how they are doing so. Governments are the stewards of health resources. This stewardship has been defined as "a function of a government responsible for the welfare of the population and concerned about the trust and legitimacy with which its activities are viewed by the citizenry". The careful and responsible management of population well-being is the very essence of good government. With regard to risks to health, therefore, governments must take a long-term view and have the vision to tackle major, common and complex risks, even if they do not have high public appeal. Governments should not respond disproportionately to risks that are controversial and newsworthy, but rare, yet must still respond appropriately to highly uncertain or unknown risks.

Recommended actions

This report offers a unique opportunity for governments. They can use it to take bold and determined actions against only a relatively few major risks to health, in the knowledge that the likely result within the next ten years will be large gains in healthy life expectancy for their citizens. The potential benefits apply equally to poor countries and rich countries, even if some of the risk factors are different.

Bold policies are required. They may, for example, have to focus on increased taxes on tobacco; legislation to reduce the proportion of salt and other unhealthy components in foods; stricter environmental controls and ambitious energy policies; and stronger health promotion and health safety campaigns.

At the same time, governments will need to strengthen the scientific and empirical evidence bases for their policies. They will have to improve public dialogue and communications; develop greater levels of trust for risk prevention among all interested parties; and consider carefully a range of ethical and other issues.

This is undoubtedly a radical approach. It requires governments to see the value of shifting the main focus from the minority of high-risk individuals to include preventive measures that can be applied to the whole population.

For many of the main risk factors there is likely to be good agreement between the general public and public health experts on what needs to be done once a dialogue begins. In some countries, risk understanding may need to be strengthened among the general public, politicians and public health practitioners.

Recommended actions that governments can take in risk reduction have been tailored to suit high, middle and low income countries, but in general the report recommends the following.

- Governments, especially health ministries, should play a stronger role in formulating risk prevention policies, including more support for scientific research, improved surveillance systems and better access to global information.
- Countries should give top priority to developing effective, committed policies for the prevention of large risks to health. The right balance should be struck between population-wide risk reduction and aiming to reduce risk in a smaller number of high-risk individuals. The former has great, often unrealized, potential.

- Cost-effectiveness analyses should be used to identify high, medium and low priority interventions to prevent or reduce risks, with highest priority given to those interventions that are cost-effective and affordable.
- Intersectoral and international collaboration to reduce major extraneous risk to health, such as unsafe water and sanitation or a lack of education, is likely to have large health benefits and should be increased, especially in poorer countries.
- Similarly, international and intersectoral collaboration should be strengthened to improve risk management and increase public awareness and understanding of risks to health.
- A balance between government, community and individual action is necessary. For example, the great potential from community action by nongovernmental organizations, local groups, the media and others should be encouraged and expanded.

REDUCING RISKS, PROMOTING HEALTHY LIFE

In conclusion, it is clear that the world faces some large, common and certain risks to health. Over 20 major risk factors identified in this report are already responsible for about almost half of the total number of global premature deaths occurring each year. The leading 10 of them account for one-third of all deaths worldwide.

Furthermore, although many major risk factors are usually associated with high income countries, in fact over half of the total global burden of diseases they cause already occurs in low and middle income countries.

Most of these risk factors are well understood scientifically, and estimates of their risk probabilities and consequences are available. Many cost-effective interventions are also known and prevention strategies are potentially transferable between similar countries. Thus most of the important scientific and economic information is already available for policy decisions that could significantly improve global health.

What is now required is concerted, government-led action. The result of reducing risks and promoting healthy life will have a wide and lasting social value, even beyond preventing death and disability, for each country.

Statistical Annex

The first five tables in this technical annex present updated information on the burden of disease, summary measures of population health and national health accounts for WHO Member States and Regions. Population health measures for 2000 have been revised to take new data into account and differ from those published in The World Health Report 2001 *for many Member States. The work leading to these annex tables was undertaken mostly by the WHO Global Programme on Evidence for Health Policy and the Department of Health Financing and Stewardship in collaboration with counterparts from the Regional Offices of WHO. The material in these tables will be presented on an annual basis in each* World Health Report. *This annex also contains tables on the selection of risk factors considered in this report, with ranges of uncertainty for global estimates of their attributable burden. The prevalence of risk factors, attributable mortality, attributable years of life lost and attributable DALYs is also given. The risk factors have been grouped under seven separate headings. These are childhood and maternal undernutrition, other diet-related risk factors, sexual and reproductive health, addictive substances, environmental risks, occupational risks, and other risks to health.*

STATISTICAL ANNEX

EXPLANATORY NOTES

The tables in this technical annex present updated information on the burden of disease, summary measures of population health and national health accounts for WHO Member States and Regions. Population health measures for 2000 have been revised to take new data into account and differ from those published in *The World Health Report 2001* for many Member States. The work leading to these annex tables was undertaken mostly by the WHO Global Programme on Evidence for Health Policy and the Department of Health Financing and Stewardship in collaboration with counterparts from the Regional Offices of WHO. The material in these tables will be presented on an annual basis in each *World Health Report*. Working papers have been prepared which provide details on the concepts, methods and results that are only briefly mentioned here. The footnotes to these technical notes include a complete listing of the detailed working papers.

As with any innovative approach, methods and data sources can be refined and improved. It is hoped that careful scrutiny and use of the results will lead to progressively better measurement of health attainment and health expenditure data in the coming *World Health Reports*. All the main health results are reported with uncertainty intervals in order to communicate to the user the plausible range of estimates for each country on each measure. Where data are presented by country, initial WHO estimates and technical explanations were sent to Member States for comment. Comments or data provided in response were discussed with them and incorporated where possible. The estimates reported here should still be interpreted as the best estimates of WHO rather than the official viewpoint of Member States.

ANNEX TABLE 1

To assess overall levels of health achievement, it is crucial to develop the best possible assessment of the life table for each country. New life tables have been developed for all 191 Member States starting with a systematic review of all available evidence from surveys, censuses, sample registration systems, population laboratories and vital registration on levels and trends in child mortality and adult mortality.[1] This review benefited greatly from the work undertaken on child mortality by UNICEF[2] and on general mortality by the United States Census Bureau[3] and the UN Population Division 2000 demographic assessment.[4] All estimates of population size and structure for 2000 and 2001 are based on the 2000 and 2001 demographic assessments prepared by the United Nations Population Division.[4] UN estimates refer to the de facto resident population, and not the de jure population in each Member State. To aid in demographic, cause of death and burden of disease analyses, the

191 Member States have been divided into five mortality strata on the basis of their level of child and adult male mortality. The matrix defined by the six WHO Regions and the five mortality strata leads to 14 subregions, since not every mortality stratum is represented in every Region. These subregions are defined in the List of Member States by WHO Region and mortality stratum and used in Annex Tables 2 and 3 for presentation of results.

Because of increasing heterogeneity of patterns of adult and child mortality, WHO has developed a model life table system of two-parameter logit life tables using a global standard, with additional age-specific parameters to correct for systematic biases in the application of a two-parameter system.[5] This system of model life tables has been used extensively in the development of life tables for those Member States without adequate vital registration and in projecting life tables to 2000 and 2001 when the most recent data available are from earlier years.

Demographic techniques (Preston–Coale method, Brass Growth–Balance method, Generalized Growth–Balance method and Bennett–Horiuchi method) have been applied, as appropriate, to assess the level of completeness of recorded mortality data for Member States with vital registration systems. For Member States without national vital registration systems, all available survey, census and vital registration data were assessed, adjusted and averaged to estimate the probable trend in child mortality over the past few decades. This trend was projected to estimate child mortality levels in 2000 and 2001. In addition, adult sibling survival data from available population surveys was analysed to obtain additional information on adult mortality.

The World Health Organization uses a standard method to estimate and project life tables for all Member States with comparable data. This may lead to minor differences compared with official life tables prepared by Member States. Life expectancies for the year 2000 for many Member States have been revised from those published in *The World Health Report 2001* to take into account more recently available mortality data.

To capture the uncertainty due to sampling, indirect estimation technique or projection to 2000, a total of 1000 life tables have been developed for each Member State. Ninety-five per cent uncertainty bounds are reported in Annex Table 1 by giving key life table values at the 2.5th percentile and the 97.5th percentile. This uncertainty analysis was facilitated by the development of new methods and software tools.[6] In countries with a substantial HIV epidemic, recent estimates of the level and uncertainty range of the magnitude of the HIV epidemic have been incorporated into the life table uncertainty analysis.[7]

ANNEX TABLES 2 AND 3

Causes of death for the 14 subregions and the world have been estimated based on data from national vital registration systems that capture about 18.6 million deaths annually. In addition, information from sample registration systems, population laboratories and epidemiological analyses of specific conditions has been used to improve estimates of the cause of death patterns.[8] WHO is intensifying efforts with Member States to obtain and verify recent vital registration data on causes of death.

Cause of death data have been carefully analysed to take into account incomplete coverage of vital registration in countries and the likely differences in cause of death patterns that would be expected in the uncovered and often poorer subpopulations. Techniques to undertake this analysis have been developed based on the global burden of disease study[9] and further refined using a much more extensive database and more robust modelling techniques.[10]

Special attention has been paid to problems of misattribution or miscoding of causes of death in cardiovascular diseases, cancer, injuries and general ill-defined categories. A correction algorithm for reclassifying ill-defined cardiovascular codes has been developed.[11] Cancer mortality by site has been evaluated using both vital registration data and population-based cancer incidence registries. The latter have been analysed using a complete age, period cohort model of cancer survival in each region.[12]

Annex Table 3 provides estimates of the burden of disease using disability-adjusted life years (DALYs) as a measure of the health gap in the world in 2001. DALYs along with healthy life expectancy are summary measures of population health.[13, 14] One DALY can be thought of as one lost year of "healthy" life and the burden of disease as a measurement of the gap between the current health of a population and an ideal situation where everyone in the population lives to old age in full health. DALYs for a disease or health condition are calculated as the sum of the years of life lost due to premature mortality (YLL) in the population and the years lost due to disability (YLD) for incident cases of the health condition. For a review of the development of the DALY and recent advances in the measurement of the burden of disease, see Murray & Lopez.[15] For a more comprehensive review of the conceptual and other issues underlying summary measures of population health, see Murray et al.[14] DALYs for 2001 have been estimated based on cause of death information for each Region and regional assessments of the epidemiology of major disabling conditions. For this report, burden of disease estimates have been updated for many of the cause categories included in the Global Burden of Disease 2000 study, based on the wealth of data on major diseases and injuries available to WHO technical programmes and through collaboration with scientists worldwide.[8] Examples are the extensive data sets on tuberculosis, maternal conditions, injuries, diabetes, cancer, and sexually transmitted infections. These data, together with new and revised estimates of deaths by cause, age and sex, for all Member States, have been used to develop internally consistent estimates of incidence, prevalence, duration and DALYs for over 130 major causes, for 14 subregions of the world.

ANNEX TABLE 4

Annex Table 4 reports the average level of population health for WHO Member States in terms of healthy life expectancy. Based on more than 15 years of work, WHO introduced disability-adjusted life expectancy (DALE) as a summary measure of the level of health attained by populations in *The World Health Report 2000*.[16,17] To better reflect the inclusion of all states of health in the calculation of healthy life expectancy, the name of the indicator used to measure healthy life expectancy has been changed from disability-adjusted life expectancy (DALE) to health-adjusted life expectancy (HALE). HALE is based on life expectancy at birth (see Annex Table 1) but includes an adjustment for time spent in poor health. It is most easily understood as the equivalent number of years in full health that a newborn can expect to live based on current rates of ill-health and mortality.

The measurement of time spent in poor health is based on combining condition-specific estimates from the Global Burden of Disease 2000 study with estimates of the prevalence of different health states by age and sex derived from health surveys.[17, 18] As noted above, for this year's *World Health Report*, burden of disease estimates of prevalences for specific diseases, injuries and their sequelae have been updated for many of the cause categories included in the Global Burden of Disease (GBD) 2000 study. [8]

Analyses of over 50 national health surveys for the calculation of healthy life expectancy in *The World Health Report 2000* identified severe limitations in the comparability of self-reported health status data from different populations, even when identical survey instruments and methods are used.[19, 20] The WHO Household Survey Study[21] carried out 69 representative household surveys in 60 Member States in 2000 and 2001 using a new health status instrument based on the International Classification of Functioning, Disability and Health,[22] which seeks information from a representative sample of respondents on their current states of health according to six core domains. These domains were identified from an extensive review of the currently available health status measurement instruments. To overcome the problem of comparability of self-report health data, the WHO survey instrument used performance tests and vignettes to calibrate self-reported health on selected domains such as cognition, mobility and vision. WHO has developed several statistical methods for correcting biases in self-reported health using these data, based on the hierarchical ordered probit (HOPIT) model.[23-25] The calibrated responses are used to estimate the true prevalence of different states of health by age and sex.

Annex Table 4 reports average HALE at birth for Member States for 2000 and 2001, and for 2001 the following additional information: HALE at age 60, expected lost healthy years (LHE) at birth, per cent of total life expectancy lost, and 95% uncertainty intervals. LHE is calculated as life expectancy (LE) minus HALE and is the expected equivalent number of years of full health lost through living in health states of less than full health. The percentage of total life expectancy lost is LHE expressed as a percentage of total LE and represents the proportion of total life expectancy that is lost through living in health states of less than full health. HALEs for 2000 differ from those published in *The World Health Report 2001* for many Member States, as they incorporate new epidemiological information, new data from health surveys, and new information on mortality rates, as well as improvements in survey analysis methods.[24]

The uncertainty ranges for healthy life expectancy given in Annex Table 4 are based on the 2.5th percentile and 97.5th percentile of the relevant uncertainty distributions.[6] The ranges thus define 95% uncertainty intervals around the estimates. HALE uncertainty is a function of the uncertainty in age-specific mortality measurement for each country, of the uncertainty in burden of disease based estimates of country-level disability prevalence, and of uncertainty in the health state prevalences derived from health surveys.

ANNEX TABLE 5

Sources and methods

The estimates for the six years 1995–2000 exhibited in Annex 5 have been submitted for comments to the national authorities of Member States. They remain, however, WHO estimates. As in every developmental work of this kind, some estimates change from the previous exhibit, i.e. Annex Table 5 of *The World Health Report 2001*. The resulting synthesis of expenditure on health trends represents a measurement of the state-of-the-art in the middle of 2002 and orders of magnitude, that extends beyond what was achieved in the previous exercise.

Content

The indicators selected emphasize the financing agents facet. Macroeconomic and social accounting processes are multidimensional in nature, consisting in monitoring the origin of funds and the operations of managers that mobilize these funds. This monitoring also includes the allocation to providers of care and other interventions necessary for a health system to operate, the use of the resources delivered, and the benefits that accrue to different population segments. Several hundred rows of statistical data and calculations for each health system are thus necessary.

The table shown tracks the details of two groups of entities: general government and private agents. General government comprises the central or federal government, regional/ state/provincial authorities, municipal and local authorities, and autonomous trust funds or boards implementing government policies, principally social protection agencies or social security schemes. In many countries, subnational authorities obtain their resources from the national taxation system and other intragovernment transfer mechanisms. This implies that a simple addition of the various layers of government would lead to double counting. The deconsolidation procedure in the absence of detailed records also entails, however, a risky procedure: national and subnational authorities or autonomous funds dealing with the health system do not systematically adhere to the same accounting conventions.

External resources earmarked for health programmes, a financing source, is also included, comprising concessional loans and grants for medical care and medical goods channelled through the Ministry of Health or via the Ministry of Finance or Central Bank.

General government expenditure on health (GGHE) is the sum of outlays on health paid for by taxes, social security contributions and external resources (without double-counting the government transfers to social security and extrabudgetary funds). Social security and extrabudgetary funds on health include the expenditure to purchase health goods and services by schemes that are compulsory, under governmental control, and covering a sizeable segment of the population. A major hurdle has consisted in verifying that no double counting occurs and that no cash benefits for sickness and/or loss of employment are included in the estimates, as these are classified as income maintenance expenditure.

The private sector comprises four types of entities: those that pool resources in order to purchase medical goods and services and, sometimes, to finance delivery facilities; these prepaid private risk-pooling plans include the outlays of private social insurance schemes, commercial and non-profit (mutual) insurance schemes, health maintenance organizations and other agents managing prepaid medical and paramedical benefits, including the operating costs of these schemes. Non-financial corporations provide medical and paramedical goods and services to their employees on top of compulsory social insurance or resource pooling entities. Nongovernmental organizations and non-profit institutions use resources to purchase health goods and services that are not allowed to be a source of income, profit or other financial gain for the units that establish, control or finance them. Households share out-of-pocket in the costs of many publicly funded programmes, top-up benefits accessible through private pooling, and initiate self-diagnose and self-care without intervention of the health system which they belong. Included are gratuities and payments in-kind made to health practitioners and to suppliers of pharmaceuticals and therapeutic appliances.

In Annex Table 5, the general government and private expenditure on health flows are expressed as ratios. The denominators are the gross domestic product (GDP), which corresponds to the total sum of expenditure (consumption and investment) of the private and government agents of the economy, and general government expenditure (GGE), which corresponds to the consolidated outlays of all levels of government (territorial authorities: central/federal, provincial/regional/state/district, municipal/local), social security institutions, and extrabudgetary funds, including capital outlays. The per capita figures reported here are calculated using population data supplied by the UN Population Division (for non-OECD Member States) and the OECD (for OECD countries). UN estimates refer to the de facto resident population rather than the de jure population. These figures are not necessarily the official estimates of all Member States, and the per capita expenditures reported here may differ from offical estimates of Member States accordingly. Per capita figures are expressed in US$ at exchange rates, as the observed annual average number of units at which a currency is traded in the banking system, or in international dollar estimates, derived by dividing local currency units by an estimate of their purchasing power parity (PPP) compared to US$, i.e. a rate or measure that eliminates the consequences of differences in price levels existing between countries.

Sources of data

A modelling process is inherent to the construction of any accounting system, private or public, but for all 191 countries part of the health accounting construct rests on national information. Only a minority of Member States have released health accounts data for all years from 1995–2000 contained in Annex Table 5.

The International Monetary Fund at the level of 101 nations has pioneered in releasing a "functional" breakdown of central government expenditure, which has served as a pilot to track government expenditure. When no national source was accessed, the IMF *Government finance statistics yearbook 2001,* Washington 2001, has been the source that served as a base. An exception relates to the OECD Member countries for which OECD *Health data 2002* served as the reference, requiring a few extrapolations to the year 2000 for a small number of cases or missed-out figures for the mid-1990s.

For the remainder, sources included United Nations national accounts, both for public and/or private expenditure on health; World Bank Development indicators; national statistical yearbooks and other reports containing estimates consistent with the principles underlying the data lifted from the sources quoted; household surveys; WHO secretariat estimates and correspondence with officials in Member States; and partial entries have had to be supplemented. As with all accounts constructed in the world, this set of accounts comprises numbers of imputations of missing cells: the foundations are the statistical series of what countries release about their health systems, statements which are rarely comprehensive, consistent, or timely.

The Development Assistance Committee of the OECD has a huge database of the commitments made by the principal external financing countries; it cross-classifies these by country in favour of which programmes are earmarked and by purpose. By courtesy of the OECD secretariat, a file has been processed from the data stored by that institution. Appropriations for external assistance are not spent overnight but vary according to the absorptive capacity of the recipient country and the nature and size of the programme. The funds are typically spent between two and ten years after commitment. The amounts on record have been crudely distributed as spent over periods ranging usually from two to five years, an element of uncertainty that has been corrected by "importing" data from a few recipient health ministries, finance – economic development – or economic planning ministries whenever accessed.

Although standardized methods to calculate GDP have been agreed to at world level, many Member States continue to release GDP figures that are partly based on other concepts. For the purposes of *The World Health Report 2002* annex, standardized concepts are used. The GDP was obtained from United Nations National accounts, a prepublication compilation supplied by courtesy of the UN Statistics Department, or IMF International financial statistics, Yearbook 2001 and June 2002 issue, or OECD National accounts 2002, and follows the new standard of the System of National Accounts (SNA93) time series whenever the Member States' statistical agencies moved to the new concepts and definitions, or of the SNA68 for the others. General government expenditures are taken from United Nations National accounts 1995–1997, Table 1.4 extrapolated to 2000; OECD National accounts; volume II; IMF *International financial statistics*, Yearbook 2001 and June 2002 issue (central government disbursements grossed up to include where possible regional and local authorities). Exchange rates were taken from IMF *International financial statistics*, June 2002 issue. International dollars have been estimated by WHO using methods similar to those used by the World Bank. PPPs are based on price comparison studies for 1996 where they exist. For other countries they are estimated using the GDP per capita in US $, inflation trends, and various dummy variables accounting for regional differences. Forward projections to 2000 are made using the real GDP growth rate adjusted by the relative rate of inflation between the country in question and the United States.

The System of health accounts methodology pioneered by the OECD has served as an overall guideline to compile the estimates contained in Annex Table 5 and to mould hundreds of heterogeneous sources of information into a rigorous and comparative format. The estimates presented are as honest as possible a measurement of what Member States release about their health systems for one or more years. The records accessible, though intended to be those relating to executed and, preferably, audited budgets, relate sometimes only to "prospective" spending of the institutions which have health in their portfolio. These may also be accountable for other environmental and social policy goals and, in parallel, non-health ministries conduct programmes that pursue mainly the achievement of the nation's health goals.

For statistical purposes, the data for China do not include those for the Hong Kong Special Administrative Region and the Macao Special Administrative Region. For Jordan, data for territory under occupation since 1967 by Israel are excluded.

The following section gives a list of all the risk factors considered in this report according to the groupings that have been used, with ranges of uncertainty for global estimates of attributable burden. The prevalence of risk factors, attributable mortality, attributable years of life lost and attributable DALYs is also given.

The risk factors have been grouped under seven separate headings. The first, childhood and maternal undernutrition, includes underweight, deficiencies in iron, vitamin A and zinc. The second group, referring to other diet-related risk factors, consists of high blood pressure, high cholesterol, overweight, low fruit and vegetable intake, and also physical inactivity. The third group is concerned with sexual and reproductive health and consists of unsafe sex and lack of contraception. The fourth group comprises addictive substances, which includes smoking and oral tobacco use, alcohol use and illicit drug use. The fifth group, on environmental risks, consists of unsafe water, sanitation and hygiene, urban air pollution, indoor smoke from solid fuels, lead exposure and climate change. The sixth group is a selection of occupational risks, namely work-related risk factors for injuries, and work-related carcinogens, airborne particulates, ergonomic stressors and noise. The seventh group comprises other selected risks to health of unsafe medical injections and childhood sexual abuse. A full description of the methods used is contained in the Explanatory Notes of the Statistical Annex on *The World Health Report 2002* web site (www.who.int/whr).

[1] Lopez AD, Ahmad O, Guillot M, Ferguson BD, Salomon JA, Murray CJL, Hill KH (2002). *World Mortality in 2000: Life Tables for 191 Countries.* Geneva, World Health Organization.

[2] Hill K, Rohini PO, Mahy M, Jones G (1999). *Trends in child mortality in the developing world: 1960 to 1996.* New York, UNICEF.

[3] United States Bureau of the Census: International database available at http://www.census.gov/ipc/www/idbnew.html

[4] *World population prospects: the 2000 revision* (2001). New York , United Nations.

[5] Murray CJL, Ferguson B, Lopez AD, Guillot M, Salomon JA, Ahmad O (2001). *Modified-logit life table system: principles, empirical validation and application.* Geneva, World Health Organization (GPE Discussion Paper No. 39).

[6] Salomon JA, Mathers CD, Murray CJL, Ferguson B (2001). *Methods for life expectancy and healthy life expectancy uncertainty analysis.* Geneva, World Health Organization (GPE Discussion Paper No. 10).

[7] Salomon JA, Murray CJL (2001). Modelling HIV/AIDS epidemics in sub-Saharan Africa using seroprevalence data from antenatal clinics. *Bulletin of the World Health Organization* 79(7): 596-607.

[8] Mathers CD, Stein C, Tomijima N, Ma Fat D, Rao C, Inoue M, Lopez AD, Murray CJL. (2002). *Global Burden of Disease 2000: Version 2 methods and results.* Geneva, World Health Organization (GPE Discussion Paper No. 50).

[9] Murray CJL, Lopez AD, eds (1996). *The global burden of disease: a comprehensive assessment of mortality and disability from diseases, injuries and risk factors in 1990 and projected to 2020.* Cambridge, MA, Harvard School of Public Health on behalf of the World Health Organization and the World Bank (Global Burden of Disease and Injury Series, Vol. 1).

[10] Salomon JA, Murray CJL (2000). *The epidemiological transition revisited: new compositional models for mortality by age, sex and cause.* Geneva, World Health Organization (GPE Discussion Paper No. 11, revised edition).

[11] Lozano R, Murray CJL, Lopez AD, Satoh T (2001). *Miscoding and misclassification of ischaemic heart disease mortality.* Geneva, World Health Organization (GPE Discussion Paper No. 12).

[12] Mathers CD, Murray CJL, Lopez AD, Boschi-Pinto C (2001). *Cancer incidence, mortality and survival by site for 14 regions of the world.* Geneva, World Health Organization (GPE Discussion Paper No. 13).

[13] Murray CJL, Salomon JA, Mathers CD (2000). A critical examination of summary measures of population health. *Bulletin of the World Health Organization,* 78: 981-994.

[14] Murray CJL, Salomon JA, Mathers CD, Lopez AD, eds (2002). *Summary measures of population health: concepts, ethics, measurement and applications.* Geneva, World Health Organization.

[15] Murray CJL, Lopez AD (2000). Progress and directions in refining the global burden of disease approach: response to Williams. *Health Economics,* 9: 69-82.

[16] World Health Organization (2000). *The World Health Report 2000 – Health systems: improving performance.* Geneva, World Health Organization.

[17] Mathers CD, Sadana R, Salomon JA, Murray CJL, Lopez AD (2001). Healthy life expectancy in 191 countries, 1999. *Lancet,* 357(9269): 1685-1691.

[18] Mathers CD, Murray CJL, Lopez AD, Salomon JA, Sadana R, Tandon A, Üstün TB, Chatterji S. (2001). *Estimates of healthy life expectancy for 191 countries in the year 2000: methods and results.* Geneva, World Health Organization (GPE discussion paper No. 38).

[19] Sadana R, Mathers CD, Lopez AD, Murray CJL (2000). *Comparative analysis of more than 50 household surveys on health status.* Geneva, World Health Organization (GPE Discussion Paper No. 15).

[20] Murray CJL, Tandon A, Salomon JA, Mathers CD; Sadana R (2002). *Cross-population comparability of evidence for health policy.* Geneva, World Health Organization (GPE Discussion Paper No. 46).

[21] Üstün TB, Chatterji S, Villanueva M, Bendib L, Sadana R, Valentine N, Mathers CD, Ortiz J, Tandon A, Salomon J, Yang C, Xie Wan J, Murray CJL. *WHO Multi-country Household Survey Study on Health and Responsiveness, 2000-2001* (2001). Geneva, World Health Organization (GPE discussion paper No. 37).

[22] World Health Organization (2001). *International classification of functioning, disability and health (ICF).* Geneva, World Health Organization.

[23] Murray CJL, Tandon A, Salomon JA, Mathers CD (2000). *Enhancing cross-population comparability of survey results.* Geneva, World Health Organization (GPE Discussion Paper No. 35).

[24] Tandon A, Murray CJL, Salomon JA, King G (2002). *Statistical models for enhancing cross-population comparability.* Geneva, World Health Organization (GPE Discussion Paper No. 42).

[25] Sadana R, Tandon A, Murray CJL, Serdobova I, Cao Y, Jun Xie W, Chatterji S, Ustün BL (2002). *Describing population health in six domains: comparable results from 66 household surveys.* Geneva, World Health Organization (GPE Discussion Paper No. 43).

[26] Poullier J-P, Hernandez P, Kawabata K (2001). *National health accounts: concepts, data sources and methodology.* Geneva, World Health Organization (GPE Discussion Paper No. 47).

Annex Table 1 Basic indicators for all Member States

These figures were produced by WHO using the best available evidence. They are not necessarily the official statistics of Member States.

	Member State	POPULATION ESTIMATES									LIFE EXPECTANCY AT BIRTH (YEARS)	
		Total population (000)	Annual growth rate (%)	Dependency ratio (per 100)		Percentage of population aged 60+ years		Total fertility rate		Both sexes	
		2001	1991–2001	1991	2001	1991	2001	1991	2001	2000	2001
1	Afghanistan	22 473	4.5	88	86	4.7	4.7	7.1	6.8	42.8	42.3
2	Albania	3 144	-0.5	61	55	7.9	9.2	2.9	2.4	69.4	69.5
3	Algeria	30 841	1.9	82	62	5.7	6.0	4.3	2.9	68.9	69.4
4	Andorra	90	5.0	51	50	19.4	21.1	1.5	1.3	79.5	79.6
5	Angola	13 527	3.2	100	104	4.7	4.5	7.2	7.2	36.4	36.1
6	Antigua and Barbuda	65	0.3	63	56	9.1	10.0	1.9	1.6	70.9	71.0
7	Argentina	37 487	1.3	65	59	13.0	13.4	2.9	2.5	73.7	73.9
8	Armenia	3 787	0.5	57	46	10.4	13.2	2.2	1.2	69.2	69.7
9	Australia	19 338	1.2	49	48	15.6	16.5	1.9	1.8	79.8	80.0
10	Austria	8 074	0.4	48	47	20.0	21.1	1.5	1.3	78.6	79.0
11	Azerbaijan	8 095	1.1	62	54	8.2	10.5	2.7	1.6	62.3	63.6
12	Bahamas	307	1.7	58	53	6.7	8.1	2.6	2.3	71.7	71.9
13	Bahrain	651	2.6	51	44	3.7	4.8	3.6	2.4	72.9	72.7
14	Bangladesh	140 368	2.2	81	71	4.7	5.0	4.5	3.6	61.6	61.8
15	Barbados	268	0.4	56	44	15.1	13.2	1.6	1.5	74.4	74.4
16	Belarus	10 146	-0.1	51	46	16.8	18.8	1.8	1.2	69.0	68.5
17	Belgium	10 263	0.3	50	52	20.7	22.2	1.6	1.5	77.8	78.0
18	Belize	230	2.0	93	72	6.0	5.9	4.3	3.0	69.9	70.0
19	Benin	6 445	3.0	106	95	4.7	4.2	6.6	5.8	52.1	52.1
20	Bhutan	2 141	2.2	86	87	6.0	6.5	5.8	5.2	61.3	61.6
21	Bolivia	8 516	2.4	81	77	5.9	6.2	4.9	4.1	62.2	62.7
22	Bosnia and Herzegovina	4 066	-0.2	43	40	10.7	15.1	1.6	1.3	72.6	72.8
23	Botswana	1 553	2.0	93	81	3.6	4.6	5.0	4.1	41.1	39.1
24	Brazil[a]	172 558	1.4	63	50	6.8	8.0	2.6	2.2	68.4	68.7
25	Brunei Darussalam	334	2.4	58	53	4.0	5.2	3.2	2.6	74.1	74.4
26	Bulgaria	7 866	-1.0	50	46	19.5	21.7	1.6	1.1	71.6	71.5
27	Burkina Faso	11 855	2.5	107	108	5.2	4.8	7.2	6.8	42.8	42.9
28	Burundi	6 501	1.2	94	100	4.7	4.3	6.8	6.8	40.8	40.4
29	Cambodia	13 440	3.0	92	85	4.4	4.4	5.5	4.9	55.7	56.2
30	Cameroon	15 202	2.4	95	87	5.6	5.6	5.8	4.8	50.5	49.7
31	Canada	31 014	1.0	47	46	15.7	16.9	1.7	1.6	79.1	79.3
32	Cape Verde	436	2.3	92	77	6.8	6.3	4.1	3.3	69.2	69.5
33	Central African Republic	3 781	2.3	91	89	6.2	6.1	5.6	5.0	42.7	42.7
34	Chad	8 134	3.1	96	99	5.2	4.9	6.7	6.7	48.2	48.6
35	Chile	15 401	1.5	57	55	9.1	10.4	2.6	2.4	76.1	76.3
36	China	1 292 378	0.9	49	45	8.6	10.0	2.1	1.8	70.8	71.2
37	Colombia	42 802	1.8	67	59	6.3	7.0	3.1	2.7	70.7	70.7
38	Comoros	726	3.0	97	83	4.0	4.2	6.0	5.1	61.6	61.8
39	Congo	3 109	3.1	95	99	5.3	5.0	6.3	6.3	52.7	52.9
40	Cook Islands	20	0.7	70	64	5.8	6.9	4.1	3.3	71.7	71.9
41	Costa Rica	4 112	2.7	68	59	6.4	7.6	3.1	2.7	76.4	76.1
42	Côte d'Ivoire	16 348	2.3	96	81	4.3	5.0	6.1	4.8	46.2	45.9
43	Croatia	4 654	0.3	47	48	17.3	20.5	1.6	1.7	72.9	72.9
44	Cuba[a]	11 236	0.5	45	44	11.8	14.0	1.7	1.6	76.8	76.9
45	Cyprus	790	1.3	58	52	14.8	15.9	2.4	1.9	76.8	76.9
46	Czech Republic	10 260	0.0	51	43	17.8	18.6	1.7	1.2	75.1	75.4
47	Democratic People's Republic of Korea	22 427	1.0	47	48	7.8	10.4	2.4	2.1	66.1	66.1
48	Democratic Republic of the Congo	52 521	3.2	100	108	4.6	4.5	6.7	6.7	44.0	43.8
49	Denmark	5 332	0.3	48	50	20.3	20.2	1.7	1.7	76.9	77.2
50	Djibouti	643	2.2	82	87	4.1	5.7	6.3	5.9	49.0	49.3
51	Dominica	71	-0.1	63	56	9.1	10.0	2.1	1.8	73.7	73.8
52	Dominican Republic	8 506	1.7	71	60	5.5	6.7	3.3	2.8	66.8	67.0
53	Ecuador	12 879	2.1	74	62	6.2	7.0	3.7	2.9	69.7	70.3
54	Egypt	69 079	1.9	77	64	6.1	6.3	4.0	3.0	66.3	66.5

	LIFE EXPECTANCY AT BIRTH (YEARS)				PROBABILITY OF DYING (PER 1000)							
					Under age 5 years				Between ages 15 and 59 years			
	Males		Females		Males		Females		Males		Females	
	2001	Uncertainty	2001	Uncertainty	2001	Uncertainty	2001	Uncertainty	2001	Uncertainty	2001	Uncertainty
1	41.1	33.1 - 48.6	43.7	34.8 - 52.6	252	205 - 298	249	195 - 298	527	331 - 772	418	215 - 645
2	66.3	64.9 - 67.7	73.2	72.4 - 74.2	35	31 - 39	30	22 - 42	177	147 - 207	98	81 - 113
3	67.7	66.5 - 68.8	71.1	70.0 - 72.4	55	44 - 65	44	34 - 53	164	147 - 180	129	113 - 145
4	76.2	74.9 - 80.8	82.9	81.5 - 88.0	5	3 - 7	5	3 - 6	113	87 - 140	46	36 - 57
5	34.1	28.1 - 40.1	38.3	30.1 - 44.0	306	269 - 343	279	250 - 310	660	499 - 810	527	369 - 735
6	68.7	67.4 - 70.2	73.5	72.2 - 74.9	25	11 - 35	21	10 - 31	197	175 - 215	128	113 - 142
7	70.1	69.8 - 70.3	77.7	77.5 - 77.9	22	20 - 23	17	16 - 19	183	178 - 188	92	90 - 95
8	66.2	65.5 - 67.0	73.0	72.0 - 74.1	44	37 - 53	32	29 - 36	216	197 - 234	99	86 - 112
9	77.4	77.1 - 77.6	82.6	82.4 - 82.9	7	6 - 7	5	5 - 6	94	92 - 97	54	52 - 56
10	75.9	75.7 - 76.2	81.8	81.4 - 82.2	5	5 - 6	5	4 - 5	119	116 - 123	61	57 - 64
11	60.7	59.1 - 62.1	66.6	65.0 - 68.1	100	87 - 116	88	74 - 106	253	209 - 296	132	102 - 161
12	68.8	67.8 - 69.6	75.0	74.2 - 75.5	14	13 - 17	11	10 - 15	249	224 - 269	152	142 - 162
13	72.2	70.7 - 73.5	73.4	72.1 - 74.6	9	5 - 14	7	5 - 12	123	105 - 145	89	75 - 109
14	61.9	60.6 - 63.1	61.7	60.4 - 63.0	82	73 - 90	84	76 - 92	251	223 - 279	258	233 - 284
15	70.5	69.4 - 71.4	78.2	77.7 - 78.7	15	14 - 18	11	10 - 14	192	172 - 213	103	94 - 111
16	62.9	62.2 - 63.7	74.2	73.5 - 74.8	14	12 - 18	11	10 - 13	368	336 - 395	134	122 - 149
17	74.8	74.5 - 75.1	81.2	80.9 - 81.5	6	5 - 7	5	4 - 6	128	123 - 132	67	65 - 70
18	67.7	66.6 - 68.9	72.7	71.9 - 73.6	39	30 - 50	30	22 - 38	191	173 - 210	124	118 - 130
19	51.0	45.4 - 56.5	53.3	46.2 - 60.3	160	159 - 161	149	148 - 150	407	258 - 567	348	184 - 532
20	60.5	54.6 - 67.7	62.7	55.8 - 71.4	90	70 - 109	90	74 - 107	270	113 - 426	224	59 - 408
21	61.1	55.1 - 67.8	64.3	56.5 - 73.5	84	76 - 92	76	68 - 84	266	115 - 427	212	35 - 399
22	69.3	68.0 - 70.7	76.4	75.3 - 77.5	19	14 - 24	15	11 - 18	194	167 - 222	91	78 - 105
23	39.3	37.4 - 41.6	38.6	36.8 - 40.4	110	90 - 129	107	94 - 131	797	748 - 837	767	730 - 798
24	65.5	64.5 - 66.3	72.0	71.2 - 72.8	47	35 - 63	40	30 - 54	247	232 - 264	134	118 - 147
25	73.2	72.5 - 73.8	75.9	74.5 - 77.2	14	13 - 16	14	12 - 18	127	117 - 137	95	77 - 117
26	68.4	67.7 - 69.1	74.8	74.2 - 75.4	18	15 - 22	16	13 - 19	221	204 - 240	99	90 - 108
27	42.2	37.4 - 47.2	43.5	38.0 - 49.0	216	199 - 232	205	187 - 222	571	444 - 705	513	378 - 651
28	38.4	34.6 - 42.1	42.3	36.3 - 48.1	193	159 - 228	180	143 - 219	704	631 - 785	586	469 - 704
29	53.3	47.6 - 58.8	59.0	52.4 - 67.8	130	120 - 140	114	104 - 123	385	245 - 544	268	80 - 438
30	48.9	44.2 - 54.2	50.5	45.4 - 56.8	150	137 - 162	141	130 - 152	489	357 - 616	438	304 - 560
31	76.6	76.3 - 76.8	81.9	81.8 - 82.1	6	6 - 6	5	5 - 6	98	95 - 101	59	58 - 61
32	65.7	63.7 - 67.1	72.0	70.9 - 73.0	49	39 - 61	35	26 - 47	218	198 - 248	127	116 - 139
33	42.0	37.4 - 46.5	43.3	37.7 - 49.1	197	166 - 227	183	153 - 210	608	500 - 712	556	436 - 691
34	47.0	40.9 - 52.7	50.2	42.8 - 57.1	191	158 - 223	170	141 - 201	466	323 - 626	391	236 - 563
35	73.2	72.4 - 73.8	79.5	79.2 - 79.7	10	9 - 11	8	8 - 9	139	129 - 152	70	67 - 73
36	69.8	69.2 - 70.3	72.7	72.1 - 73.4	34	31 - 38	40	36 - 44	157	148 - 167	106	98 - 116
37	66.7	65.9 - 67.4	74.8	74.1 - 75.4	26	21 - 32	21	17 - 25	247	230 - 263	115	105 - 125
38	59.8	53.4 - 67.4	63.8	57.5 - 73.0	90	71 - 107	80	64 - 97	288	112 - 452	217	46 - 367
39	51.8	46.5 - 57.7	53.8	47.4 - 59.8	115	88 - 143	106	82 - 130	466	348 - 593	415	289 - 561
40	69.9	68.7 - 71.2	74.0	73.0 - 75.4	23	11 - 33	18	10 - 26	174	162 - 188	122	112 - 132
41	73.8	73.1 - 74.5	78.6	78.1 - 79.2	13	11 - 16	10	9 - 12	134	123 - 145	78	71 - 84
42	45.0	39.4 - 51.3	47.0	41.1 - 54.1	178	144 - 213	161	129 - 193	551	421 - 683	493	360 - 624
43	68.9	68.5 - 69.3	77.1	76.7 - 77.5	8	7 - 9	7	6 - 9	186	177 - 194	74	69 - 80
44	74.7	74.3 - 75.1	79.2	78.9 - 79.6	11	9 - 12	8	7 - 9	142	136 - 148	90	86 - 94
45	74.6	73.8 - 75.4	79.2	77.9 - 80.3	7	6 - 8	7	6 - 8	110	100 - 121	58	47 - 70
46	71.9	71.5 - 72.2	78.8	78.5 - 79.1	5	5 - 6	4	4 - 5	168	160 - 176	73	68 - 76
47	64.0	61.9 - 66.6	68.3	66.0 - 70.9	54	27 - 77	52	27 - 77	250	224 - 278	169	145 - 191
48	42.1	35.7 - 48.4	45.5	37.2 - 53.4	216	160 - 271	203	159 - 256	566	430 - 708	459	288 - 637
49	74.8	74.4 - 75.1	79.5	79.2 - 79.8	6	5 - 7	5	4 - 6	122	117 - 128	77	74 - 81
50	47.9	42.1 - 53.0	50.4	43.5 - 57.0	181	151 - 214	165	139 - 192	459	343 - 598	394	250 - 554
51	71.6	70.5 - 72.6	76.0	74.4 - 77.2	13	10 - 16	14	10 - 20	202	183 - 223	121	96 - 154
52	64.1	63.1 - 65.0	70.5	69.5 - 71.5	48	41 - 55	44	37 - 51	259	236 - 284	152	133 - 171
53	67.6	66.9 - 68.3	73.2	72.5 - 73.9	36	31 - 41	31	26 - 37	217	204 - 231	134	121 - 145
54	65.3	64.5 - 66.0	67.8	66.8 - 68.9	46	41 - 52	44	39 - 51	230	213 - 248	160	139 - 183

Annex Table 1 Basic indicators for all Member States

These figures were produced by WHO using the best available evidence. They are not necessarily the official statistics of Member States.

| | Member State | POPULATION ESTIMATES | | | | | | | | | | LIFE EXPECTANCY AT BIRTH (YEARS) | |
| | | Total population (000) | Annual growth rate (%) | Dependency ratio (per 100) | | Percentage of population aged 60+ years | | Total fertility rate | | | Both sexes | |
		2001	1991–2001	1991	2001	1991	2001	1991	2001		2000	2001
55	El Salvador	6 399	2.1	80	68	6.6	7.2	3.6	3.0		69.0	69.5
56	Equatorial Guinea	469	2.7	87	91	6.3	5.9	5.9	5.9		53.5	53.7
57	Eritrea	3 815	2.0	88	88	4.4	4.7	6.2	5.4		44.7	53.6
58	Estonia	1 376	-1.3	51	46	17.5	20.3	1.8	1.2		71.0	71.2
59	Ethiopia	64 458	2.8	90	93	4.5	4.7	6.9	6.8		47.5	48.0
60	Fiji	822	1.2	68	58	4.9	5.8	3.4	3.0		69.6	69.7
61	Finland	5 177	0.3	49	49	18.6	20.2	1.8	1.6		77.7	77.9
62	France	59 452	0.4	52	53	19.3	20.5	1.7	1.8		79.1	79.3
63	Gabon	1 261	2.7	76	86	9.1	8.6	5.1	5.4		59.1	59.3
64	Gambia	1 337	3.3	80	76	4.8	5.2	5.8	4.9		58.3	58.5
65	Georgia	5 238	-0.4	52	50	15.3	18.9	2.0	1.4		68.7	68.9
66	Germany	82 006	0.3	45	47	20.5	23.7	1.4	1.3		78.0	78.2
67	Ghana	19 733	2.4	92	78	4.6	5.1	5.5	4.3		57.3	57.4
68	Greece	10 623	0.4	49	49	20.4	23.7	1.4	1.3		78.0	78.1
69	Grenada	94	0.3	63	56	9.1	10.0	4.1	3.5		67.1	67.2
70	Guatemala	11 686	2.7	96	88	5.1	5.3	5.5	4.6		65.9	66.2
71	Guinea	8 273	2.7	94	88	4.4	4.5	6.5	6.0		51.4	51.9
72	Guinea-Bissau	1 226	2.4	86	89	5.9	5.6	6.0	6.0		47.3	47.3
73	Guyana	762	0.4	69	54	6.7	6.9	2.6	2.4		63.8	64.0
74	Haiti	8 269	1.6	92	78	5.7	5.6	5.1	4.1		53.0	50.0
75	Honduras	6 574	2.7	92	81	4.5	5.1	5.1	3.9		67.1	67.3
76	Hungary	9 916	-0.4	50	46	19.1	19.9	1.8	1.3		71.5	71.7
77	Iceland	281	0.9	55	53	14.6	15.1	2.2	1.9		79.6	79.8
78	India	1 025 095	1.8	68	62	6.9	7.7	3.8	3.1		60.6	60.8
79	Indonesia	214 839	1.5	65	54	6.3	7.8	3.2	2.4		65.4	65.9
80	Iran, Islamic Republic of	71 368	1.8	89	66	4.7	5.3	4.8	2.9		68.3	68.6
81	Iraq	23 583	2.9	88	79	4.5	4.6	5.8	4.9		60.4	60.7
82	Ireland	3 840	0.9	62	48	15.2	15.3	2.1	2.0		76.3	76.5
83	Israel	6 171	2.9	67	61	12.5	13.1	3.0	2.8		78.5	78.5
84	Italy	57 502	0.1	45	48	21.5	24.3	1.3	1.2		79.1	79.3
85	Jamaica	2 598	0.9	73	62	10.0	9.6	2.8	2.4		72.6	72.7
86	Japan[a]	127 334	0.3	43	48	18.0	23.8	1.5	1.4		81.3	81.4
87	Jordan	5 050	3.9	96	75	4.6	4.6	5.7	4.4		70.7	70.8
88	Kazakhstan	16 094	-0.4	60	50	9.7	11.2	2.6	2.0		62.5	63.0
89	Kenya	31 292	2.5	107	84	4.1	4.2	5.8	4.3		49.7	48.9
90	Kiribati	84	1.4	69	76	6.0	6.9	4.4	4.6		63.2	63.6
91	Kuwait	1 970	-0.6	63	47	2.1	4.8	3.4	2.7		75.4	75.3
92	Kyrgyzstan	4 986	1.2	74	65	8.3	8.9	3.6	2.5		63.8	64.1
93	Lao People's Democratic Republic	5 402	2.5	91	85	6.0	5.6	6.0	5.0		54.6	54.6
94	Latvia	2 405	-1.0	51	46	17.9	21.1	1.8	1.1		70.5	70.7
95	Lebanon	3 555	2.5	66	58	8.2	8.5	3.1	2.2		69.6	69.8
96	Lesotho	2 057	1.8	80	77	6.0	6.6	5.1	4.5		41.9	40.0
97	Liberia	3 107	4.0	122	83	5.2	4.4	6.8	6.8		45.6	46.2
98	Libyan Arab Jamahiriya	5 407	2.1	83	58	4.3	5.6	4.6	3.5		70.0	70.4
99	Lithuania	3 688	-0.1	51	48	16.4	18.8	1.9	1.3		72.6	72.9
100	Luxembourg	441	1.4	45	49	19.0	19.4	1.6	1.7		78.2	78.5
101	Madagascar	16 436	2.9	92	91	4.8	4.7	6.2	5.8		54.7	54.8
102	Malawi	11 571	1.8	99	97	4.3	4.7	7.3	6.5		36.6	36.3
103	Malaysia	22 632	2.2	67	61	5.8	6.7	3.7	3.0		71.7	71.7
104	Maldives	299	3.0	99	88	5.3	5.2	6.3	5.5		63.4	64.0
105	Mali	11 676	2.6	98	101	5.3	5.8	7.0	7.0		45.0	45.2
106	Malta	391	0.8	51	48	14.8	17.2	2.0	1.8		77.9	78.1
107	Marshall Islands	52	1.4	69	76	6.0	6.9	5.5	5.7		62.0	62.4
108	Mauritania	2 746	3.0	93	90	4.9	4.7	6.1	6.0		51.9	52.0
109	Mauritius	1 170	0.9	53	46	8.3	9.1	2.3	1.9		71.3	71.1

	LIFE EXPECTANCY AT BIRTH (YEARS)				PROBABILITY OF DYING (PER 1000)							
					Under age 5 years				Between ages 15 and 59 years			
	Males		Females		Males		Females		Males		Females	
	2001	Uncertainty	2001	Uncertainty	2001	Uncertainty	2001	Uncertainty	2001	Uncertainty	2001	Uncertainty
55	66.3	65.0 - 67.4	72.7	71.8 - 73.4	35	28 - 43	32	26 - 41	268	236 - 298	146	133 - 160
56	52.3	45.9 - 59.0	55.1	47.9 - 63.3	154	129 - 181	141	122 - 162	378	219 - 548	315	138 - 496
57	52.3	47.6 - 57.8	55.0	48.1 - 62.8	123	112 - 133	107	99 - 118	440	273 - 585	383	188 - 591
58	65.7	64.4 - 67.0	76.5	75.7 - 77.4	12	9 - 15	10	8 - 13	312	263 - 360	111	96 - 127
59	46.8	41.2 - 52.6	49.2	41.3 - 55.8	185	148 - 221	170	139 - 195	484	353 - 619	420	267 - 596
60	67.8	66.8 - 68.7	71.8	70.9 - 72.8	27	24 - 30	24	22 - 27	212	193 - 232	152	134 - 167
61	74.5	74.1 - 74.8	81.2	80.9 - 81.5	5	4 - 5	4	3 - 4	139	134 - 145	61	58 - 64
62	75.6	75.3 - 75.9	82.9	82.8 - 83.1	5	5 - 6	4	4 - 5	134	129 - 139	60	58 - 62
63	58.0	52.4 - 63.8	60.5	53.9 - 70.7	93	85 - 101	86	79 - 93	335	203 - 479	284	100 - 438
64	56.2	53.8 - 59.0	61.0	58.9 - 63.1	121	103 - 140	108	92 - 123	329	263 - 388	231	191 - 276
65	65.4	64.0 - 66.9	72.4	70.5 - 74.1	33	27 - 39	26	21 - 32	250	211 - 287	108	84 - 138
66	75.1	74.7 - 75.5	81.1	81.0 - 81.2	5	5 - 6	4	4 - 5	121	116 - 127	61	60 - 63
67	55.8	50.5 - 62.1	58.9	52.2 - 66.6	111	95 - 127	97	84 - 110	360	212 - 493	303	147 - 462
68	75.5	75.2 - 75.7	80.8	80.5 - 81.0	7	6 - 8	6	6 - 7	119	115 - 122	50	48 - 53
69	65.8	64.7 - 66.8	68.7	67.7 - 69.7	25	19 - 31	21	15 - 27	263	240 - 288	225	207 - 243
70	63.6	62.2 - 65.1	69.0	67.7 - 70.1	55	47 - 65	45	38 - 52	277	233 - 320	168	134 - 207
71	50.1	43.8 - 56.0	53.8	46.9 - 61.2	172	155 - 188	153	139 - 167	407	249 - 578	327	167 - 500
72	45.9	40.4 - 51.3	48.7	42.0 - 55.8	213	194 - 233	195	178 - 213	457	305 - 618	382	199 - 556
73	61.3	58.7 - 64.0	66.7	63.9 - 69.5	62	32 - 92	51	25 - 78	302	270 - 333	206	174 - 237
74	45.6	43.1 - 52.2	54.7	51.1 - 60.7	118	90 - 143	103	75 - 128	615	454 - 661	397	296 - 458
75	64.4	62.7 - 66.0	70.3	68.5 - 71.8	44	39 - 49	41	37 - 47	261	237 - 295	151	135 - 171
76	67.3	66.7 - 67.8	76.1	75.7 - 76.5	11	10 - 12	9	7 - 10	275	257 - 293	118	111 - 126
77	78.2	77.5 - 78.8	81.3	80.8 - 81.9	4	4 - 6	3	3 - 4	84	77 - 91	57	52 - 63
78	60.0	59.2 - 60.6	61.7	60.9 - 62.5	89	84 - 95	98	90 - 107	291	267 - 315	222	203 - 243
79	64.4	63.6 - 65.3	67.4	66.6 - 68.1	50	45 - 55	40	36 - 44	246	229 - 262	213	198 - 229
80	66.4	65.3 - 67.7	71.1	70.1 - 72.1	45	35 - 54	39	31 - 47	209	191 - 228	137	124 - 148
81	58.7	55.0 - 62.5	62.9	59.2 - 67.1	122	71 - 170	111	66 - 154	258	230 - 290	180	151 - 203
82	73.8	73.3 - 74.2	79.2	78.8 - 79.6	7	6 - 9	6	4 - 8	118	111 - 124	64	60 - 69
83	76.1	75.6 - 76.7	80.9	80.6 - 81.1	7	6 - 8	6	5 - 6	115	108 - 122	55	52 - 57
84	76.2	75.8 - 76.6	82.2	81.9 - 82.4	6	5 - 6	5	5 - 6	100	95 - 105	51	49 - 53
85	71.0	69.8 - 72.4	74.5	73.6 - 75.4	16	13 - 19	15	12 - 17	164	140 - 188	123	108 - 137
86	77.9	77.5 - 78.2	84.7	84.5 - 84.9	5	4 - 5	4	4 - 4	97	93 - 101	47	46 - 49
87	68.6	67.5 - 69.7	73.5	72.7 - 74.3	27	21 - 34	24	18 - 30	193	174 - 215	122	113 - 130
88	58.8	58.2 - 59.8	67.2	66.2 - 68.1	59	51 - 67	45	40 - 50	375	319 - 437	209	182 - 238
89	48.2	44.3 - 52.6	49.6	45.5 - 55.2	119	111 - 129	109	101 - 117	560	457 - 653	513	409 - 616
90	61.7	58.7 - 64.9	65.8	63.3 - 68.4	82	72 - 93	66	56 - 77	255	186 - 321	196	143 - 253
91	74.9	73.7 - 76.1	75.9	73.6 - 78.1	12	9 - 15	10	7 - 14	87	77 - 98	66	51 - 88
92	60.1	58.9 - 61.3	68.2	67.0 - 69.3	72	63 - 84	55	47 - 64	334	291 - 375	168	142 - 200
93	53.5	50.7 - 56.2	55.6	53.3 - 58.5	153	119 - 188	137	108 - 166	342	279 - 398	309	272 - 348
94	65.2	64.2 - 66.4	76.0	75.0 - 76.9	14	10 - 18	12	9 - 15	312	268 - 353	116	100 - 134
95	67.6	66.4 - 68.9	72.0	71.2 - 72.8	34	31 - 37	28	25 - 30	204	177 - 230	140	125 - 156
96	40.1	37.1 - 43.2	39.8	36.0 - 44.4	155	126 - 181	147	120 - 172	724	666 - 788	692	618 - 771
97	44.6	38.0 - 50.8	48.0	41.2 - 55.3	203	164 - 242	185	146 - 223	517	373 - 665	425	275 - 561
98	68.3	67.1 - 69.5	73.1	72.1 - 74.4	31	25 - 37	29	23 - 34	194	177 - 211	118	107 - 129
99	67.7	66.7 - 68.6	77.9	77.3 - 78.5	10	9 - 12	10	9 - 11	270	241 - 301	96	87 - 106
100	74.9	74.6 - 75.2	81.8	81.4 - 82.1	4	4 - 6	4	4 - 5	122	117 - 127	61	57 - 66
101	53.3	46.9 - 59.5	56.4	48.7 - 64.3	155	134 - 177	142	125 - 158	345	187 - 508	279	98 - 452
102	35.7	31.0 - 40.0	36.9	31.7 - 42.5	261	227 - 291	240	210 - 267	695	592 - 802	636	515 - 763
103	69.2	68.8 - 69.7	74.4	74.0 - 74.7	13	12 - 14	11	10 - 12	194	184 - 204	108	103 - 114
104	63.9	62.9 - 64.6	64.4	63.7 - 65.0	42	34 - 50	48	37 - 60	276	248 - 311	213	193 - 236
105	44.2	38.1 - 50.6	46.2	38.2 - 53.4	229	209 - 253	218	197 - 240	480	303 - 651	410	225 - 600
106	75.8	75.0 - 76.5	80.3	79.8 - 80.8	8	7 - 9	6	5 - 8	89	82 - 97	48	44 - 52
107	60.7	59.3 - 62.1	64.3	63.0 - 65.6	48	36 - 59	37	28 - 47	347	318 - 376	292	268 - 315
108	50.9	44.2 - 57.0	53.1	45.7 - 61.5	174	150 - 195	167	145 - 187	378	207 - 560	317	116 - 501
109	67.5	66.6 - 68.3	74.9	74.4 - 75.5	23	19 - 26	16	12 - 20	229	208 - 250	116	108 - 124

Annex Table 2 Deaths by cause, sex and mortality stratum in WHO Regions,[a] estimates for 2001

These figures were produced by WHO using the best available evidence. They are not necessarily the official statistics of Member States.

Cause[b]	SEX						AFRICA		THE AMERICAS		
	Both sexes		Males		Females		Mortality stratum		Mortality stratum		
							High child, high adult	High child, very high adult	Very low child, very low adult	Low child, low adult	High child, high adult
Population (000)	6 122 210		3 083 884		3 038 327		301 878	353 598	328 176	437 142	72 649
	(000)	% total	(000)	% total	(000)	% total	(000)	(000)	(000)	(000)	(000)
II. Noncommunicable conditions	33 077	58.5	16 726	56.5	16 352	60.7	1 098	1 264	2 400	1 810	288
Malignant neoplasms	7 115	12.6	3 952	13.3	3 163	11.7	241	303	645	392	74
Mouth and oropharynx cancers	326	0.6	226	0.8	100	0.4	12	22	10	11	1
Oesophagus cancer	438	0.8	278	0.9	160	0.6	6	21	16	14	1
Stomach cancer	850	1.5	522	1.8	328	1.2	20	17	18	43	15
Colon/rectum cancer	615	1.1	317	1.1	298	1.1	12	15	75	29	4
Liver cancer	616	1.1	423	1.4	193	0.7	30	34	15	18	6
Pancreas cancer	225	0.4	119	0.4	107	0.4	3	5	34	16	2
Trachea/bronchus/lung cancers	1 213	2.1	882	3.0	331	1.2	9	14	176	48	3
Melanoma and other skin cancers	66	0.1	35	0.1	31	0.1	4	5	12	6	1
Breast cancer	479	0.8	3	0.0	476	1.8	14	24	55	31	4
Cervix uteri cancer	258	0.5	…	…	258	1.0	21	38	6	19	5
Corpus uteri cancer	74	0.1	…	…	74	0.3	1	2	9	10	4
Ovary cancer	131	0.2	…	…	131	0.5	3	7	16	7	1
Prostate cancer	269	0.5	269	0.9	…	…	25	20	42	29	6
Bladder cancer	183	0.3	129	0.4	54	0.2	8	6	16	7	1
Lymphomas, multiple myeloma	333	0.6	171	0.6	162	0.6	20	19	46	17	4
Leukaemia	260	0.5	145	0.5	115	0.4	8	12	27	18	4
Other neoplasms	147	0.3	73	0.2	74	0.3	1	2	15	10	1
Diabetes mellitus	895	1.6	401	1.4	495	1.8	20	35	78	137	15
Nutritional/endocrine disorders	247	0.4	110	0.4	136	0.5	17	19	30	24	5
Neuropsychiatric disorders	1 023	1.8	523	1.8	500	1.9	36	44	150	53	10
Unipolar depressive disorders	12	0.0	6	0.0	7	0.0	0	0	1	0	0
Bipolar affective disorder	1	0.0	0	0.0	1	0.0	0	0	0	0	0
Schizophrenia	24	0.0	12	0.0	12	0.0	0	0	1	0	0
Epilepsy	109	0.2	63	0.2	46	0.2	10	14	2	6	2
Alcohol use disorders	87	0.2	74	0.2	13	0.0	3	8	8	14	2
Alzheimer and other dementias	368	0.7	132	0.4	236	0.9	2	3	86	8	0
Parkinson disease	92	0.2	45	0.2	47	0.2	2	2	17	4	1
Multiple sclerosis	15	0.0	6	0.0	9	0.0	0	0	3	1	0
Drug use disorders	68	0.1	56	0.2	12	0.0	2	0	5	2	1
Post-traumatic stress disorder	0	0.0	0	0.0	0	0.0	0	0	0	0	0
Obsessive–compulsive disorder	0	0.0	0	0.0	0	0.0	0	0	0	0	0
Panic disorder	0	0.0	0	0.0	0	0.0	0	0	0	0	0
Insomnia (primary)	0	0.0	0	0.0	0	0.0	0	0	0	0	0
Migraine	0	0.0	0	0.0	0	0.0	0	0	0	0	0
Sense organ disorders	4	0.0	2	0.0	3	0.0	0	0	0	0	0
Glaucoma	0	0.0	0	0.0	0	0.0	0	0	0	0	0
Cataracts	1	0.0	0	0.0	1	0.0	0	0	0	0	0
Hearing loss, adult onset	0	0.0	0	0.0	0	0.0	0	0	0	0	0
Cardiovascular diseases	16 585	29.3	7 962	26.9	8 623	32.0	482	503	1 106	773	100
Rheumatic heart disease	338	0.6	140	0.5	197	0.7	14	15	5	6	0
Hypertensive heart disease	874	1.5	397	1.3	477	1.8	25	29	48	69	14
Ischaemic heart disease	7 181	12.7	3 756	12.7	3 425	12.7	169	164	622	310	35
Cerebrovascular disease	5 454	9.6	2 499	8.4	2 956	11.0	143	164	199	229	26
Inflammatory heart disease	375	0.7	192	0.6	183	0.7	16	18	37	29	1

Cause[b]	EASTERN MEDITERRANEAN Mortality stratum		EUROPE Mortality stratum			SOUTH-EAST ASIA Mortality stratum		WESTERN PACIFIC Mortality stratum	
	Low child, Low adult	High child, high adult	Very low child, very low adult	Low child, low adult	Low child, high adult	Low child, low adult	High child, high adult	Very low child, very low adult	Low child, low adult
	141 835	351 256	412 512	219 983	241 683	297 525	1 262 285	154 919	1 546 770
	(000)	(000)	(000)	(000)	(000)	(000)	(000)	(000)	(000)
II. Noncommunicable conditions	475	1 454	3 643	1 664	3 048	1 275	5 913	939	7 805
Malignant neoplasms	80	199	1 059	293	515	231	882	343	1 859
Mouth and oropharynx cancers	3	18	25	9	18	16	128	6	48
Oesophagus cancer	3	10	29	7	14	4	76	12	224
Stomach cancer	11	10	67	30	75	9	56	55	425
Colon/rectum cancer	5	10	142	29	64	24	34	44	130
Liver cancer	4	10	39	11	14	31	34	35	336
Pancreas cancer	2	3	53	12	21	5	14	21	33
Trachea/bronchus/lung cancers	11	19	206	62	103	35	127	62	337
Melanoma and other skin cancers	0	1	15	4	6	1	2	3	4
Breast cancer	5	23	92	22	40	24	66	13	66
Cervix uteri cancer	4	8	8	7	12	14	85	3	30
Corpus uteri cancer	0	1	16	5	11	2	3	3	6
Ovary cancer	1	4	25	6	13	7	19	5	16
Prostate cancer	2	6	71	10	14	7	19	11	8
Bladder cancer	3	19	38	10	14	5	27	6	23
Lymphomas, multiple myeloma	7	15	55	12	10	14	76	14	24
Leukaemia	4	13	37	11	15	11	32	9	60
Other neoplasms	2	12	28	4	5	24	15	10	18
Diabetes mellitus	16	36	90	30	21	62	176	17	162
Nutritional/endocrine disorders	5	23	28	3	3	16	19	9	45
Neuropsychiatric disorders	16	57	175	24	40	53	210	21	134
Unipolar depressive disorders	0	1	2	0	0	0	9	0	0
Bipolar affective disorder	0	0	0	0	0	0	0	0	0
Schizophrenia	0	1	1	0	1	1	13	0	4
Epilepsy	2	8	6	4	5	4	29	1	17
Alcohol use disorders	1	1	13	3	8	4	10	1	11
Alzheimer and other dementias	1	9	89	3	5	21	79	9	53
Parkinson disease	1	1	21	2	1	3	8	4	25
Multiple sclerosis	0	0	4	1	2	0	1	0	1
Drug use disorders	4	17	6	2	7	1	19	1	4
Post-traumatic stress disorder	0	0	0	0	0	0	0	0	0
Obsessive–compulsive disorder	0	0	0	0	0	0	0	0	0
Panic disorder	0	0	0	0	0	0	0	0	0
Insomnia (primary)	0	0	0	0	0	0	0	0	0
Migraine	0	0	0	0	0	0	0	0	0
Sense organ disorders	0	1	0	0	0	0	1	0	0
Glaucoma	0	0	0	0	0	0	0	0	0
Cataracts	0	0	0	0	0	0	0	0	0
Hearing loss, adult onset	0	0	0	0	0	0	0	0	0
Cardiovascular diseases	280	757	1 760	1 111	2 171	571	3 226	395	3 350
Rheumatic heart disease	3	21	11	8	15	9	123	3	105
Hypertensive heart disease	35	56	68	67	40	63	75	9	276
Ischaemic heart disease	147	376	738	500	1 185	232	1 740	136	827
Cerebrovascular disease	47	171	456	296	728	193	877	163	1 763
Inflammatory heart disease	6	23	29	27	31	12	66	8	74

Annex Table 2 Deaths by cause, sex and mortality stratum in WHO Regions,[a] estimates for 2001

These figures were produced by WHO using the best available evidence. They are not necessarily the official statistics of Member States.

Cause[b]	SEX Both sexes (000)	% total	Males (000)	% total	Females (000)	% total	AFRICA Mortality stratum High child, high adult (000)	High child, very high adult (000)	THE AMERICAS Mortality stratum Very low child, very low adult (000)	Low child, low adult (000)	High child, high adult (000)
Population (000)	6 122 210		3 083 884		3 038 327		301 878	353 598	328 176	437 142	72 649
Respiratory diseases	3 560	6.3	1 818	6.1	1 742	6.5	105	129	186	163	20
Chronic obstructive pulmonary disease	2 672	4.7	1 355	4.6	1 317	4.9	53	63	133	84	5
Asthma	226	0.4	111	0.4	114	0.4	9	15	6	10	2
Digestive diseases	1 987	3.5	1 108	3.7	879	3.3	92	108	98	149	34
Peptic ulcer disease	262	0.5	155	0.5	108	0.4	7	9	6	11	3
Cirrhosis of the liver	796	1.4	507	1.7	289	1.1	33	37	30	59	15
Appendicitis	22	0.0	12	0.0	10	0.0	1	1	0	2	1
Diseases of the genitourinary system	825	1.5	450	1.5	375	1.4	57	64	60	52	16
Nephritis/nephrosis	625	1.1	332	1.1	294	1.1	38	42	41	41	13
Benign prostatic hypertrophy	36	0.1	36	0.1	...	...	3	4	1	2	0
Skin diseases	67	0.1	29	0.1	38	0.1	10	12	4	6	2
Musculoskeletal diseases	113	0.2	38	0.1	74	0.3	6	7	15	10	2
Rheumatoid arthritis	24	0.0	7	0.0	18	0.1	1	1	3	2	1
Osteoarthritis	4	0.0	1	0.0	3	0.0	0	0	1	0	0
Congenital abnormalities	507	0.9	257	0.9	249	0.9	29	38	13	40	9
Oral diseases	2	0.0	1	0.0	1	0.0	0	0	0	0	0
Dental caries	0	0.0	0	0.0	0	0.0	0	0	0	0	0
Periodontal disease	0	0.0	0	0.0	0	0.0	0	0	0	0	0
Edentulism	0	0.0	0	0.0	0	0.0	0	0	0	0	0
III. Injuries	5 103	9.0	3 374	11.4	1 729	6.4	298	437	176	324	57
Unintentional	3 508	6.2	2 251	7.6	1 257	4.7	218	251	117	170	43
Road traffic accidents	1 194	2.1	848	2.9	346	1.3	79	100	49	78	14
Poisoning	343	0.6	216	0.7	127	0.5	16	21	14	2	1
Falls	385	0.7	229	0.8	156	0.6	9	10	18	12	1
Fires	309	0.5	129	0.4	181	0.7	19	17	4	4	1
Drowning	403	0.7	277	0.9	126	0.5	50	42	4	16	4
Other unintentional injuries	874	1.5	553	1.9	321	1.2	45	61	28	58	22
Intentional	1 594	2.8	1 123	3.8	472	1.8	80	186	59	154	14
Self-inflicted	849	1.5	521	1.8	328	1.2	11	17	37	25	3
Violence	500	0.9	383	1.3	117	0.4	45	71	19	120	11
War	230	0.4	207	0.7	23	0.1	24	98	3	8	0

[a] See the List of Member States by WHO Region and mortality stratum.

[b] Estimates for specific causes may not sum to broader cause groupings due to omission of residual categories.

[c] Does not include liver cancer and cirrhosis deaths resulting from chronic hepatitis virus infection.

... Data not available or not applicable.

Cause[b]	EASTERN MEDITERRANEAN Mortality stratum		EUROPE Mortality stratum			SOUTH-EAST ASIA Mortality stratum		WESTERN PACIFIC Mortality stratum	
	Low child, Low adult	High child, high adult	Very low child, very low adult	Low child, low adult	Low child, high adult	Low child, low adult	High child, high adult	Very low child, very low adult	Low child, low adult
	141 835	*351 256*	*412 512*	*219 983*	*241 683*	*297 525*	*1 262 285*	*154 919*	*1 546 770*
	(000)	(000)	(000)	(000)	(000)	(000)	(000)	(000)	(000)
Respiratory diseases	19	125	213	80	126	130	693	59	1 513
Chronic obstructive pulmonary disease	10	78	140	49	96	66	548	23	1 324
Asthma	3	15	13	11	16	21	66	6	33
Digestive diseases	20	121	187	78	118	100	407	45	429
Peptic ulcer disease	3	10	18	9	14	20	76	5	72
Cirrhosis of the liver	8	52	67	41	58	42	172	15	168
Appendicitis	0	1	1	0	1	1	7	0	5
Diseases of the genitourinary system	16	60	62	27	27	53	138	28	164
Nephritis/nephrosis	9	52	41	21	15	40	115	24	133
Benign prostatic hypertrophy	1	2	1	1	2	2	11	0	5
Skin diseases	1	3	8	0	3	5	8	1	2
Musculoskeletal diseases	1	3	19	2	5	11	8	5	19
Rheumatoid arthritis	0	0	4	1	3	0	2	2	5
Osteoarthritis	0	0	2	0	0	0	0	0	0
Congenital abnormalities	18	57	11	13	14	20	129	4	112
Oral diseases	0	0	0	0	0	0	1	0	0
Dental caries	0	0	0	0	0	0	0	0	0
Periodontal disease	0	0	0	0	0	0	0	0	0
Edentulism	0	0	0	0	0	0	0	0	0
III. Injuries	**106**	**295**	**197**	**113**	**453**	**275**	**1 188**	**84**	**1 098**
Unintentional	87	196	141	79	286	215	909	48	748
Road traffic accidents	41	62	47	22	56	139	214	14	278
Poisoning	3	15	6	6	92	8	87	2	71
Falls	5	18	49	9	23	17	104	7	102
Fires	7	24	3	3	30	9	169	2	18
Drowning	5	22	4	7	26	12	79	6	126
Other unintentional injuries	26	55	32	31	60	30	256	17	153
Intentional	19	99	57	33	167	60	278	36	351
Self inflicted	10	25	51	22	95	35	199	35	283
Violence	6	16	4	8	58	14	63	1	64
War	2	57	1	2	13	12	8	0	3

Annex Table 3 Burden of disease in DALYs by cause, sex and mortality stratum in WHO Regions,[a] estimates for 2001

These figures were produced by WHO using the best available evidence. They are not necessarily the official statistics of Member States.

Cause[b]	SEX						AFRICA		THE AMERICAS		
							Mortality stratum		Mortality stratum		
	Both sexes		Males		Females		High child, high adult	High child, very high adult	Very low child, very low adult	Low child, low adult	High child, high adult
Population (000)	6 122 210		3 083 884		3 038 327		301 878	353 598	328 176	437 142	72 649
	(000)	% total	(000)	% total	(000)	% total	(000)	(000)	(000)	(000)	(000)
TOTAL DALYs	1 467 257	100	768 131	100	699 126	100	147 899	209 985	46 520	81 270	17 427
I. Communicable diseases, maternal and perinatal conditions and nutritional deficiencies	615 737	42.0	304 269	39.6	311 468	44.6	105 097	156 359	3 250	17 105	6 761
Infectious and parasitic diseases	359 377	24.5	184 997	24.1	174 380	24.9	71 903	117 144	1 422	7 424	3 709
Tuberculosis	36 040	2.5	22 629	2.9	13 411	1.9	3 987	4 954	15	532	397
STDs excluding HIV	12 404	0.8	4 804	0.6	7 600	1.1	2 287	2 854	73	484	78
Syphilis	5 400	0.4	2 984	0.4	2 416	0.3	1 398	1 842	2	65	32
Chlamydia	3 494	0.2	295	0.0	3 199	0.5	373	434	53	235	14
Gonorrhoea	3 320	0.2	1 437	0.2	1 883	0.3	516	577	16	178	30
HIV/AIDS	88 429	6.0	45 457	5.9	42 973	6.1	12 513	54 947	465	1 161	1 141
Diarrhoeal diseases	62 451	4.3	31 633	4.1	30 818	4.4	8 058	13 466	102	1 860	832
Childhood diseases	48 268	3.3	24 102	3.1	24 166	3.5	14 476	10 522	52	191	247
Pertussis	12 464	0.8	6 224	0.8	6 240	0.9	3 479	2 790	50	176	229
Poliomyelitis	164	0.0	84	0.0	80	0.0	11	4	2	6	1
Diphtheria	185	0.0	96	0.0	89	0.0	24	24	0	2	7
Measles	26 495	1.8	13 235	1.7	13 260	1.9	8 863	6 261	0	0	0
Tetanus	8 960	0.6	4 462	0.6	4 497	0.6	2 098	1 444	0	6	10
Meningitis	6 420	0.4	3 458	0.5	2 961	0.4	472	492	48	458	190
Hepatitis B[c]	1 684	0.1	1 079	0.1	605	0.1	123	150	21	61	43
Hepatitis C[c]	844	0.1	531	0.1	313	0.0	64	77	60	30	9
Malaria	42 280	2.9	20 024	2.6	22 256	3.2	18 255	17 757	0	88	20
Tropical diseases	12 994	0.9	8 741	1.1	4 252	0.6	3 138	3 113	11	576	218
Trypanosomiasis	1 598	0.1	1 029	0.1	568	0.1	802	755	0	0	0
Chagas disease	649	0.0	333	0.0	316	0.0	0	0	8	440	200
Schistosomiasis	1 760	0.1	1 081	0.1	678	0.1	666	754	1	72	10
Leishmaniasis	2 357	0.2	1 410	0.2	946	0.1	228	175	1	54	5
Lymphatic filariasis	5 644	0.4	4 317	0.6	1 327	0.2	921	1 012	0	8	1
Onchocerciasis	987	0.1	571	0.1	416	0.1	521	417	0	1	2
Leprosy	177	0.0	98	0.0	79	0.0	8	8	0	18	0
Dengue	653	0.0	287	0.0	366	0.1	2	4	0	24	66
Japanese encephalitis	767	0.1	367	0.0	400	0.1	0	0	0	0	0
Trachoma	3 997	0.3	1 082	0.1	2 915	0.4	708	818	0	0	0
Intestinal nematode infections	4 706	0.3	2 410	0.3	2 296	0.3	297	377	11	511	102
Ascariasis	1 181	0.1	604	0.1	577	0.1	49	72	3	144	26
Trichuriasis	1 649	0.1	849	0.1	800	0.1	52	72	5	240	47
Hookworm disease	1 825	0.1	932	0.1	893	0.1	195	231	3	127	20
Respiratory infections	94 037	6.4	49 591	6.5	44 446	6.4	13 111	16 761	425	2 139	965
Lower respiratory infections	90 748	6.2	47 902	6.2	42 846	6.1	12 830	16 400	373	1 980	891
Upper respiratory infections	1 815	0.1	934	0.1	881	0.1	150	189	15	48	52
Otitis media	1 474	0.1	755	0.1	719	0.1	132	172	38	110	21
Maternal conditions	30 943	2.1	0	0.0	30 943	4.4	4 783	6 546	189	1 158	496
Perinatal conditions	98 422	6.7	53 777	7.0	44 645	6.4	11 091	10 829	739	5 257	1 100
Nutritional deficiencies	32 958	2.2	15 905	2.1	17 054	2.4	4 209	5 079	476	1 127	490
Protein–energy malnutrition	16 680	1.1	8 491	1.1	8 190	1.2	2 635	2 946	33	731	257
Iodine deficiency	2 502	0.2	1 741	0.2	761	0.1	216	642	5	65	22
Vitamin A deficiency	981	0.1	402	0.1	579	0.1	386	439	0	0	0
Iron-deficiency anaemia	12 039	0.8	4 918	0.6	7 121	1.0	959	1 049	434	294	207

Cause[b]	EASTERN MEDITERRANEAN Mortality stratum		EUROPE Mortality stratum			SOUTH-EAST ASIA Mortality stratum		WESTERN PACIFIC Mortality stratum	
	Low child, low adult	High child, high adult	Very low child, very low adult	Low child, low adult	Low child, high adult	Low child, low adult	High child, high adult	Very low child, very low adult	Low child, low adult
	141 835	*351 256*	*412 512*	*219 983*	*241 683*	*297 525*	*1 262 285*	*154 919*	*1 546 770*
	(000)	(000)	(000)	(000)	(000)	(000)	(000)	(000)	(000)
TOTAL DALYs	23 007	113 214	53 075	38 936	59 212	61 290	357 554	16 430	241 438
I. Communicable diseases, maternal and perinatal conditions and nutritional deficiencies	5 691	61 446	2 579	7 029	4 999	20 403	167 749	1 064	56 205
Infectious and parasitic diseases	2 227	32 514	958	2 388	2 530	11 018	82 977	358	22 805
Tuberculosis	175	2 813	57	469	1 152	3 549	12 419	46	5 472
STDs excluding HIV	139	1 184	79	151	130	464	3 854	34	593
Syphilis	3	584	3	6	7	45	1 283	1	128
Chlamydia	96	296	60	94	79	250	1 199	25	286
Gonorrhoea	37	287	15	42	39	165	1 236	7	174
HIV/AIDS	15	1 698	208	43	657	1 850	11 758	7	1 966
Diarrhoeal diseases	683	10 101	109	584	138	1 128	21 249	44	4 097
Childhood diseases	59	7 129	65	298	30	1 529	11 431	35	2 203
Pertussis	42	2 383	63	60	26	159	2 545	34	429
Poliomyelitis	4	15	1	7	1	10	54	0	47
Diphtheria	0	16	0	1	1	7	96	0	7
Measles	9	3 039	1	227	2	1 151	5 771	1	1 169
Tetanus	4	1 676	0	3	0	202	2 964	0	551
Meningitis	110	963	64	281	96	422	2 162	13	649
Hepatitis B[c]	35	136	18	48	24	143	471	21	388
Hepatitis C[c]	16	68	30	30	14	63	192	33	158
Malaria	49	2 001	2	18	0	353	3 327	0	409
Tropical diseases	51	1 004	0	8	0	247	4 144	4	480
Trypanosomiasis	0	40	0	0	0	0	0	0	0
Chagas disease	0	0	0	0	0	0	0	0	0
Schistosomiasis	28	174	0	0	0	2	1	0	51
Leishmaniasis	20	258	0	6	0	6	1 580	0	25
Lymphatic filariasis	4	485	0	2	0	239	2 563	4	404
Onchocerciasis	0	46	0	0	0	0	0	0	0
Leprosy	0	16	0	0	0	18	101	0	7
Dengue	9	76	0	0	0	79	281	0	112
Japanese encephalitis	0	81	0	0	0	25	322	0	340
Trachoma	238	364	0	0	0	81	167	2	1 619
Intestinal nematode infections	48	219	0	8	0	487	1 063	6	1 576
Ascariasis	20	42	0	7	0	113	156	1	547
Trichuriasis	1	36	0	0	0	196	233	2	766
Hookworm disease	27	138	0	0	0	177	657	2	246
Respiratory infections	1 115	10 615	677	2 056	893	2 497	30 407	394	11 983
Lower respiratory infections	1 050	10 327	614	1 973	814	2 358	29 619	372	11 147
Upper respiratory infections	24	175	26	48	53	58	449	10	518
Otitis media	40	113	37	34	25	81	338	13	318
Maternal conditions	446	3 684	156	329	266	1 404	8 623	59	2 805
Perinatal conditions	1 289	11 174	489	1 666	712	3 828	35 667	127	14 453
Nutritional deficiencies	615	3 460	299	591	599	1 656	10 075	125	4 158
Protein–energy malnutrition	178	1 981	25	115	57	691	5 107	17	1 907
Iodine deficiency	90	398	2	162	311	57	417	0	115
Vitamin A deficiency	0	45	0	1	0	3	96	0	11
Iron-deficiency anaemia	345	933	267	288	204	821	4 050	105	2 083

Annex Table 3 Burden of disease in DALYs by cause, sex and mortality stratum in WHO Regions,[a] estimates for 2001

These figures were produced by WHO using the best available evidence. They are not necessarily the official statistics of Member States.

Cause[b]	SEX Both sexes (000)	% total	Males (000)	% total	Females (000)	% total	AFRICA High child, high adult (000)	High child, very high adult (000)	THE AMERICAS Very low child, very low adult (000)	Low child, low adult (000)	High child, high adult (000)
Population (000)	6 122 210		3 083 884		3 038 327		301 878	353 598	328 176	437 142	72 649
II. Noncommunicable conditions	672 865	45.9	346 575	45.1	326 290	46.7	30 030	36 075	38 642	50 328	8 432
Malignant neoplasms	76 716	5.2	40 943	5.3	35 772	5.1	2 956	3 881	5 555	4 513	883
Mouth and oropharynx cancers	3 734	0.3	2 693	0.4	1 041	0.1	132	284	101	128	14
Oesophagus cancer	4 191	0.3	2 712	0.4	1 478	0.2	60	238	133	134	8
Stomach cancer	8 149	0.6	5 067	0.7	3 082	0.4	214	204	139	398	141
Colon/rectum cancer	5 762	0.4	3 089	0.4	2 673	0.4	144	166	593	287	38
Liver cancer	7 317	0.5	5 132	0.7	2 185	0.3	431	500	127	180	63
Pancreas cancer	1 948	0.1	1 099	0.1	849	0.1	34	52	249	143	22
Trachea/bronchus/lung cancers	11 258	0.8	8 065	1.0	3 194	0.5	98	157	1 400	474	26
Melanoma and other skin cancers	671	0.0	377	0.0	294	0.0	38	59	123	61	11
Breast cancer	6 317	0.4	23	0.0	6 294	0.9	187	300	666	427	60
Cervix uteri cancer	3 827	0.3	…	…	3 827	0.5	288	505	94	300	77
Corpus uteri cancer	937	0.1	…	…	937	0.1	13	20	88	170	54
Ovary cancer	1 605	0.1	…	…	1 605	0.2	47	91	149	95	16
Prostate cancer	1 495	0.1	1 495	0.2	…	…	149	125	212	159	32
Bladder cancer	1 548	0.1	1 059	0.1	490	0.1	74	65	109	52	6
Lymphomas, multiple myeloma	4 360	0.3	2 403	0.3	1 957	0.3	353	362	376	230	51
Leukaemia	4 660	0.3	2 670	0.3	1 989	0.3	145	232	252	360	88
Other neoplasms	1 773	0.1	904	0.1	869	0.1	31	44	104	136	22
Diabetes mellitus	15 446	1.1	7 328	1.0	8 118	1.2	358	460	1 388	1 798	226
Nutritional/endocrine disorders	8 232	0.6	3 763	0.5	4 469	0.6	754	897	802	1 181	252
Neuropsychiatric disorders	191 260	13.0	93 488	12.2	97 772	14.0	7 868	9 412	13 845	18 598	2 927
Unipolar depressive disorders	65 911	4.5	26 279	3.4	39 632	5.7	1 939	2 258	5 152	5 687	887
Bipolar affective disorder	13 708	0.9	6 932	0.9	6 776	1.0	767	899	516	1 037	176
Schizophrenia	15 891	1.1	8 117	1.1	7 774	1.1	755	871	522	1 237	208
Epilepsy	6 787	0.5	3 617	0.5	3 171	0.5	455	690	173	729	147
Alcohol use disorders	19 843	1.4	16 623	2.2	3 221	0.5	251	752	2 497	3 435	344
Alzheimer and other dementias	12 437	0.8	5 393	0.7	7 043	1.0	287	324	1 472	774	59
Parkinson disease	1 599	0.1	771	0.1	828	0.1	31	38	230	51	7
Multiple sclerosis	1 442	0.1	624	0.1	818	0.1	52	41	113	102	16
Drug use disorders	7 116	0.5	5 556	0.7	1 560	0.2	590	642	786	806	233
Post-traumatic stress disorder	3 266	0.2	906	0.1	2 360	0.3	143	167	181	203	32
Obsessive–compulsive disorder	4 819	0.3	2 074	0.3	2 745	0.4	380	447	223	543	87
Panic disorder	6 636	0.5	2 254	0.3	4 383	0.6	347	408	269	499	85
Insomnia (primary)	3 406	0.2	1 467	0.2	1 939	0.3	136	158	264	316	48
Migraine	7 565	0.5	2 053	0.3	5 511	0.8	187	246	500	735	148
Sense organ disorders	38 742	2.6	18 759	2.4	19 983	2.9	2 086	2 234	1 681	1 793	307
Glaucoma	1 152	0.1	456	0.1	696	0.1	158	163	15	89	6
Cataracts	8 269	0.6	3 896	0.5	4 373	0.6	863	857	40	304	118
Hearing loss, adult onset	25 873	1.8	13 185	1.7	12 688	1.8	942	1 072	1 402	1 168	149
Cardiovascular diseases	144 471	9.8	77 155	10.0	67 316	9.6	5 388	5 976	6 950	7 194	1 001
Rheumatic heart disease	6 112	0.4	2 615	0.3	3 497	0.5	359	405	42	108	11
Hypertensive heart disease	7 306	0.5	3 630	0.5	3 676	0.5	256	304	324	563	118
Ischaemic heart disease	58 725	4.0	33 826	4.4	24 899	3.6	1 614	1 644	3 523	2 688	295
Cerebrovascular disease	45 870	3.1	23 603	3.1	22 267	3.2	1 508	1 810	1 448	2 332	277
Inflammatory heart disease	5 670	0.4	3 272	0.4	2 398	0.3	358	414	400	418	24

Cause[b]	EASTERN MEDITERRANEAN Mortality stratum		EUROPE Mortality stratum			SOUTH-EAST ASIA Mortality stratum		WESTERN PACIFIC Mortality stratum	
	Low child, low adult	High child, high adult	Very low child, very low adult	Low child, low adult	Low child, high adult	Low child, low adult	High child, high adult	Very low child, very low adult	Low child, low adult
	141 835	351 256	412 512	219 983	241 683	297 525	1 262 285	154 919	1 546 770
	(000)	(000)	(000)	(000)	(000)	(000)	(000)	(000)	(000)
II. Noncommunicable conditions	13 282	39 329	46 259	27 473	42 170	31 866	144 703	13 720	150 556
Malignant neoplasms	1 084	2 824	8 554	3 330	5 486	3 027	10 630	2 743	21 248
Mouth and oropharynx cancers	43	203	277	110	216	199	1 365	58	603
Oesophagus cancer	39	106	239	78	133	43	732	92	2 155
Stomach cancer	135	131	454	296	714	97	550	404	4 273
Colon/rectum cancer	64	144	1 028	279	570	279	372	373	1 426
Liver cancer	46	129	276	106	132	363	483	276	4 205
Pancreas cancer	20	34	379	121	208	60	133	148	346
Trachea/bronchus/lung cancers	122	218	1 660	642	1 021	368	1 310	420	3 341
Melanoma and other skin cancers	4	19	140	45	66	11	27	26	41
Breast cancer	86	332	993	296	514	395	839	201	1 021
Cervix uteri cancer	54	121	105	114	163	240	1 349	35	384
Corpus uteri cancer	8	17	131	78	133	29	34	32	128
Ovary cancer	16	64	229	83	157	129	239	56	235
Prostate cancer	13	38	335	64	101	41	114	59	52
Bladder cancer	26	213	254	89	125	47	270	40	178
Lymphomas, multiple myeloma	130	292	437	168	137	203	1 107	113	400
Leukaemia	101	330	323	182	211	228	759	96	1 352
Other neoplasms	35	191	176	38	65	333	271	68	259
Diabetes mellitus	418	833	1 083	526	682	1 098	3 417	377	2 783
Nutritional/endocrine disorders	242	629	637	177	184	402	537	229	1 310
Neuropsychiatric disorders	4 234	10 555	14 727	7 015	8 858	8 538	39 553	3 757	41 373
Unipolar depressive disorders	1 211	3 623	4 091	2 587	2 612	2 874	17 299	1 005	14 685
Bipolar affective disorder	360	832	617	473	450	705	2 946	241	3 691
Schizophrenia	448	994	591	569	443	1 054	3 629	234	4 336
Epilepsy	125	479	244	191	192	335	1 879	66	1 082
Alcohol use disorders	16	178	2 129	610	1 690	570	1 435	480	5 456
Alzheimer and other dementias	172	400	3 153	452	967	446	1 681	530	1 719
Parkinson disease	25	173	287	65	80	54	190	107	261
Multiple sclerosis	33	72	156	60	86	64	272	30	346
Drug use disorders	488	606	757	180	447	124	859	246	351
Post-traumatic stress disorder	79	185	207	125	130	180	705	81	847
Obsessive–compulsive disorder	186	335	256	270	281	172	822	63	755
Panic disorder	177	408	321	245	238	363	1 470	127	1 679
Insomnia (primary)	34	155	346	117	158	116	842	130	584
Migraine	144	405	742	254	238	341	1 682	153	1 788
Sense organ disorders	879	2 457	2 234	1 024	1 819	2 995	10 585	806	7 841
Glaucoma	68	141	44	37	102	34	71	8	217
Cataracts	174	695	19	87	236	599	2 959	18	1 299
Hearing loss, adult onset	574	1 464	1 857	768	1 299	2 199	6 917	661	5 400
Cardiovascular diseases	2 935	8 855	9 201	8 495	16 440	6 104	35 427	2 391	28 115
Rheumatic heart disease	68	510	78	137	217	228	2 336	20	1 593
Hypertensive heart disease	294	537	317	515	349	593	866	41	2 229
Ischaemic heart disease	1 514	3 839	3 867	3 702	8 431	2 246	17 990	772	6 601
Cerebrovascular disease	489	1 875	2 590	2 496	5 357	1 971	7 981	1 099	14 637
Inflammatory heart disease	79	386	278	324	600	254	1 320	78	737

Annex Table 3 Burden of disease in DALYs by cause, sex and mortality stratum in WHO Regions,[a] estimates for 2001

These figures were produced by WHO using the best available evidence. They are not necessarily the official statistics of Member States.

Cause[b]	SEX						AFRICA		THE AMERICAS		
							Mortality stratum		Mortality stratum		
	Both sexes		Males		Females		High child, high adult	High child, very high adult	Very low child, very low adult	Low child, low adult	High child, high adult
Population (000)	6 122 210		3 083 884		3 038 327		301 878	353 598	328 176	437 142	72 649
	(000)	% total	(000)	% total	(000)	% total	(000)	(000)	(000)	(000)	(000)
Respiratory diseases	62 842	4.3	34 634	4.5	28 208	4.0	3 126	4 144	2 986	4 848	761
Chronic obstructive pulmonary disease	29 917	2.0	17 012	2.2	12 905	1.8	505	608	1 552	1 359	86
Asthma	15 010	1.0	8 036	1.0	6 973	1.0	943	1 300	777	1 539	282
Digestive diseases	50 173	3.4	28 303	3.7	21 869	3.1	2 864	3 506	1 705	3 759	782
Peptic ulcer disease	4 585	0.3	2 922	0.4	1 663	0.2	144	196	53	136	39
Cirrhosis of the liver	15 051	1.0	9 765	1.3	5 286	0.8	527	621	494	1 164	274
Appendicitis	418	0.0	245	0.0	173	0.0	25	33	14	37	14
Diseases of the genitourinary system	15 010	1.0	8 822	1.1	6 188	0.9	1 271	1 509	595	1 055	265
Nephritis/nephrosis	8 236	0.6	4 527	0.6	3 709	0.5	651	771	238	488	166
Benign prostatic hypertrophy	2 428	0.2	2 428	0.3	...	...	126	143	87	200	28
Skin diseases	2 171	0.1	1 183	0.2	989	0.1	335	425	73	171	42
Musculoskeletal diseases	29 798	2.0	13 007	1.7	16 792	2.4	1 037	1 144	1 923	2 178	304
Rheumatoid arthritis	4 757	0.3	1 353	0.2	3 404	0.5	127	141	324	532	83
Osteoarthritis	16 372	1.1	6 621	0.9	9 750	1.4	625	687	1 045	969	117
Congenital abnormalities	28 083	1.9	14 330	1.9	13 753	2.0	1 715	2 161	685	2 284	514
Oral diseases	8 148	0.6	3 956	0.5	4 191	0.6	242	282	352	820	147
Dental caries	4 677	0.3	2 371	0.3	2 306	0.3	180	212	180	696	129
Periodontal disease	296	0.0	150	0.0	146	0.0	14	17	13	21	3
Edentulism	3 057	0.2	1 398	0.2	1 659	0.2	43	48	156	95	13
III. Injuries	**178 656**	**12.2**	**117 287**	**15.3**	**61 368**	**8.8**	**12 771**	**17 551**	**4 628**	**13 837**	**2 235**
Unintentional	129 853	8.9	82 378	10.7	47 475	6.8	9 403	10 886	3 053	7 288	1 679
Road traffic accidents	37 719	2.6	26 187	3.4	11 532	1.6	2 786	3 527	1 348	2 712	459
Poisoning	7 508	0.5	4 706	0.6	2 802	0.4	488	662	315	73	20
Falls	15 672	1.1	9 835	1.3	5 837	0.8	411	472	378	696	130
Fires	10 974	0.7	4 686	0.6	6 287	0.9	837	827	96	143	37
Drowning	11 778	0.8	8 150	1.1	3 628	0.5	1 648	1 353	112	478	109
Other unintentional injuries	46 202	3.1	28 814	3.8	17 389	2.5	3 233	4 045	804	3 186	926
Intentional	48 802	3.3	34 910	4.5	13 893	2.0	3 369	6 666	1 575	6 549	555
Self-inflicted	19 923	1.4	11 579	1.5	8 345	1.2	284	461	808	635	99
Violence	20 167	1.4	15 831	2.1	4 336	0.6	2 248	2 895	684	5 653	452
War	8 309	0.6	7 193	0.9	1 116	0.2	836	3 309	70	236	4

[a] See the List of Member States by WHO Region and mortality stratum.

[b] Estimates for specific causes may not sum to broader cause groupings due to omission of residual categories.

[c] Does not include liver cancer and cirrhosis deaths resulting from chronic hepatitis virus infection.

... Data not available or not applicable.

Cause[b]	EASTERN MEDITERRANEAN Mortality stratum		EUROPE Mortality stratum			SOUTH-EAST ASIA Mortality stratum		WESTERN PACIFIC Mortality stratum	
	Low child, low adult	High child, high adult	Very low child, very low adult	Low child, low adult	Low child, high adult	Low child, low adult	High child, high adult	Very low child, very low adult	Low child, low adult
	141 835	*351 256*	*412 512*	*219 983*	*241 683*	*297 525*	*1 262 285*	*154 919*	*1 546 770*
	(000)	(000)	(000)	(000)	(000)	(000)	(000)	(000)	(000)
Respiratory diseases	674	3 125	3 195	1 699	2 149	2 366	14 042	1 053	18 674
Chronic obstructive pulmonary disease	178	828	1 777	737	1 201	895	6 441	380	13 372
Asthma	304	999	706	369	290	543	3 630	375	2 952
Digestive diseases	545	3 622	2 447	2 027	2 682	2 523	12 791	706	10 214
Peptic ulcer disease	38	235	133	153	219	258	1 712	35	1 234
Cirrhosis of the liver	133	940	922	687	1 014	854	4 206	201	3 015
Appendicitis	7	20	16	9	21	27	96	5	94
Diseases of the genitourinary system	349	1 114	549	565	725	823	2 729	225	3 236
Nephritis/nephrosis	120	757	195	273	220	479	1 865	99	1 915
Benign prostatic hypertrophy	67	133	121	64	76	116	526	50	690
Skin diseases	21	145	88	37	133	241	309	19	133
Musculoskeletal diseases	485	1 203	2 448	1 468	1 902	1 564	5 085	982	8 077
Rheumatoid arthritis	99	218	423	271	359	117	855	142	1 065
Osteoarthritis	227	577	1 489	930	1 210	931	2 474	649	4 442
Congenital abnormalities	962	3 121	566	679	697	1 191	7 616	221	5 670
Oral diseases	419	655	353	393	347	661	1 712	141	1 623
Dental caries	201	367	200	192	164	251	1 062	76	767
Periodontal disease	5	19	16	11	13	15	98	6	46
Edentulism	210	262	134	189	169	389	517	58	775
III. Injuries	**3 960**	**12 439**	**4 237**	**4 434**	**12 042**	**9 021**	**45 102**	**1 646**	**34 677**
Unintentional	3 296	9 033	3 121	3 371	7 614	7 032	36 900	994	26 184
Road traffic accidents	1 312	2 273	1 251	651	1 615	3 934	7 245	323	8 286
Poisoning	66	367	128	132	1 860	172	1 662	42	1 521
Falls	350	1 098	635	547	853	713	4 939	185	4 266
Fires	242	1 013	62	165	668	307	6 008	26	542
Drowning	154	690	76	176	603	329	2 201	66	3 781
Other unintentional injuries	1 171	3 592	969	1 700	2 017	1 577	14 844	350	7 787
Intentional	738	3 406	1 116	1 063	4 428	1 989	8 203	653	8 493
Self-inflicted	291	690	947	512	1 995	864	5 768	617	5 952
Violence	324	618	144	320	1 916	521	1 978	35	2 378
War	113	2 040	24	211	490	600	246	0	130

Annex Table 5 Selected National Health Accounts indicators for all Member States, estimates for 1995 to 2000[a]

These figures were produced by WHO using the best available evidence. They are not necessarily the official statistics of Member States.

Member State	Total expenditure on health as % of GDP						Private expenditure on health as % of total expenditure on health						General government expenditure on health as % of total expenditure on health					
	1995	1996	1997	1998	1999	2000	1995	1996	1997	1998	1999	2000	1995	1996	1997	1998	1999	2000
56 Equatorial Guinea	4.2	4.7	3.6	4.2	3.4	3.4	34.8	44.4	44	40.6	32.4	32.4	65.2	55.6	56	59.4	67.6	67.6
57 Eritrea	3.4	3.9	4.4	5.4	4.1	4.3	14.9	12.9	34.2	33.9	35.7	34.4	85.1	87.1	65.8	66.1	64.3	65.6
58 Estonia	8.6	7.2	6.3	6	6.6	6.1	8.6	10.2	11.5	13.7	19.6	23.3	91.4	89.8	88.5	86.3	80.4	76.7
59 Ethiopia	3.8	3.8	4.4	4.9	4.6	4.6	62.7	60.8	62.1	57.1	60.2	60.6	37.3	39.2	37.9	42.9	39.8	39.4
60 Fiji	3.8	3.9	3.9	4.1	3.7	3.9	35	33.8	33.3	34.6	34.8	34.8	65	66.2	66.7	65.4	65.2	65.2
61 Finland	7.5	7.7	7.3	6.9	6.9	6.6	24.5	24.2	23.9	23.7	24.7	24.9	75.5	75.8	76.1	76.3	75.3	75.1
62 France	9.6	9.6	9.4	9.3	9.4	9.5	23.9	23.9	23.8	24	23.9	24	76.1	76.1	76.2	76	76.1	76
63 Gabon	3.1	3	2.9	3.2	3.3	3	33.8	33.7	33.5	36.5	38.8	31.4	66.2	66.3	66.5	63.5	61.2	68.6
64 Gambia	3.9	3.6	3.5	3.8	4.2	4.1	18.6	18.6	18.2	17.9	17.1	17.6	81.4	81.4	81.8	82.1	82.9	82.4
65 Georgia	4.6	6.9	6.9	7.1	6.9	7.1	87.1	86.1	85.3	86.7	89.8	89.5	12.9	13.9	14.7	13.3	10.2	10.5
66 Germany	10.6	10.9	10.7	10.6	10.7	10.6	23.3	23.2	24.7	25.2	25.2	24.9	76.7	76.8	75.3	74.8	74.8	75.1
67 Ghana	4.2	4.1	3.9	4.1	4.2	4.2	56.6	56	55.2	48.5	48.1	46.5	43.4	44	44.8	51.5	51.9	53.5
68 Greece	8.9	8.9	8.7	8.7	8.7	8.3	45.5	44.8	44.8	45.6	45.7	44.5	54.5	55.2	55.2	54.4	54.3	55.5
69 Grenada	4.4	4.8	4.7	4.8	4.8	4.8	33.4	31.7	33.9	34.2	30.3	29.9	66.6	68.3	66.1	65.8	69.7	70.1
70 Guatemala	4.1	4.1	4.3	4.5	4.7	4.7	56.2	57.6	55.1	52.9	51.7	52.1	43.8	42.4	44.9	47.1	48.3	47.9
71 Guinea	3.5	3.5	3.6	3.6	3.8	3.4	45.7	45.6	42.8	39.6	37.5	42.9	54.3	54.4	57.2	60.4	62.5	57.1
72 Guinea-Bissau	3.6	4.3	3.9	4	3.9	3.9	37.9	36.1	36	34.9	34.2	34.6	62.1	63.9	64	65.1	65.8	65.4
73 Guyana	4.7	4.5	4.8	4.8	5	5.1	17.6	17.5	16.5	16.6	16	17.3	82.4	82.5	83.5	83.4	84	82.7
74 Haiti	5.8	5.1	4.9	5.1	4.9	4.9	43.2	47.7	48.3	50.1	49	50.7	56.8	52.3	51.7	49.9	51	49.3
75 Honduras	6.8	6.8	6.1	6.6	6.3	6.8	47.5	45.5	42.4	35	38.4	36.9	52.5	54.5	57.6	65	61.6	63.1
76 Hungary	7.5	7.2	7	6.9	6.8	6.8	16	18.4	18.7	20.4	21.8	24.3	84	81.6	81.3	79.6	78.2	75.7
77 Iceland	8.2	8.2	8	8.3	8.7	8.9	15.5	16.1	16.3	16.1	15.2	15.6	84.5	83.9	83.7	83.9	84.8	84.4
78 India	5	5.2	5.3	5	5.1	4.9	83.8	84.4	84.3	81.6	82.1	82.2	16.2	15.6	15.7	18.4	17.9	17.8
79 Indonesia	1.7	2.3	2.4	2.5	2.6	2.7	62.7	72.1	76.3	72.8	72	76.3	37.3	27.9	23.7	27.2	28	23.7
80 Iran, Islamic Republic of	5.6	5.4	5.7	5.6	5.4	5.5	54.4	51.8	54	54.5	53.8	53.7	45.6	48.2	46	45.5	46.2	46.3
81 Iraq	4.9	4.6	5	4.4	3.7	3.7	40.7	41.8	41.1	40.9	40	40.1	59.3	58.2	58.9	59.1	60	59.9
82 Ireland	7.3	7	6.9	6.8	6.8	6.7	27.5	26.7	24.1	23.8	23.7	24.2	72.5	73.3	75.9	76.2	76.3	75.8
83 Israel	9.9	10.2	10.1	10	10.9	10.9	25.6	21.4	21.3	23	22.3	24.1	74.4	78.6	78.7	77	77.7	75.9
84 Italy	7.4	7.5	7.7	7.7	7.8	8.1	27.8	28.2	27.8	28	27.7	26.3	72.2	71.8	72.2	72	72.3	73.7
85 Jamaica	4.5	4.5	4.9	5.3	5.8	5.5	53.8	53.4	52.1	50.2	50.2	53	46.2	46.6	47.9	49.8	49.8	47
86 Japan[b]	7	7	7.2	7.1	7.4	7.8	21.8	19.7	20.5	22.6	22	23.3	78.2	80.3	79.5	77.4	78	76.7
87 Jordan	9.6	9.9	8.8	8.8	8	8.1	50.2	49.8	43.1	43.1	44.7	48.2	49.8	50.2	56.9	56.9	55.3	51.8
88 Kazakhstan	6	6	6.2	5.1	4.2	3.7	18.2	23.7	23.6	29.4	29.1	26.8	81.8	76.3	76.4	70.6	70.9	73.2
89 Kenya	8.1	8.1	8.3	8.4	8.4	8.3	73.4	72.7	73.8	73.8	73.5	77.8	26.6	27.3	26.2	26.2	26.5	22.2
90 Kiribati	9	8.8	9	8.4	8.3	8.1	0.9	0.9	0.9	0.8	0.8	1.3	99.1	99.1	99.1	99.2	99.2	98.7
91 Kuwait	3.6	3.1	3.3	3.9	3.5	3	10	13	12.6	12.9	13.2	12.8	90	87	87.4	87.1	86.8	87.2
92 Kyrgyzstan	7.8	6.7	6.4	6.8	6.1	6	11.9	19.2	20.3	28.1	33.4	38.3	88.1	80.8	79.7	71.9	66.6	61.7
93 Lao People's Democratic Republic	2.8	2.9	3.5	3.3	3.4	3.4	52.9	58	61.5	64	63	62	47.1	42	38.5	36	37	38
94 Latvia	6.5	6.3	6.2	6.6	6.4	5.9	34.6	36.9	38.2	38.9	37.1	40	65.4	63.1	61.8	61.1	62.9	60
95 Lebanon	10.8	10.9	11.3	11.6	11.7	11.8	72	71.6	72.3	72.5	72.5	72.2	28	28.4	27.7	27.5	27.5	27.8
96 Lesotho	6.2	5.6	5.3	5.9	6.4	6.3	21.3	22	24	21.7	18.8	17.7	78.7	78	76	78.3	81.2	82.3
97 Liberia	2.9	3	3.2	3.5	3.9	4	31.1	32.1	30.9	26.6	23.5	23.8	68.9	67.9	69.1	73.4	76.5	76.2
98 Libyan Arab Jamahiriya	3.6	3.6	3.5	3.7	3.3	3.3	59.5	58.1	50	50	50.9	51.4	40.5	41.9	50	50	49.1	48.6
99 Lithuania	5.2	5.5	5.9	6.3	6.1	6	13.7	23.1	22.3	23.3	24.9	27.6	86.3	76.9	77.7	76.7	75.1	72.4
100 Luxembourg	6.4	6.4	5.9	5.8	6	5.8	7.6	7.2	7.6	7.6	7.1	8.1	92.4	92.8	92.4	92.4	92.9	91.9
101 Madagascar	2.7	2.7	2	2.8	3	3.5	40.4	39.1	19.3	38.1	34.6	28.2	59.6	60.9	80.7	61.9	65.4	71.8
102 Malawi	6.1	6.5	7.3	6.8	6.9	7.6	50.6	54.8	49.4	49.7	50.2	52.2	49.4	45.2	50.6	50.3	49.8	47.8
103 Malaysia	2.2	2.3	2.3	2.5	2.5	2.5	43.9	41.7	42.4	42.3	40.2	41.2	56.1	58.3	57.6	57.7	59.8	58.8
104 Maldives	5.9	6.4	6.5	6.4	6.8	7.6	16.2	15.5	18.1	18.2	17.5	16.6	83.8	84.5	81.9	81.8	82.5	83.4
105 Mali	3.2	3.3	4.2	4.5	4.7	4.9	46.9	50.4	54.2	53.5	53.2	54.5	53.1	49.6	45.8	46.5	46.8	45.5
106 Malta	8.3	8.4	8.6	8.4	8.4	8.8	28.6	30	32.1	30.7	32.5	31.5	71.4	70	67.9	69.3	67.5	68.5
107 Marshall Islands	7.8	8.8	9.2	9.5	9.8	9.4	38.8	38.3	38.1	38.4	38.9	38.6	61.2	61.7	61.9	61.6	61.1	61.4
108 Mauritania	3.2	3.2	3.3	3.8	4.2	4.3	25.5	24	26.7	27.2	24.1	20.7	74.5	76	73.3	72.8	75.9	79.3
109 Mauritius	3.6	3.6	3.5	3.4	3.6	3.4	45.9	47	46.7	46.2	43.3	43.7	54.1	53	53.3	53.8	56.7	56.3
110 Mexico	5.6	5.3	5.3	5.3	5.4	5.4	58.5	57.5	56.7	52	52.7	53.6	41.5	42.5	43.3	48	47.3	46.4

		General government expenditure on health as % of total general government expenditure						External resources for health as % of general government expenditure on health						Social security expenditure on health as % of general government expenditure on health					
		1995	1996	1997	1998	1999	2000	1995	1996	1997	1998	1999	2000	1995	1996	1997	1998	1999	2000
56	Equatorial Guinea	11.2	10.4	7.9	8.3	11.6	14.3	10.4	10.2	19	24.2	23.6	19.6	0	0	0	0	0	0
57	Eritrea	4.1	5.3	5.3	4.5	3.9	4	32.8	24.7	63.3	31.7	46.2	60.7	0	0	0	0	0	0
58	Estonia	18.8	15.9	14.6	13.3	12.7	12.4	0.6	0.9	1.1	1.7	4.4	0.5	68.8	70.6	72.2	77.1	82.1	86
59	Ethiopia	5.8	6.2	6.9	8.2	5.9	5.5	17.9	21.7	16.9	22.3	29.4	35.6	0.6	0.6	0.6	0.5	0.6	0.6
60	Fiji	8.5	8.1	7.4	6.9	6.9	7.5	7.2	6.5	6.4	19.1	18.3	19.4	0	0	0	0	0	0
61	Finland	9.5	9.7	9.8	9.9	10	10.2	0	0	0	0	0	0	17.7	18.3	18.7	19.4	19.8	20.4
62	France	13.2	13.1	13.1	13.2	13.3	13.5	0	0	0	0	0	0	96.9	96.9	96.8	96.8	96.7	96.8
63	Gabon	6.4	6.4	6.2	6.4	6.4	8.9	3.7	3.8	6.1	4.6	5.7	5.8	0	0	0	0	0	0
64	Gambia	13.7	12.7	14.3	14.7	12.1	12.1	31.5	23.2	29.3	35.1	41.1	37.5	0	0	0	0	0	0
65	Georgia	1.6	4.6	4.8	4.5	3.3	3.4	11.9	8.5	9.4	14.2	11.1	9.7	11.3	10.3	15.6	15	20.2	14.6
66	Germany	14.5	16.6	16.3	16.3	16.3	17.3	0	0	0	0	0	0	86.3	88.1	90.7	91.4	91.5	91.7
67	Ghana	8.3	8.1	8.4	8.2	8.1	7.9	15.8	14.3	17.1	14.6	14.7	24.1	0	0	0	0	0	0
68	Greece	9.5	9.8	9.9	9.8	9.6	9.2	0	0	0	0	0	0	23.6	25.2	28	38.6	38.4	36.9
69	Grenada	10.4	10	10.6	11.3	12.3	12.3	5.6	4.8	1.5	1.3	0	0	0	0	0	0	0	0
70	Guatemala	17.2	16.9	15.5	14	15.5	16.4	6.5	6.4	6.4	11.4	10.9	9.5	58.6	55.6	57.7	55.3	54.8	56.7
71	Guinea	9.2	9.2	9.7	12.9	11.9	11.9	5.3	7.4	8.5	9.6	9	16.2	0	0	0	0	0	0
72	Guinea-Bissau	9.6	10.1	10.4	13.9	11.1	8.4	11.3	13.3	36	33.1	33	39.3	0	0	0	0	0	0
73	Guyana	9.6	9.2	9.3	9.3	9.1	9.3	4.8	4.3	5.6	4.4	4.8	3.8	0	0	0	0	0	0
74	Haiti	28.1	19.8	19.6	19	20.9	22.1	40.4	45.7	29.3	41.3	46.1	67	0	0	0	0	0	0
75	Honduras	17.3	18.1	17	20.8	18.2	18.3	11.9	20.3	18.5	13.5	14.7	12.1	9.7	9.6	9.7	8.9	9.8	10.2
76	Hungary	11.3	11.4	11.4	10.2	11.5	11.8	0	0	0	0	0	0	80	82.4	82.8	82.8	83.5	83.2
77	Iceland	17.5	17.6	18.9	21	20.3	20.4	0	0	0	0	0	0	34.9	35.7	31.5	29.8	28.7	28.8
78	India	4.7	4.7	4.7	5.6	5.7	5.3	13.2	12.8	14.8	13.1	12.5	12.4	0	0	0	0	0	0
79	Indonesia	3.6	3.5	2.8	3.2	3.2	3.1	3.2	3.7	15	30.7	30.1	28.5	11.4	10.6	14.1	9	7.3	7.5
80	Iran, Islamic Republic of	10.5	12.3	10.5	10.9	11.3	11.8	0	0	0	0	0	1	40.2	37.4	36.9	39.1	39.5	39.3
81	Iraq	10.7	10.5	12.5	13.5	15.2	15.1	0	0	0	0	0	0	0	0	0	0	0	0
82	Ireland	12.8	12.9	14	14.8	14.8	16	0	0	0	0	0	0	9.7	9.2	8.3	9	11.7	12.9
83	Israel	15.7	16.8	14.6	14.3	15.9	15.7	0	0	0	0	0.3	0.4	23.8	24.9	25.6	26.3	24.3	25.8
84	Italy	10	10.1	10.9	11.1	11.6	12.7	0	0	0	0	0	0	0.4	0.4	0.4	0.1	0.1	0.1
85	Jamaica	8	5.8	7.2	7.5	7.6	7	7.9	5.5	6.1	5.8	5	4.4	0	0	0	0	0	0
86	Japan[b]	15.1	15.2	16.2	13.2	15.3	15.4	0	0	0	0	0	0	84.7	84.4	89	84.8	84	89.1
87	Jordan	12.2	12.3	12.3	12.3	12.3	12.4	2	2.1	3.6	4.1	4.2	4.3	0	0	0	0	0	0
88	Kazakhstan	15	16.1	17.4	13.4	13.4	12.3	0.4	0.3	0.3	0.4	9.3	2.4	10.2	9.5	26.9	28.3	28.7	26.4
89	Kenya	6.6	7.2	8	8.1	8.1	8.1	32.3	26.1	26.9	29.8	32.3	38.3	13.4	13	13.3	13.1	12.8	15.2
90	Kiribati	16.4	14.5	14.5	14	13.8	13.2	1.6	1.5	1.5	1.7	0.5	0.5	0	0	0	0	0	0
91	Kuwait	6.8	7.9	8.4	8	8.2	8.9	0	0	0	0	0	0	0	0	0	0	0	0
92	Kyrgyzstan	21.5	23.7	21.8	21.3	20.2	18.8	1.5	4.7	6.7	8.5	15.5	20.4	0	0	0.3	2.5	4.9	5.8
93	Lao People's Democratic Republic	6.3	5.1	5.9	4.9	4.6	5	29.4	29	33.2	46.8	72.9	73.7	0.7	0.8	0.7	0.8	0.4	0.4
94	Latvia	11	10.3	10.1	10.3	9.9	9.7	0.1	0.1	0.1	0.7	0.6	0.7	51.4	48.6	49.9	50.5	57.1	65.4
95	Lebanon	8.5	8.1	7.3	9.8	9.9	9.8	2.2	2.3	2	1.7	1.6	1.6	48	47.6	49.7	45.6	45.9	45.5
96	Lesotho	9.6	8.6	8.1	9.3	10.4	10.8	5.5	6.3	10.4	7.9	5.9	6.8	0	0	0	0	0	0
97	Liberia	9.5	9	9.3	10.1	10.8	10.7	31.4	48.3	39	37.3	36.8	40.5	0	0	0	0	0	0
98	Libyan Arab Jamahiriya	2.2	2.3	2.6	2.7	2.4	2.4	0	0	0	0	0	0	0	0	0	0	0	0
99	Lithuania	12.1	12.3	13.6	14.8	11.7	13.9	0	0	0	0	0	0	17.2	19	82.7	89.9	92.2	90.7
100	Luxembourg	13	13.1	12.5	12.7	13.3	13.3	0	0	0	0	0	0	83.4	84.3	86	82.7	88.5	90.9
101	Madagascar	9.2	9.6	10.3	10.3	11.2	15.1	36.3	29.3	30.6	36.9	37	26.9	0	0	0	0	0	0
102	Malawi	11.3	11.7	14.6	14.5	14.6	14.6	50.2	42.2	42.7	74.4	71.8	86.7	0	0	0	0	0	0
103	Malaysia	5	5.7	5.6	6	5.8	5.8	2.2	1.7	1.8	2.3	2	1.8	0	0	0	0	0	0
104	Maldives	9.2	11.3	10.9	10.1	10.4	10.2	8.5	7	6.3	7.5	6.5	6.6	0	0	0	0	0	0
105	Mali	6.9	6.6	7.8	8.3	8.3	8.3	39.6	44.1	32.4	33.6	26.4	27.3	0	0	0	0	0	0
106	Malta	13	12.3	11.7	11.9	11.8	13.2	0	0	0	0	0	0	61.5	56.5	64.5	68.9	68	59.9
107	Marshall Islands	8	7.5	9.7	10	10.6	10.8	26.4	25	24	23.6	63.6	64.8	0	0	0	0	0	0
108	Mauritania	9.5	9.9	9.3	12.5	14.6	16.3	23.7	28.6	29	33.6	43	46.6	0	0	0	0	0	0
109	Mauritius	8.9	8.4	7.9	8.3	8.4	8.4	3.4	2.6	3	3	2.6	2.5	0	0	0	0	0	0
110	Mexico	11.3	11.5	11.6	13.6	16.5	15.6	0.8	0.8	0.6	1.8	1.6	1.4	77.9	73	73.6	70.4	72.4	71.1

Annex Table 5 Selected National Health Accounts indicators for all Member States, estimates for 1995 to 2000[a]

These figures were produced by WHO using the best available evidence. They are not necessarily the official statistics of Member States.

	Member State	Total expenditure on health as % of GDP						Private expenditure on health as % of total expenditure on health						General government expenditure on health as % of total expenditure on health					
		1995	1996	1997	1998	1999	2000	1995	1996	1997	1998	1999	2000	1995	1996	1997	1998	1999	2000
111	Micronesia, Federated States of	12.1	11.4	11.4	11.2	10.9	10.5	42.9	44	43.3	44.7	45.4	46.3	57.1	56	56.7	55.3	54.6	53.7
112	Monaco	7.1	7.3	7	7.2	7.4	7.4	50	50	50	50.7	51.4	51.9	50	50	50	49.3	48.6	48.1
113	Mongolia	4.2	5.2	5	6.2	6.1	6.6	31	36.9	37.3	34.6	33.5	29.7	69	63.1	62.7	65.4	66.5	70.3
114	Morocco	4.6	4.5	4.4	4.3	4.4	4.5	71.3	71	70.5	71.8	70.6	70.4	28.7	29	29.5	28.2	29.4	29.6
115	Mozambique	4.9	5	4.6	4.3	4.1	4.3	38.9	37.2	37	37.2	38.1	36.6	61.1	62.8	63	62.8	61.9	63.4
116	Myanmar	2.1	2.2	2.1	2	2	2.2	81	82.7	85.7	89.4	88.3	82.9	19	17.3	14.3	10.6	11.7	17.1
117	Namibia	8.2	7.4	7.4	7.6	7.3	7.1	43	49	48.4	48.3	40.8	40.7	57	51	51.6	51.7	59.2	59.3
118	Nauru	10	10.6	11.7	11.8	11.4	11.3	1.1	1.1	1.1	1.1	1.1	1.1	98.9	98.9	98.9	98.9	98.9	98.9
119	Nepal	5.1	5.2	5.5	5.7	5.5	5.4	73.6	74	69.4	67.4	71.1	70.7	26.4	26	30.6	32.6	28.9	29.3
120	Netherlands	8.4	8.3	8.2	8.1	8.2	8.1	29	33.8	32.2	32.2	33.5	32.5	71	66.2	67.8	67.8	66.5	67.5
121	New Zealand	7.2	7.2	7.5	7.9	7.9	8	22.8	23.3	22.7	23	22.5	22	77.2	76.7	77.3	77	77.5	78
122	Nicaragua	6.4	6	5.2	4.8	4.7	4.4	21.7	25.6	46.2	39.7	47.2	48.3	78.3	74.4	53.8	60.3	52.8	51.7
123	Niger	3.8	3.8	3.8	3.9	3.8	3.9	54.9	57.2	56.3	55.3	54.6	55.1	45.1	42.8	43.7	44.7	45.4	44.9
124	Nigeria	2.8	2.6	2.4	2.5	2.4	2.2	85.5	88.3	86.4	81.1	77.1	79.2	14.5	11.7	13.6	18.9	22.9	20.8
125	Niue	7.4	7.9	7.6	6.7	8.2	7.6	3.2	2.6	2.7	3.3	2.9	3.8	96.8	97.4	97.3	96.7	97.1	96.2
126	Norway	8	8	7.9	8.6	8.8	7.8	15.8	15.8	15.7	15.3	14.8	14.8	84.2	84.2	84.3	84.7	85.2	85.2
127	Oman	3	2.9	2.7	3.1	2.9	2.8	20.5	19.9	21.2	21.7	20.5	17.1	79.5	80.1	78.8	78.3	79.5	82.9
128	Pakistan	4.2	4	4	4	4.1	4.1	75.2	77	77.1	76.4	78.1	77.1	24.8	23	22.9	23.6	21.9	22.9
129	Palau	7.5	6.5	6.1	6.4	6.5	6.4	11.4	12.3	12.5	12	11.8	11.5	88.6	87.7	87.5	88	88.2	88.5
130	Panama	7.8	8	7.4	7.4	7.6	7.6	29.8	29	31.6	29.7	30.1	30.8	70.2	71	68.4	70.3	69.9	69.2
131	Papua New Guinea	2.9	2.7	3.2	3.9	4.2	4.1	8.4	10.1	10.6	9.1	10.1	11.4	91.6	89.9	89.4	90.9	89.9	88.6
132	Paraguay	7.8	7.2	7.6	7.3	7.9	7.9	72.5	64	67.2	62.6	60.6	61.7	27.5	36	32.8	37.4	39.4	38.3
133	Peru	4.6	4.5	4.5	4.7	4.9	4.8	44.1	41.7	42.6	42.3	40.4	40.8	55.9	58.3	57.4	57.7	59.6	59.2
134	Philippines	3.4	3.5	3.6	3.6	3.6	3.4	60.1	58.6	56.6	57.6	53.5	54.3	39.9	41.4	43.4	42.4	46.5	45.7
135	Poland	6	6.4	6.1	6.4	6.2	6	27.1	26.6	28	34.6	28.9	30.3	72.9	73.4	72	65.4	71.1	69.7
136	Portugal	8.3	8.5	8.6	8.3	8.4	8.2	38.3	35.3	35.2	32.5	29.3	28.8	61.7	64.7	64.8	67.5	70.7	71.2
137	Qatar	4.8	4.8	4	4.5	4.1	3.2	26.1	23.4	23.7	23.4	22.7	22.5	73.9	76.6	76.3	76.6	77.3	77.5
138	Republic of Korea	4.7	4.9	5	5.1	5.6	6	63.5	61.2	59	53.8	56.9	55.9	36.5	38.8	41	46.2	43.1	44.1
139	Republic of Moldova	6.2	7.1	6.4	4.7	3.4	3.5	7.2	5.7	6.3	9.2	15.2	17.6	92.8	94.3	93.7	90.8	84.8	82.4
140	Romania	2.8	4.5	4	3.5	3.3	2.9	34	27.8	37.1	43.1	40.7	36.2	66	72.2	62.9	56.9	59.3	63.8
141	Russian Federation	5.5	5.4	5.8	5.9	5.6	5.3	18.5	21.9	27.1	31.1	35.3	27.5	81.5	78.1	72.9	68.9	64.7	72.5
142	Rwanda	6.2	6.1	5.5	5	5.4	5.2	52.4	50.1	52.1	48.7	46.6	48.7	47.6	49.9	47.9	51.3	53.4	51.3
143	Saint Kitts and Nevis	4.7	5.1	4.7	4.7	4.9	5.2	33.9	33.9	32.5	31.9	36.5	40.8	66.1	66.1	67.5	68.1	63.5	59.2
144	Saint Lucia	3.8	4	4.2	4.3	4.1	4.3	38.8	36.9	37.7	34.4	34.7	37.9	61.2	63.1	62.3	65.6	65.3	62.1
145	Saint Vincent and the Grenadines	5.8	5.7	6.1	5.9	6.1	6.3	34	32.9	36.2	37.5	38.5	34.6	66	67.1	63.8	62.5	61.5	65.4
146	Samoa	5.3	5.6	5.4	5.7	6.4	6.6	24.8	24.5	24.1	24.3	23.6	23.8	75.2	75.5	75.9	75.7	76.4	76.2
147	San Marino	10.8	10.9	10.9	11.9	11.6	11.7	14.3	15.4	15.6	14	14.2	14.3	85.7	84.6	84.4	86	85.8	85.7
148	Sao Tome and Principe	3.3	3.5	3	2.9	2.3	2.3	30.6	28.6	33.3	32.1	32.1	32.2	69.4	71.4	66.7	67.9	67.9	67.8
149	Saudi Arabia	5.3	5.1	5.1	5.7	5.4	5.3	21.3	22	21.5	20.9	20.7	20.9	78.7	78	78.5	79.1	79.3	79.1
150	Senegal	4.7	4.9	4.9	4.7	4.7	4.6	47.1	46.8	46.6	44	43.9	43.4	52.9	53.2	53.4	56	56.1	56.6
151	Seychelles	6.2	6.4	6.6	6.7	6.5	6.2	31.5	30.9	27.9	30.6	31.2	33.1	68.5	69.1	72.1	69.4	68.8	66.9
152	Sierra Leone	2.8	2.6	2.8	3	3.5	4.3	59	59	61	58	50	40	41	41	39	42	50	60
153	Singapore	3.7	3.7	3.6	4.1	4	3.5	58.2	59.8	60.5	58	61.2	64.3	41.8	40.2	39.5	42	38.8	35.7
154	Slovakia	7	7.5	6.1	5.9	5.8	5.9	17.9	18.8	8.3	8.4	10.6	10.4	82.1	81.2	91.7	91.6	89.4	89.6
155	Slovenia	9.1	8.8	8.9	8.7	8.7	8.6	21.9	20.6	20.7	21.3	21.4	21.1	78.1	79.4	79.3	78.7	78.6	78.9
156	Solomon Islands	4.3	4.2	4.6	5.3	5.6	5.9	3.8	3.8	4.7	4.2	2.7	5.5	96.2	96.2	95.3	95.8	97.3	94.5
157	Somalia	2.6	2.3	2.4	2	1.6	1.3	57.1	54.6	37.5	37.6	21.1	28.6	42.9	45.4	62.5	62.4	78.9	71.4
158	South Africa	8.4	9.2	9	8.7	8.8	8.8	51.3	53.1	53.9	57.6	57.4	57.8	48.7	46.9	46.1	42.4	42.6	42.2
159	Spain	7.7	7.7	7.6	7.6	7.7	7.7	29.1	28.9	28.9	29.5	29.8	30.1	70.9	71.1	71.1	70.5	70.2	69.9
160	Sri Lanka	3.4	3.3	3.2	3.4	3.6	3.6	51.9	50.4	50.8	49	51.3	51	48.1	49.6	49.2	51	48.7	49
161	Sudan	3.8	3.5	3.3	4.2	4.2	4.7	71.4	71.4	79.1	75.9	75.9	78.8	28.6	28.6	20.9	24.1	24.1	21.2
162	Suriname	8.3	8.8	9.1	9.9	9.7	9.8	23.8	28.9	35.4	38.4	39.3	43.9	76.2	71.1	64.6	61.6	60.7	56.1
163	Swaziland	3.3	3.9	3.3	3.7	4	4.2	27.2	27	28.4	28	30.1	27.9	72.8	73	71.6	72	69.9	72.1
164	Sweden	8.1	8.4	8.1	7.9	8.6	8.4	14.8	15.2	15.7	16.2	22.2	22.7	85.2	84.8	84.3	83.8	77.8	77.3
165	Switzerland	10	10.4	10.4	10.6	10.7	10.7	46.2	45.3	44.8	45.1	44.7	44.4	53.8	54.7	55.2	54.9	55.3	55.6

		General government expenditure on health as % of total general government expenditure						External resources for health as % of general government expenditure on health						Social security expenditure on health as % of general government expenditure on health					
		1995	1996	1997	1998	1999	2000	1995	1996	1997	1998	1999	2000	1995	1996	1997	1998	1999	2000
111	Micronesia, Federated States of	9.8	10.2	10.9	10.4	10.4	10.5	7.3	0	0	0	17.9	17.9	0	0	0	0	0	0
112	Monaco	17.6	17.8	17.8	17.9	18.4	18.5	0	0	0	0	0	0	93.3	93.8	93.8	94.1	94.4	94.6
113	Mongolia	16.3	17.4	13.4	14.7	15.2	14	10.9	5.8	6.6	13.8	28.4	24.4	17.8	14.3	36.8	39.9	39.3	40.2
114	Morocco	3.9	4.4	4.3	3.9	4	3.9	6.4	8.8	9.3	8.7	6.7	7.7	9.1	8.2	8.4	9.2	9.1	9.3
115	Mozambique	12.4	17.3	14.8	13.8	13	13.7	55.5	69.7	69.9	68.7	66.8	68.5	0	0	0	0	0	0
116	Myanmar	2.9	2.8	3.2	3.6	4.2	6.5	0.2	3.2	2.5	4.2	2.9	2.3	0.9	1.4	3.1	0.9	1.8	1.8
117	Namibia	12.9	10.2	10.3	10.4	11.3	11.1	3.7	4.4	4.2	5.2	5.7	5.7	0	0	0	0	0	0
118	Nauru	27.1	27.5	27.6	28.6	28.2	29.5	0	0	0	0	0	0	0	0	0	0	0	0
119	Nepal	7.6	7.2	9.3	9.9	9	9	37.1	36	33.9	29.8	34.4	27.5	0	0	0	0	0	0
120	Netherlands	10.6	11.1	11.5	11.7	11.5	12.1	0	0	0	0	0	0	93.6	93.7	93.6	93.8	93.8	94.1
121	New Zealand	12.2	11.5	12.7	13.5	13.9	14.5	0	0	0	0	0	0	0	0	0	0	0	0
122	Nicaragua	28.9	26.6	17	17.9	12.6	10.3	11.9	21.1	19.6	26.5	30.3	30.5	14.4	15.4	24.3	23	27.9	29.7
123	Niger	5	6.4	6.5	6.6	6.5	6.6	30.1	34	40	33.5	34.9	36.7	5.3	4.3	4.5	3.7	4	4
124	Nigeria	1.7	1.3	2.1	2.9	3.2	3	22.4	23	12	37.8	39.6	32.2	0	0	0	0	0	0
125	Niue	12	13.3	13	12.6	15.9	15.6	0	0	0	0	0	0	0	0	0	0	0	0
126	Norway	13.2	13.8	14.3	14.7	15.3	15.8	0	0	0	0	0	0	0	0	0	0	0	0
127	Oman	5.3	6	5.6	5.9	6.1	6.7	0	0	0	0	0	0	0	0	0	0	0	0
128	Pakistan	4.3	3.6	3.8	4.1	4	4	8.8	10.7	10.7	8.1	9.7	8.2	55.1	55	55.1	55.2	55.2	50
129	Palau	8.4	9.3	8.9	9.1	9.3	9.6	20	19.7	21.4	26.2	22.9	22.3	0	0	0	0	0	0
130	Panama	16.9	15.7	18.7	18.5	18.5	18.4	2.1	2	2.1	1.9	1.8	1.7	70.1	69.5	60.6	66.2	58.9	66.4
131	Papua New Guinea	8.7	8.7	9.6	12.3	13.3	12.9	15.2	24.9	30.1	31.9	20.5	24.6	0	0	0	0	0	0
132	Paraguay	11.8	14.9	13.6	14.9	17.4	16.8	0.3	4.8	5	5.1	4.9	5.1	42.1	39	47.8	44.9	46.7	48.3
133	Peru	10.9	11.6	11.7	11.9	12	11.7	3.5	3.2	3.1	3.1	3.7	3.7	42.6	45.4	44	43.5	43.9	44
134	Philippines	6.3	6.5	6.7	6.6	7.1	6.7	6.9	4	3.1	7.6	5.3	6.9	11.4	12.2	11.8	8.8	9	9.9
135	Poland	9.1	10	9.5	9.4	10.6	10.2	0	0	0	0	0	0	0	0	0	0	0	0
136	Portugal	11.4	12	12.5	12.9	13.1	13.1	0	0	0	0	0	0	7.2	6.6	6.7	7.7	7	7.2
137	Qatar	7.8	7.4	7.6	7.8	8.3	6.6	0	0	0	0	0	0	0	0	0	0	0	0
138	Republic of Korea	8.6	9.1	9.4	9.6	10.2	11.2	0	0	0	0	0	0	69.6	71	71.9	74.5	75.2	77.3
139	Republic of Moldova	15.8	18.4	14.9	13	10.2	11	0.4	0.5	0.5	1.7	7.5	13.9	0	0	0	0	0	0
140	Romania	5.3	9.6	7.5	5.5	5.1	5	0.1	0.1	1	0.9	1.5	1.1	30.7	14.5	18.7	21.6	17.5	13.3
141	Russian Federation	11.7	10.4	10.6	12.3	11.9	14.5	0.3	0.4	0.5	1.7	5.8	4.4	28.1	31.5	33.8	36.3	36.9	24.5
142	Rwanda	14	13.3	13.3	13.5	12.9	12.9	29.9	41.4	60.8	53.8	54.2	48.2	0.8	0.7	0.6	0.6	0.7	0.8
143	Saint Kitts and Nevis	9.7	9.7	10.9	10.9	10.6	10.6	13.1	11.4	10.8	10.3	10.1	9.3	0	0	0	0	0	0
144	Saint Lucia	8	8.9	9	8.8	7.9	7.8	1.2	1	1	0.8	0.8	0.8	0	0	0	0	0	0
145	Saint Vincent and the Grenadines	13.1	12.1	9.2	8.7	9	9.7	3.1	3	2.8	2.7	2.5	2.2	0	0	0	0	0	0
146	Samoa	16.4	16.9	18.2	19.7	19.5	19.3	14.2	10.8	9.5	13.6	15	32.2	0	0	0	0	0	0
147	San Marino	24.2	24.2	22.7	26.4	25.6	26.2	0	0	0	0	0	0	25.1	26	26.5	25.2	26.5	27
148	Sao Tome and Principe	2.9	3.7	2.9	3.6	3.6	3.6	44.9	36.4	71.3	75.1	89.8	71.8	0	0	0	0	0	0
149	Saudi Arabia	13.3	14	12.2	11.1	13.9	14.6	0	0	0	0	0	0	0	0	0	0	0	0
150	Senegal	13.1	13.2	13.1	13.1	13.1	13	18.4	10.8	11.8	10.7	13.3	14.3	0	0	0	0	0	0
151	Seychelles	8.2	7.8	8.7	7.9	8	6.8	1.3	1.3	4.9	5.6	5.7	5.7	0	0	0	0	0	0
152	Sierra Leone	7.1	7.2	6.5	9	8.3	9.2	19.8	23.6	19.1	27.9	22	26.7	0	0	0	0	0	0
153	Singapore	9.4	6.9	6.7	8.7	8.2	6.7	0	0	0	0	0	0	19.1	19.6	20.2	17.5	19.1	23.3
154	Slovakia	15.8	18.2	18.3	18.6	18.5	19.4	0	0	0	0.1	0	0	87.9	96.9	96.7	96.6	96.7	96.8
155	Slovenia	16.4	16.5	16.3	15.6	15.4	15.4	0	0	0	0	0	0.8	74.5	76.8	77	80.7	79.8	82
156	Solomon Islands	8.9	9	11.4	11.4	11.1	11.4	12.5	11.6	7.7	8.3	7.6	17.7	0	0	0	0	0	0
157	Somalia	4.1	3.8	5.6	4.5	4.4	3.3	22.5	14.7	7.4	10.5	5.1	1.3	0	0	0	0	0	0
158	South Africa	12.6	12.6	12.4	11.3	11.1	11.2	0.1	0.2	0.2	0.2	0.2	0.2	0	0	0	0	0	0
159	Spain	12.2	12.6	12.9	12.9	13.2	13.5	0	0	0	0	0	0	23.8	20.2	13.5	11.6	9.2	0
160	Sri Lanka	5.4	5.7	6	5.8	5.7	6.1	4.6	6.7	6.4	5.5	5.6	5.5	0	0	0	0	0	0
161	Sudan	5	4.4	3	4.2	4.2	4.2	2.6	2.5	4.2	4.5	6.8	6	0	0	0	0	0	0
162	Suriname	19.4	19	20.3	18.2	17.6	16.5	20.6	14.4	11.4	18.6	42.7	25.2	24	28.9	25.8	25	24.4	22.7
163	Swaziland	8	7.9	7.9	8.1	8	8.6	5.5	4.7	6.6	6.3	3.7	3.4	0	0	0	0	0	0
164	Sweden	10.2	10.8	10.8	10.9	11	11.3	0	0	0	0	0	0	0	0	0	0	0	0
165	Switzerland	14.5	15.2	15.3	15.4	11.9	12.7	0	0	0	0	0	0	70	70.5	71.6	72.3	72.1	72.7

Annex Table 5 Selected National Health Accounts indicators for all Member States, estimates for 1995 to 2000[a]

These figures were produced by WHO using the best available evidence. They are not necessarily the official statistics of Member States.

	Member State	Total expenditure on health as % of GDP						Private expenditure on health as % of total expenditure on health						General government expenditure on health as % of total expenditure on health					
		1995	1996	1997	1998	1999	2000	1995	1996	1997	1998	1999	2000	1995	1996	1997	1998	1999	2000
166	Syrian Arab Republic	2	2	2.1	2.3	2.5	2.5	23.9	28.1	31.2	33.4	35.2	36.6	76.1	71.9	68.8	66.6	64.8	63.4
167	Tajikistan	2	2.9	3	2.5	2.8	2.5	39.5	36.9	34	35	15.4	19.2	60.5	63.1	66	65	84.6	80.8
168	Thailand	3.4	3.6	3.7	3.9	3.7	3.7	51.1	48.9	42.8	38.6	41.7	42.6	48.9	51.1	57.2	61.4	58.3	57.4
169	The former Yugoslav Republic of Macedonia	5.2	5.8	6.1	7.6	5.9	6	9.4	13	16.1	12.9	15.9	15.5	90.6	87	83.9	87.1	84.1	84.5
170	Togo	2.9	2.6	3.1	2.7	2.7	2.8	52.4	58.4	51.5	44.8	42.9	45.7	47.6	41.6	48.5	55.2	57.1	54.3
171	Tonga	7.5	7.3	7.9	7.7	7.8	7.5	56.7	56.7	53.2	53.9	54.1	53.2	43.3	43.3	46.8	46.1	45.9	46.8
172	Trinidad and Tobago	4.5	4.6	4.8	5.3	5.3	5.2	49.5	51.2	52.5	49.1	49	49.3	50.5	48.8	47.5	50.9	51	50.7
173	Tunisia	6.8	6.6	6.4	6.8	7	7	43.9	32.5	22.3	20.9	21.2	21.8	56.1	67.5	77.7	79.1	78.8	78.2
174	Turkey	3.4	3.9	4.2	4.8	4.9	5	29.7	30.8	28.4	28.1	28.9	28.9	70.3	69.2	71.6	71.9	71.1	71.1
175	Turkmenistan	2.4	2.8	4	5	5.3	5.4	22.9	18.6	25.5	18.9	17.4	15.1	77.1	81.4	74.5	81.1	82.6	84.9
176	Tuvalu	8.9	8.3	8.4	8.6	8.8	7.8	29.1	31.3	30.2	29.3	29.3	28.6	70.9	68.8	69.8	70.7	70.7	71.4
177	Uganda	3.5	3.4	3.4	3.7	4	3.9	60.5	56.7	54.8	62	58.1	62	39.5	43.3	45.2	38	41.9	38
178	Ukraine	5.8	5	5.4	5.1	4.3	4.1	16	20.4	25	28.9	31.9	29.9	84	79.6	75	71.1	68.1	70.1
179	United Arab Emirates	3.4	3.2	3.7	4.1	3.7	3.2	20.1	20.6	20.7	20.3	21.4	22.3	79.9	79.4	79.3	79.7	78.6	77.7
180	United Kingdom	7	7	6.8	6.8	7.1	7.3	16.1	17.1	20.1	20.1	19.8	19	83.9	82.9	79.9	79.9	80.2	81
181	United Republic of Tanzania	5.3	5.1	5.2	5	5.5	5.9	44.6	51.2	51.9	51.3	56.6	53	55.4	48.8	48.1	48.7	43.4	47
182	United States of America	13.3	13.2	13	12.9	13	13	54.7	54.5	54.8	55.5	55.7	55.7	45.3	45.5	45.2	44.5	44.3	44.3
183	Uruguay	9.2	9.6	10	10.2	10.8	10.9	50.5	53	54.1	53.6	51.3	53.5	49.5	47	45.9	46.4	48.7	46.5
184	Uzbekistan	4.8	4.8	4.5	3.9	3.9	3.7	22.7	17.5	17.9	15.3	21.2	22.5	77.3	82.5	82.1	84.7	78.8	77.5
185	Vanuatu	3.3	2.8	3.3	3.5	3.9	3.9	33.9	42.4	35.8	34.6	39.7	39.1	66.1	57.6	64.2	65.4	60.3	60.9
186	Venezuela, Bolivarian Republic of	4.6	3.9	4.3	5	4.6	4.7	47.7	47.7	45.4	48.4	47.4	42.6	52.3	52.3	54.6	51.6	52.6	57.4
187	Viet Nam	3.9	4.6	4.5	4.7	5.5	5.2	59.6	65.2	68.8	70.9	75.6	74.2	40.4	34.8	31.2	29.1	24.4	25.8
188	Yemen	5.1	4.4	4.6	5.2	5	5	77.7	71.6	69.8	64	67.8	68	22.3	28.4	30.2	36	32.2	32
189	Yugoslavia	6.5	7.1	6.7	5.6	5.6	5.6	42.1	42.6	41.4	49.1	49.1	49	57.9	57.4	58.6	50.9	50.9	51
190	Zambia	5.2	5.8	6	5.6	5.2	5.6	46.9	46.8	44.9	43.1	40.7	37.9	53.1	53.2	55.1	56.9	59.3	62.1
191	Zimbabwe	7.1	7.5	9.3	11.4	8.1	7.3	49	45.4	40.9	44.1	51.1	57.4	51	54.6	59.1	55.9	48.9	42.6

[a] A zero does not always mean "not applicable"; when no information has been collated to estimate an entry, say private insurance and other prepaid plans, that entry is shown as zero.

[b] There is a break in the series for Japan between 1997 and 1998. Since 1998, data have been based on new Japanese national health accounts, estimated as a pilot implementation of the OECD manual *A System of Health Accounts*. Consequently, the comparability of data over time is limited. In addition, the data for the year 2000 have been largely developed by WHO and are not endorsed by the Government of Japan.

		General government expenditure on health as % of total general government expenditure						External resources for health as % of general government expenditure on health						Social security expenditure on health as % of general government expenditure on health					
		1995	1996	1997	1998	1999	2000	1995	1996	1997	1998	1999	2000	1995	1996	1997	1998	1999	2000
166	Syrian Arab Republic	5.4	5.2	5.2	5.1	5.2	6	0.7	0.5	1.1	0.8	0.5	0.4	0	0	0	0	0	0
167	Tajikistan	4.9	10.1	9.4	9.6	11.4	11.3	28.1	10.3	11.3	13.7	4.4	19.5	0	0	0	0	0	0
168	Thailand	8.1	9.6	10.9	13.3	11.4	11.4	0.2	0.6	0.5	0.7	0.9	0.9	26.5	27.9	30.2	25.8	26.3	26.4
169	The former Yugoslav Republic of Macedonia	12.6	13.6	14.5	19	14.8	15.6	1.4	2.8	3.1	3	3.4	3.7	98	95.1	96.3	96.8	93.8	87.5
170	Togo	4.9	3.8	5.4	5.3	5.7	5.2	31.9	39.8	27.5	30.9	25.6	28	0	0	0	0	0	0
171	Tonga	12	12.2	13.1	14.2	14.2	14	2.9	2.8	9.3	9.2	8.2	16.8	0	0	0	0	0	0
172	Trinidad and Tobago	7.9	8	7.9	8	8.1	8	0.1	0.1	10.1	8.2	7.9	7.6	16.7	16.9	16.8	16.6	16.6	16.7
173	Tunisia	11.5	13.5	15.7	16.9	17.3	17.2	1.2	0.9	0.9	0.7	0.6	0.7	37.2	42.2	45.3	47.1	47.8	47.6
174	Turkey	10.7	10	10.8	11.5	9.1	9	0.9	0.9	0.6	0.5	0.1	0.1	33.8	29.7	38.8	43.8	28.4	28.4
175	Turkmenistan	7.9	13.9	11.7	16.7	19.5	20.2	0.8	1.7	3.3	3.2	1.9	0.8	8.4	6.3	9.9	14	21.1	18.9
176	Tuvalu	12.6	13.4	5.6	6.5	7.9	6.8	6.5	5.6	5.4	5.9	5.3	5.5	0	0	0	0	0	0
177	Uganda	9.2	9.2	9.2	9.2	10.8	9.5	84	80.4	81.9	49	75.1	96	0	0	0	0	0	0
178	Ukraine	11.4	9.8	9.3	8	8.3	7.6	0.3	0.4	0.8	0.5	0.2	0	0	0	0	0	0	0
179	United Arab Emirates	6.5	7.2	7.9	7.4	7.2	6.3	0	0	0	0	0	0	0	0	0	0	0	0
180	United Kingdom	13.1	13.5	13.2	13.7	14.6	14.9	0	0	0	0	0	0	11.3	11.3	11.9	12.2	11.6	11.2
181	United Republic of Tanzania	14.7	15.1	15.5	12.5	12.2	11.4	31.7	34.4	39.2	44.2	48.5	41.9	0	0	0	0	0	0
182	United States of America	16.8	17	17.2	16.8	16.7	16.7	0	0	0	0	0	0	32.1	32.8	32.2	33.4	33.3	33.7
183	Uruguay	14.8	15.3	13.7	14.2	15.1	14.8	1.9	1.5	1.3	1.3	1.3	1	70.1	63.6	51.7	53	36.9	34.8
184	Uzbekistan	9.7	9.5	11.1	10	9.9	9.6	0.7	0.8	1.2	1.5	1.7	1.3	0	0	0	0	0	0
185	Vanuatu	8	6.3	8.8	7.3	9.3	9.4	32.3	41.8	32.2	46.6	45.1	46.8	0	0	0	0	0	0
186	Venezuela, Bolivarian Republic of	10.7	10	9.4	10.9	10.9	10.9	4.3	4.1	3	2.4	2.4	0.9	18.6	33.1	27.7	28.6	31.4	31.3
187	Viet Nam	6.6	6.7	6.2	6.8	6.4	6.5	6.6	10.8	13.7	15.6	12.5	12.3	0.8	1	1.2	1.3	1.6	1.5
188	Yemen	5	4.1	4.1	4.8	5.4	5.4	6.1	8.9	8.1	7.8	9.1	8.1	0	0	0	0	0	0
189	Yugoslavia	18.3	13	13.8	10.5	10.5	10.5	0	0	0	0.2	0.8	6.2	0	0	0	0	0	0
190	Zambia	11.5	14.6	13.1	12.5	12.3	11.2	22	34.7	40.3	43.2	21.3	24.8	0	0	0	0	0	0
191	Zimbabwe	10.1	11.6	15.4	17.9	10	6.3	16.4	13.4	8.6	6.8	12	17.4	0	0	0	0	0	0

Annex Table 5 Selected National Health Accounts indicators for all Member States, estimates for 1995 to 2000[a]

These figures were produced by WHO using the best available evidence. They are not necessarily the official statistics of Member States.

	Member State	Out-of-pocket expenditure % of total expenditure on health						Prepaid plans as % of private expenditure on health						Per capita total expenditure on health at average exchange rate (US$)					
		1995	1996	1997	1998	1999	2000	1995	1996	1997	1998	1999	2000	1995	1996	1997	1998	1999	2000
1	Afghanistan	50	50	47.4	42.3	43.1	36.5	0	0	0	0	0	0	13	5	6	8	9	8
2	Albania	19.6	17.8	20.2	21.1	21.2	23.8	12.8	43.2	43.1	41.1	40	36.4	26	31	23	33	40	41
3	Algeria	20.7	18.8	19.7	19.3	18.3	17.4	0	0	0	0	0	0	73	73	69	72	69	64
4	Andorra	13.3	13.3	13.4	11	13.2	13.5	0	0	0	0	0	0	1330	1246	1218	1434	1120	953
5	Angola	50.5	48.5	54.8	60.2	55.8	44.1	0	0	0	0	0	0	22	22	25	18	16	24
6	Antigua and Barbuda	36.4	38.2	38.1	37.5	38.7	40.1	0	0	0	0	0	0	438	477	484	506	533	562
7	Argentina	28.3	30.2	32.3	33.5	33.4	34.1	27.8	27	26	25.1	24.6	24.2	610	612	643	662	656	658
8	Armenia	60.3	56.6	58.5	57.1	58.7	57.7	0	0	0	0	0	0	27	33	34	37	37	38
9	Australia	15.9	16.5	16	18.4	17.6	16.8	32.7	31.9	29.9	27	26.3	25.9	1686	1884	1879	1683	1796	1698
10	Austria	14.6	15.2	17.3	16.8	18.2	18.6	28.1	25.1	26.6	25.6	23.8	23.2	2508	2489	2016	2096	2085	1872
11	Azerbaijan	22.3	28	26.6	26.9	51.1	55.8	0	0	0	0	0	0	9	9	11	13	14	14
12	Bahamas	43.7	41.2	44.4	42.4	43.7	44.5	0	0	0	0	0	0	587	650	701	752	790	880
13	Bahrain	21.2	22	20.9	21.2	21.5	21.6	24.2	25.2	25.4	26.2	26	26.3	464	462	502	501	504	512
14	Bangladesh	66.1	62.1	60.7	59.7	59.6	59.7	0	0	0	0	0	0	9	11	11	12	13	14
15	Barbados	24.6	24.2	26.6	27.7	27.7	27.1	24.2	24.2	24.2	23.7	23	23	445	462	489	504	542	606
16	Belarus	15.2	15.1	12.5	14.8	17.5	17.2	0	0	0	0	0	0	58	77	85	80	68	57
17	Belgium	13.4	13.5	13.7	13.9	13.6	16	6	7	6.8	6.9	6.9	6.8	2368	2341	2034	2095	2120	1936
18	Belize	57.8	59.1	57.1	54.1	55.2	54.5	0	0	0	0	0	0	111	108	118	126	147	158
19	Benin	48.8	50.4	51.4	50.5	50.2	50	0	0	0	0	0	0	11	12	11	12	12	11
20	Bhutan	9.7	11.7	9.6	9.7	10.4	9.4	0	0	0	0	0	0	5	6	7	8	8	9
21	Bolivia	26.3	24.5	27.2	29.5	29	22.7	13.2	13.3	9.1	7.8	8.1	9.5	40	45	46	53	53	67
22	Bosnia and Herzegovina	53.8	47.1	44.6	42.9	37.3	31	0	0	0	0	0	0	27	33	37	43	47	50
23	Botswana	12.6	13.1	11.4	12.1	12.1	11	29.3	24.9	24.1	23.8	22.8	21.6	168	164	177	168	176	191
24	Brazil	39	40.9	37.8	37.5	38.3	38.5	32	31.4	33.1	33.1	32.9	35.1	319	355	365	351	248	267
25	Brunei Darussalam	20	19.4	20.6	18.7	20.6	20	0	0	0	0	0	0	459	475	432	467	490	490
26	Bulgaria	18.1	19.2	18.9	20.6	21.1	22.4	0	0	0	0	0	0	69	46	54	60	63	59
27	Burkina Faso	39	33.7	31.6	31	28.4	29.3	0	0	0	0	0	0	7	9	8	9	9	8
28	Burundi	52.1	47	48.5	47.6	47.3	46.9	0	0	0	0	0	0	6	5	4	4	3	3
29	Cambodia	79	76.7	77	76.5	76.2	75.5	0	0	0	0	0	0	18	20	21	19	19	19
30	Cameroon	70.4	70.3	69.7	68.7	67	66.3	0	0	0	0	0	0	27	28	26	29	25	24
31	Canada	15.8	16.1	16.8	16.2	16.1	15.5	71.9	73.1	73.7	77.2	76.4	70.7	1821	1831	1868	1839	1939	2058
32	Cape Verde	22.2	28.6	30.7	31	31.1	31.5	0	0	0	0	0	0	31	33	31	35	34	30
33	Central African Republic	39	39.9	38.3	39.5	43.4	41.6	0	0	0	0	0	0	7	6	7	7	8	8
34	Chad	20.7	20	20.7	21.4	21.4	20.2	0	0	0	0	0	0	6	7	7	7	6	6
35	Chile	42.7	41.9	41.2	40	38.8	34.3	33.8	33.8	33.7	33.8	34.5	40.2	307	329	371	369	331	336
36	China	50.2	54.3	56.5	57.3	58.9	60.4	0	0	0.4	0.6	0.4	0.4	22	28	33	36	40	45
37	Colombia	32.3	28	25.9	27.7	28.4	29	23.8	31.5	38.9	38.6	38.6	34.4	178	218	247	226	202	186
38	Comoros	32.6	31.6	31.8	28.2	28.3	28.4	0	0	0	0	0	0	17	16	13	15	15	13
39	Congo	31.9	31.8	35.4	43.7	32.7	29.8	0	0	0	0	0	0	27	26	24	24	22	22
40	Cook Islands	21.1	33.3	32.9	31.7	36.6	37.2	0	0	0	0	0	0	329	270	273	237	208	188
41	Costa Rica	26.6	27.6	28.4	28.9	26.8	27.5	8	7.7	6.9	6.4	6.9	6.3	206	200	214	236	246	273
42	Côte d'Ivoire	45.8	49.3	50.3	50	55.5	55	18.6	16	14.9	14	12.9	12.9	20	21	19	20	19	16
43	Croatia	19.1	18.2	19.5	18.2	17.2	15.4	0	0	0	0	0	0	348	382	354	408	369	353
44	Cuba	9.8	10.5	12.5	12.4	11.4	10.8	0	0	0	0	0	0	112	121	131	138	157	169
45	Cyprus	44.6	48	48.7	46.9	46.7	46.2	0	0	0	0	0	0	839	911	913	933	925	888
46	Czech Republic	7.3	7.5	8.3	8.1	8.5	8.6	0	0	0	0	0	0	367	395	364	392	380	358
47	Democratic People's Republic of Korea	20.1	19.5	16.5	16.5	17.6	22.7	0	0	0	0	0	0	8	14	14	14	14	18
48	Democratic Republic of the Congo	35.7	30	25.9	25.9	26.2	26.3	0	0	0	0	0	0	11	9	26	14	19	9
49	Denmark	16.3	16.2	16.3	16.6	16.2	16.4	6.7	7.7	7.9	8.2	8.8	8.9	2830	2885	2639	2737	2791	2512
50	Djibouti	14.9	15	16.5	16	15.4	15.6	0	0	0	0	0	0	45	44	39	41	42	41
51	Dominica	26.9	26.6	23.7	24.1	24.5	24.4	16.7	16.7	17.6	16.7	16.1	16.1	194	207	216	221	246	247
52	Dominican Republic	57	55.9	54.7	54.6	53.6	55.6	12.7	14.2	13.1	14.2	13	12.8	98	111	122	126	134	151
53	Ecuador	32.6	28.9	25.8	29	36.5	37.5	14.1	12.4	10.5	10.5	9.4	8.5	72	83	77	70	43	26
54	Egypt	51	50.4	49.5	49.5	49.3	49.6	0.4	0.5	0.5	0.6	0.5	0.5	36	41	46	48	52	51
55	El Salvador	58.3	57.6	59.5	55.5	56.2	55.4	1.2	2	2.7	3.3	2.7	2.7	111	135	153	164	172	184

		Per capita total expenditure on health in international dollars						Per capita government expenditure on health at average exchange rate (US$)						Per capita government expenditure on health in international dollars					
		1995	1996	1997	1998	1999	2000	1995	1996	1997	1998	1999	2000	1995	1996	1997	1998	1999	2000
1	Afghanistan	17	8	8	10	10	9	6	3	3	5	5	5	9	4	4	6	6	5
2	Albania	89	108	91	104	117	129	20	21	15	21	26	26	68	73	58	66	75	80
3	Algeria	158	149	146	163	162	142	58	59	55	58	56	53	125	121	117	131	132	117
4	Andorra	1915	1725	1874	2143	1654	1639	1154	1081	1055	1277	973	824	1661	1496	1622	1908	1436	1418
5	Angola	58	52	55	49	46	52	11	11	11	7	7	13	29	27	25	19	21	29
6	Antigua and Barbuda	480	513	523	540	578	629	279	295	300	316	327	337	305	317	324	338	354	377
7	Argentina	886	906	977	1037	1067	1091	372	359	363	366	365	362	539	532	551	574	595	600
8	Armenia	142	154	161	164	178	192	11	14	14	16	15	16	56	67	67	70	74	81
9	Australia	1765	1855	1951	2059	2141	2213	1132	1255	1287	1175	1277	1229	1185	1236	1336	1437	1523	1601
10	Austria	1831	1936	1869	1965	2063	2171	1801	1756	1430	1497	1460	1305	1315	1366	1326	1404	1445	1513
11	Azerbaijan	49	41	44	51	57	57	7	6	8	9	7	6	38	29	33	37	28	25
12	Bahamas	677	772	828	921	1033	1137	331	382	389	434	445	488	381	454	460	531	582	631
13	Bahrain	683	686	728	747	705	641	326	318	354	350	349	354	480	473	513	521	488	443
14	Bangladesh	34	40	42	42	46	47	3	4	4	4	5	5	11	14	15	15	17	17
15	Barbados	782	760	765	741	795	915	300	314	317	321	347	393	528	517	496	472	509	593
16	Belarus	290	297	380	363	405	430	49	66	74	68	56	47	246	252	332	309	334	356
17	Belgium	1900	1981	2011	2006	2142	2269	1648	1682	1435	1480	1507	1379	1322	1423	1419	1417	1524	1616
18	Belize	188	184	207	223	254	273	47	44	50	58	66	72	79	75	89	102	114	124
19	Benin	21	22	23	25	26	27	6	6	6	6	6	6	11	11	11	12	13	14
20	Bhutan	34	42	48	52	54	64	4	5	7	7	7	8	31	38	43	47	48	58
21	Bolivia	94	104	99	115	120	158	26	31	31	35	35	48	61	70	67	75	79	114
22	Bosnia and Herzegovina	109	127	156	230	271	319	12	18	20	25	30	34	50	67	86	131	170	221
23	Botswana	245	269	272	276	315	358	88	85	100	98	104	120	128	139	154	160	187	226
24	Brazil	476	503	531	533	566	631	136	143	159	154	106	109	203	203	231	234	243	257
25	Brunei Darussalam	461	480	529	576	615	618	367	383	343	380	389	392	369	387	420	468	488	495
26	Bulgaria	241	191	204	192	196	198	56	37	43	48	49	46	197	154	165	153	155	154
27	Burkina Faso	22	27	30	31	37	37	4	6	6	6	7	6	13	18	21	22	26	26
28	Burundi	17	14	12	14	13	16	3	2	2	2	2	2	8	8	6	7	7	8
29	Cambodia	79	93	105	105	105	111	4	5	5	4	5	5	16	22	24	25	25	27
30	Cameroon	46	48	50	49	52	55	6	6	6	6	6	6	9	10	11	11	12	13
31	Canada	2114	2092	2184	2287	2428	2534	1299	1296	1312	1302	1373	1483	1509	1482	1535	1619	1719	1826
32	Cape Verde	63	69	70	81	87	92	24	23	21	24	23	20	49	49	49	56	60	63
33	Central African Republic	23	21	27	29	34	37	4	3	3	4	4	4	12	10	13	14	16	18
34	Chad	18	19	19	19	18	19	5	6	5	5	5	4	14	15	15	15	14	15
35	Chile	507	566	640	687	670	697	109	121	141	146	135	143	180	208	242	272	274	297
36	China	94	113	135	153	177	205	10	12	13	14	15	17	44	48	54	60	67	75
37	Colombia	452	547	598	600	610	616	103	129	142	124	109	104	260	324	344	329	328	344
38	Comoros	41	39	37	37	35	35	11	11	9	11	10	9	27	27	25	27	25	25
39	Congo	39	31	30	39	31	25	18	18	15	14	15	15	26	21	20	22	21	18
40	Cook Islands	482	400	436	447	432	426	260	180	183	162	132	118	380	267	293	305	274	267
41	Costa Rica	385	378	403	445	466	481	141	134	143	157	169	187	263	254	269	296	320	329
42	Côte d'Ivoire	40	42	43	44	44	45	9	9	8	9	7	6	17	17	18	18	16	16
43	Croatia	487	547	539	606	597	638	282	313	285	334	305	299	394	447	434	495	494	540
44	Cuba	125	141	158	165	181	186	101	108	114	121	139	150	112	126	139	144	161	166
45	Cyprus	987	1106	1217	1242	1292	1415	465	474	468	495	493	478	547	575	624	659	689	762
46	Czech Republic	902	917	930	944	972	1031	340	366	334	360	347	327	836	848	853	867	889	942
47	Democratic People's Republic of Korea	32	33	37	40	38	33	6	12	12	11	12	14	25	27	31	33	31	26
48	Democratic Republic of the Congo	32	31	27	28	24	21	7	7	19	10	14	6	21	22	20	21	18	16
49	Denmark	1882	2009	2106	2247	2364	2428	2335	2378	2171	2242	2295	2061	1553	1656	1733	1841	1944	1992
50	Djibouti	63	62	58	60	62	63	23	22	18	19	20	20	32	30	26	28	30	31
51	Dominica	281	297	312	321	347	340	131	141	154	157	174	175	190	202	222	228	246	241
52	Dominican Republic	187	212	289	309	331	357	26	30	35	36	41	42	49	57	84	87	101	100
53	Ecuador	148	167	157	145	122	78	40	52	46	39	21	13	82	104	95	81	60	39
54	Egypt	100	110	121	127	133	138	16	18	21	22	24	24	44	49	55	58	61	64
55	El Salvador	255	296	331	346	367	388	45	55	59	70	72	79	104	121	128	147	155	167

Annex Table 5 Selected National Health Accounts indicators for all Member States, estimates for 1995 to 2000[a]

These figures were produced by WHO using the best available evidence. They are not necessarily the official statistics of Member States.

	Member State	Out-of-pocket expenditure % of total expenditure on health						Prepaid plans as % of private expenditure on health						Per capita total expenditure on health at average exchange rate (US$)					
		1995	1996	1997	1998	1999	2000	1995	1996	1997	1998	1999	2000	1995	1996	1997	1998	1999	2000
56	Equatorial Guinea	34.8	44.4	44	40.6	32.4	32.4	0	0	0	0	0	0	18	29	41	46	50	54
57	Eritrea	14.9	12.9	34.2	33.9	35.7	34.4	0	0	0	0	0	0	6	7	9	10	9	9
58	Estonia	8.6	10	11.3	13.2	14	19.7	0	0	0	0	4.1	4.1	206	215	203	218	239	218
59	Ethiopia	57	52.7	54.4	49.1	51.5	51.6	0	0	0	0	0	0	4	4	5	5	5	5
60	Fiji	35	33.8	33.3	34.6	34.8	34.8	0	0	0	0	0	0	98	106	106	82	85	80
61	Finland	20.5	20.3	19.9	19.6	20.4	20.6	11.7	11.8	12.2	12.5	12	12	1919	1912	1745	1733	1710	1559
62	France	11.1	10.6	10.5	10.4	10.3	10.2	49.5	51.5	51.7	52.3	52.7	53.1	2566	2545	2260	2303	2282	2057
63	Gabon	33.8	33.7	33.5	36.5	38.8	31.4	0	0	0	0	0	0	140	152	138	128	122	120
64	Gambia	18.6	18.6	18.2	17.9	17.1	17.6	0	0	0	0	0	0	13	12	13	14	11	10
65	Georgia	87.1	86.1	85.3	86.7	89.8	89.5	0	0	0	0	0	0	26	40	46	49	36	41
66	Germany	10	10.1	10.8	11.2	10.9	10.6	51.6	50.4	49.8	48.8	49.7	50.3	3194	3162	2775	2773	2729	2422
67	Ghana	56.6	56	55.2	48.5	48.1	46.5	0	0	0	0	0	0	16	16	15	17	17	11
68	Greece	35.2	38.6	36.9	36.6	35.7	37.4	4.8	4.9	4.9	4.7	4.6	4.9	998	1044	1006	1002	1034	884
69	Grenada	33.4	31.7	33.9	34.2	30.3	29.9	0	0	0	0	0	0	132	152	159	180	196	212
70	Guatemala	51.9	53.2	50.9	48.7	44.3	44.8	3.8	3.7	3.8	4.4	5.4	5.2	60	64	73	79	78	79
71	Guinea	45.7	45.6	42.8	39.6	37.5	42.9	0	0	0	0	0	0	18	18	18	17	17	13
72	Guinea-Bissau	37.9	36.1	36	34.9	34.2	34.6	0	0	0	0	0	0	15	12	9	10	10	9
73	Guyana	17.6	17.5	16.5	16.6	16	17.3	0	0	0	0	0	0	39	43	48	48	44	48
74	Haiti	18.7	20.3	20.8	20.1	21.2	22	0	0	0	0	0	0	18	18	20	23	24	21
75	Honduras	47.4	45.5	42.4	34.9	38.4	36.8	0.2	0.1	0.2	0.2	0.2	0.2	48	48	49	57	54	62
76	Hungary	16	18.4	18.7	17.4	18.8	21.2	0	0	0	0.2	0.5	0.8	327	320	314	323	328	315
77	Iceland	15.5	16.1	16.3	16.1	15.2	15.6	0	0	0	0	0	0	2139	2199	2162	2476	2705	2729
78	India	83.8	84.4	84.3	81.6	82.1	82.2	0	0	0	0	0	0	20	21	23	22	23	23
79	Indonesia	43.8	58.1	73	67.9	64.5	70.1	30.1	19.5	4.3	6.7	10.4	8.2	17	26	26	11	17	19
80	Iran, Islamic Republic of	52.1	49.2	51.6	51.6	50.4	50.9	1.3	1.4	1.3	1.8	1.9	1.9	92	117	139	160	211	258
81	Iraq	40.7	41.8	41.1	40.9	40	40.1	0	0	0	0	0	0	147	163	242	286	348	375
82	Ireland	15.6	13.5	13	12.1	11.7	11	24	25.6	26.4	27.1	24.5	23.8	1354	1394	1500	1587	1707	1692
83	Israel	22.2	21.4	21.3	23	22.3	24.1	0	0	0	0	0	0	1653	1823	1819	1767	1888	2021
84	Italy	24.4	24.2	24.1	24.5	24	22.9	3.5	3.6	3.6	3.3	3.4	3.4	1415	1605	1571	1599	1605	1498
85	Jamaica	35.5	35.9	35.2	33.8	34.6	36.6	34	32.7	32.6	32.6	31	31	104	116	142	155	171	165
86	Japan[b]	20.8	19.8	16.2	17.7	17.1	19.3	0	0	0	1.3	1.3	1.4	2950	2594	2467	2213	2631	2908
87	Jordan	42.1	41.6	33.7	33.5	34.4	37.6	4.1	4.3	5.8	5.9	6.2	6.1	148	149	135	137	137	137
88	Kazakhstan	18.2	23.7	23.6	29.4	29.1	26.8	0	0	0	0	0	0	63	72	81	66	46	44
89	Kenya	52	51.5	52.8	53.1	52.8	56.4	4.5	4.5	4.6	4.5	4.4	4.5	27	27	31	33	29	28
90	Kiribati	0.9	0.9	0.9	0.8	0.8	1.3	0	0	0	0	0	0	53	56	55	47	49	44
91	Kuwait	10	13	12.6	12.9	13.2	12.8	0	0	0	0	0	0	563	571	580	564	557	586
92	Kyrgyzstan	11.9	19.2	20.3	28.1	33.4	38.3	0	0	0	0	0	0	26	26	24	23	16	16
93	Lao People's Democratic Republic	52.9	58	61.5	64	63	62	0	0	0	0	0	0	11	11	13	8	10	11
94	Latvia	34.6	36.9	38.2	38.9	37.1	40	0	0	0	0	0	0	115	129	142	164	176	174
95	Lebanon	58.1	57.9	58.5	59.6	59.3	58.6	16.6	16.5	16.7	15.4	15.8	16.4	375	431	504	534	590	590
96	Lesotho	21.3	22	24	21.7	18.8	17.7	0	0	0	0	0	0	31	28	28	27	29	28
97	Liberia	26.7	27.7	26.6	23.3	20.8	20	0	0	0	0	0	0	1	1	1	1	2	2
98	Libyan Arab Jamahiriya	59.5	58.1	50	50	50.9	51.4	0	0	0	0	0	0	334	352	328	327	241	246
99	Lithuania	13.7	23.1	22.3	23.3	24.9	27.6	0	0	0	0	0	0	84	116	154	183	176	185
100	Luxembourg	6.2	7.2	7.4	7.6	7	6.7	18.8	20.3	21.4	21.3	20.3	17.5	2812	2792	2454	2573	2732	2514
101	Madagascar	36.5	35.3	14.1	34.4	31.1	25.3	9.6	9.8	26.8	9.7	10.3	10.3	6	8	5	7	7	9
102	Malawi	10.5	19.4	17.5	17	17.6	23	2	1.6	1.6	2.2	2.2	1.8	9	15	18	12	11	11
103	Malaysia	43.9	41.7	42.4	42.3	40.2	41.2	0	0	0	0	0	0	99	116	110	84	90	101
104	Maldives	16.2	15.5	18.1	18.2	17.5	16.6	0	0	0	0	0	0	64	74	83	85	95	100
105	Mali	42.3	43.6	48.7	46.7	46.6	48.3	0	0	0	0	0	0	8	8	10	11	11	10
106	Malta	28.6	30	32.1	30.7	32.5	31.5	0	0	0	0	0	0	714	739	747	761	782	807
107	Marshall Islands	38.8	38.3	38.1	38.4	38.9	38.6	0	0	0	0	0	0	162	167	171	173	178	172
108	Mauritania	25.5	24	26.7	27.2	24.1	20.7	0	0	0	0	0	0	15	15	14	14	15	14
109	Mauritius	45.9	47	46.7	46.2	43.3	43.7	0	0	0	0	0	0	128	137	127	122	131	134
110	Mexico	55.2	54.2	53.2	47.9	48.8	49.5	2.7	2.7	2.7	4	3.8	3.8	177	189	227	234	267	311

		Per capita total expenditure on health in international dollars						Per capita government expenditure on health at average exchange rate (US$)						Per capita government expenditure on health in international dollars					
		1995	1996	1997	1998	1999	2000	1995	1996	1997	1998	1999	2000	1995	1996	1997	1998	1999	2000
56	Equatorial Guinea	48	68	67	95	89	103	11	16	23	27	34	37	31	38	38	56	60	70
57	Eritrea	17	21	26	33	25	25	5	6	6	7	6	6	15	19	17	22	16	16
58	Estonia	531	481	483	487	541	556	188	193	179	188	192	167	485	432	427	420	435	426
59	Ethiopia	11	12	15	16	16	17	1	2	2	2	2	2	4	5	6	7	6	7
60	Fiji	174	187	187	189	184	194	64	70	70	54	56	52	113	124	125	124	120	126
61	Finland	1415	1487	1549	1529	1607	1667	1450	1449	1328	1321	1288	1171	1069	1127	1179	1166	1211	1252
62	France	1970	1985	2032	2094	2211	2335	1954	1937	1722	1751	1736	1563	1500	1511	1548	1592	1683	1775
63	Gabon	175	178	185	203	196	171	93	101	92	81	75	82	116	118	123	129	120	117
64	Gambia	36	34	34	39	45	46	11	10	10	11	9	9	29	28	28	32	37	38
65	Georgia	87	149	168	181	184	199	3	6	7	6	4	4	11	21	25	24	19	21
66	Germany	2264	2341	2466	2520	2618	2754	2449	2430	2089	2075	2042	1819	1736	1799	1857	1886	1959	2067
67	Ghana	42	43	42	47	49	51	7	7	7	9	9	6	18	19	19	24	25	27
68	Greece	1131	1176	1220	1301	1368	1390	544	576	555	545	561	491	616	649	673	708	742	772
69	Grenada	223	251	264	291	324	351	88	104	105	119	137	149	148	172	175	192	226	246
70	Guatemala	143	148	159	171	187	192	26	27	33	37	38	38	62	63	72	81	90	92
71	Guinea	49	51	54	57	62	56	10	10	10	11	11	7	27	28	31	35	39	32
72	Guinea-Bissau	28	35	33	24	26	28	10	8	6	6	7	6	17	22	21	16	17	18
73	Guyana	146	155	177	175	189	197	32	35	40	40	37	40	120	127	148	146	159	163
74	Haiti	56	51	51	53	52	54	10	10	10	11	12	10	32	27	26	27	27	27
75	Honduras	149	153	144	158	146	165	25	26	28	37	33	39	78	83	83	103	90	104
76	Hungary	678	672	696	754	790	846	274	261	255	257	256	238	569	548	565	600	618	640
77	Iceland	1823	1904	1978	2196	2410	2626	1806	1845	1810	2078	2295	2304	1540	1598	1656	1843	2044	2217
78	India	54	60	65	64	71	71	3	3	4	4	4	4	9	9	10	12	13	13
79	Indonesia	50	73	81	72	75	84	6	7	6	3	5	5	18	20	19	20	21	20
80	Iran, Islamic Republic of	281	286	318	317	310	336	42	56	64	73	98	119	128	138	146	144	143	156
81	Iraq	287	295	363	410	497	573	87	95	143	169	209	225	170	172	214	243	298	344
82	Ireland	1320	1312	1518	1569	1744	1944	981	1022	1139	1209	1302	1283	957	962	1153	1196	1330	1474
83	Israel	1777	1921	1941	1966	2188	2338	1229	1432	1431	1361	1467	1534	1321	1510	1527	1515	1699	1776
84	Italy	1486	1566	1685	1776	1886	2040	1022	1153	1133	1151	1161	1103	1073	1125	1216	1279	1364	1503
85	Jamaica	166	166	179	192	213	208	48	54	68	77	85	78	77	78	86	96	106	98
86	Japan[b]	1632	1700	1831	1735	1850	2009	2308	2083	1961	1713	2053	2230	1277	1365	1455	1343	1443	1540
87	Jordan	361	370	338	341	320	325	74	75	77	78	76	71	180	186	193	194	177	168
88	Kazakhstan	268	251	275	225	212	211	51	55	62	47	32	32	219	192	210	159	150	154
89	Kenya	106	110	114	117	117	115	7	7	8	9	8	6	28	30	30	31	31	26
90	Kiribati	134	136	144	143	146	140	53	56	54	47	49	44	132	135	143	141	144	138
91	Kuwait	577	562	620	745	628	542	506	497	507	491	483	511	519	489	542	648	545	473
92	Kyrgyzstan	150	138	147	157	147	145	23	21	19	17	11	10	132	112	117	113	98	90
93	Lao People's Democratic Republic	33	36	47	45	49	52	5	5	5	3	4	4	16	15	18	16	18	20
94	Latvia	310	317	352	394	397	398	75	82	88	100	111	104	203	200	218	241	249	239
95	Lebanon	537	560	604	590	684	696	105	123	140	147	162	164	150	159	167	162	188	193
96	Lesotho	82	81	83	87	97	100	24	22	21	21	24	23	65	63	63	68	79	82
97	Liberia	2	2	2	3	3	3	1	1	1	1	1	1	1	1	2	2	2	2
98	Libyan Arab Jamahiriya	406	407	402	422	375	392	135	147	164	164	118	119	165	170	201	211	184	190
99	Lithuania	277	314	374	423	400	420	72	89	120	140	133	134	239	241	291	324	301	304
100	Luxembourg	2138	2194	2206	2363	2620	2740	2598	2592	2267	2378	2537	2310	1976	2037	2038	2184	2434	2518
101	Madagascar	22	23	17	25	27	33	4	5	4	4	5	6	13	14	14	15	18	24
102	Malawi	26	30	35	32	34	38	4	7	9	6	6	5	13	13	18	16	17	18
103	Malaysia	166	192	201	199	213	234	55	67	63	48	54	60	93	112	116	115	127	138
104	Maldives	141	163	180	190	219	254	53	63	68	70	78	84	118	138	147	155	181	212
105	Mali	17	18	24	26	29	32	4	4	5	5	5	5	9	9	11	12	13	14
106	Malta	720	740	739	758	780	803	510	517	507	527	528	553	514	518	502	525	527	550
107	Marshall Islands	338	323	306	307	321	312	99	103	106	107	109	106	207	199	189	189	196	191
108	Mauritania	33	35	36	43	49	52	11	11	10	10	11	11	25	27	27	31	37	42
109	Mauritius	258	275	290	299	326	330	69	73	68	66	74	75	140	146	155	161	185	186
110	Mexico	384	379	410	430	453	483	74	80	98	112	126	144	160	161	177	206	214	224

Annex Table 5 Selected National Health Accounts indicators for all Member States, estimates for 1995 to 2000[a]

These figures were produced by WHO using the best available evidence. They are not necessarily the official statistics of Member States.

	Member State	Out-of-pocket expenditure % of total expenditure on health						Prepaid plans as % of private expenditure on health						Per capita total expenditure on health at average exchange rate (US$)					
		1995	1996	1997	1998	1999	2000	1995	1996	1997	1998	1999	2000	1995	1996	1997	1998	1999	2000
111	Micronesia, Federated States of	14.3	14.7	14.4	14.9	15.1	16.5	0	0	0	0	0	0	228	218	210	202	199	197
112	Monaco	50	50	50	50.7	51.4	51.9	0	0	0	0	0	0	1893	1949	1690	1784	1816	1837
113	Mongolia	19.8	27.4	27.4	25.8	24.8	21.9	0	0	0	0	0	0	21	25	22	24	21	23
114	Morocco	56.3	54.9	53.2	54.3	53.5	53.6	19.6	21.2	23	22.9	22.9	22.4	55	59	53	54	53	50
115	Mozambique	15.8	14.5	15.2	15.5	15.5	15	0	0	0	0	0	0	7	9	9	9	9	9
116	Myanmar	81	82.2	85.4	89.2	88.1	82.6	0	0	0	0	0	0	51	63	80	104	140	153
117	Namibia	5.3	5.9	6.2	6	6.2	6.5	81.1	82.3	82.1	82.4	79.2	78.9	182	160	163	152	143	136
118	Nauru	1.1	1.1	1.1	1.1	1.1	1.1	0	0	0	0	0	0	376	394	385	328	339	313
119	Nepal	67	67.3	63.1	61.3	64.4	64	0	0	0	0	0	0	11	11	12	12	12	12
120	Netherlands	9.6	8.1	7.7	8.5	8.6	8.6	74	79.2	80.3	77.2	74.3	76.7	2253	2193	1977	2038	2059	1900
121	New Zealand	16.2	16.3	15.6	16.3	15.7	15.4	27.9	28.8	29.8	27.7	27.9	28.5	1203	1294	1310	1132	1163	1062
122	Nicaragua	20.7	24.5	44.9	38.5	44.4	45.4	2.5	2.3	1.5	1.7	4.8	4.8	52	52	45	44	43	43
123	Niger	50.8	49.4	49.2	47.5	46.6	47.5	0	0	0	0	0	0	7	7	6	7	6	5
124	Nigeria	85.5	88.3	86.4	81.1	77.1	79.2	0	0	0	0	0	0	5	6	6	7	7	8
125	Niue	3.2	2.6	2.7	3.3	2.9	3.8	0	0	0	0	0	0	329	400	394	303	357	297
126	Norway	15.2	15.3	15.2	14.8	14.3	14.3	0	0	0	0	0	0	2689	2860	2798	2868	3033	2832
127	Oman	10	9.8	10.6	11.1	10.2	8.4	0	0	0	0	0	0	287	284	256	249	251	295
128	Pakistan	75.2	77	77.1	76.4	78.1	77.1	0	0	0	0	0	0	20	18	18	18	18	18
129	Palau	11.4	12.3	12.5	12	11.8	11.5	0	0	0	0	0	0	342	361	332	296	264	263
130	Panama	24.3	23.7	26.2	24.4	24.7	25	18.5	18.4	17.2	18	18.2	18.7	235	245	236	250	260	268
131	Papua New Guinea	7.6	9.1	9.3	7.9	8.4	9.8	0	0	2.1	4.8	9.4	8.3	31	33	35	32	31	31
132	Paraguay	55.1	44.9	45.9	47.8	44.1	44.8	24	29.8	31.6	23.7	27.1	27.3	145	139	143	121	115	112
133	Peru	34.6	31.7	32.3	32	30.8	30.9	17.9	20.8	21.2	21.7	21	21.7	104	105	108	107	101	100
134	Philippines	50.4	48.7	46.9	48	44.7	45.1	16.2	16.9	17.1	16.8	16.5	16.9	37	42	41	32	37	33
135	Poland	24.3	23.8	28	34.6	24.9	25.9	0	0	0	0	0	0	198	238	228	264	249	246
136	Portugal	21.4	20.4	19.5	20.5	21	19.6	3.4	3.9	4.3	4.9	5.7	5.5	902	959	922	941	962	862
137	Qatar	6.7	5.7	5.8	5.7	6.1	6.2	0	0	0	0	0	0	762	830	836	842	895	940
138	Republic of Korea	51.1	49.1	46.1	41.6	43	41	9.2	10.2	11.3	12.9	13.6	16.6	508	568	523	354	486	584
139	Republic of Moldova	5.4	5.7	6.3	9.2	15.2	17.6	0	0	0	0	0	0	21	28	29	19	9	11
140	Romania	34	27.8	37.1	43.1	40.7	36.2	0	0	0	0	0	0	44	70	63	65	52	48
141	Russian Federation	15.2	17.4	21.1	25.1	29.9	23.4	5.1	7.3	6.7	5.6	4.6	4.3	126	153	167	112	71	92
142	Rwanda	38.1	37.5	38.3	32.6	28.9	29.5	0.4	0.3	0.3	0.3	0.3	0.3	16	16	18	16	14	12
143	Saint Kitts and Nevis	33.9	33.9	32.5	31.9	36.5	40.8	0	0	0	0	0	0	273	317	329	346	382	447
144	Saint Lucia	38.8	36.9	37.7	34.4	34.7	37.9	0	0	0	0	0	0	150	163	169	186	190	202
145	Saint Vincent and the Grenadines	34	32.9	36.2	37.5	38.5	34.6	0	0	0	0	0	0	139	143	161	168	180	190
146	Samoa	21.8	21.8	21.2	21.6	21	20.9	0	0	0	0	0	0	64	76	81	79	77	81
147	San Marino	14.3	15.4	15.6	14	14.2	14.3	0	0	0	0	0	0	2065	2338	2208	2456	2373	2127
148	Sao Tome and Principe	30.6	28.6	33.3	32.1	32.1	32.2	0	0	0	0	0	0	12	12	10	9	8	8
149	Saudi Arabia	4.7	4.5	4.3	6.2	4.1	3.8	7.4	7.1	7.3	7.8	8.3	7.4	397	408	411	387	394	448
150	Senegal	43	42.7	42.5	39.9	40.1	39.6	8.5	8.7	8.7	9.4	8.8	8.7	26	27	24	24	24	22
151	Seychelles	24.3	23.5	21.7	23	23.4	24.7	0	0	0	0	0	0	416	424	481	493	484	440
152	Sierra Leone	59	59	61	58	50	40	0	0	0	0	0	0	6	6	6	5	5	6
153	Singapore	56.9	59	60.1	57.5	60.7	63.7	0	0	0	0	0	0	881	930	923	890	840	814
154	Slovakia	17.9	18.8	8.3	8.4	10.6	10.4	0	0	0	0	0	0	239	277	230	235	213	210
155	Slovenia	13.2	11	10.7	10.8	10.9	10.8	39.5	46.8	48.1	49.1	48.9	48.9	853	834	811	852	873	788
156	Solomon Islands	0.4	0.4	0.3	0.3	0.2	3.2	0	0	0	0	0	0	36	38	43	38	39	38
157	Somalia	57.1	54.6	37.5	37.6	21.1	28.6	0	0	0	0	0	0	4	4	5	4	11	19
158	South Africa	12.3	11.3	10.6	12.6	12.5	12.6	71.7	76.3	78.3	76.4	76.7	76.6	318	324	322	275	269	255
159	Spain	26.1	25.7	25.7	26.2	26.4	26.6	10.1	10.8	11	11.3	11.5	11.7	1137	1190	1074	1123	1158	1073
160	Sri Lanka	50.7	49.3	49.7	48	50.2	50	1	1	1	1	1	1.1	24	25	26	29	30	31
161	Sudan	71.4	71.4	79.1	75.9	75.9	78.8	0	0	0	0	0	0	10	10	12	12	11	13
162	Suriname	6.3	7.7	13.7	14.8	13.5	14.9	2	2.6	1.7	1.4	0.6	0.2	106	161	199	196	104	186
163	Swaziland	27.2	27	28.4	28	30.1	27.9	0	0	0	0	0	0	50	56	50	51	54	56
164	Sweden	14.8	15.2	15.7	16.2	22.2	22.7	0	0	0	0	0	0	2214	2473	2193	2144	2346	2179
165	Switzerland	33	31.4	32.3	32.8	33.3	32.8	48.7	51.7	47.7	44.2	42.2	42.4	4305	4278	3724	3876	3866	3573

		Per capita total expenditure on health in international dollars						Per capita government expenditure on health at average exchange rate (US$)						Per capita government expenditure on health in international dollars					
		1995	1996	1997	1998	1999	2000	1995	1996	1997	1998	1999	2000	1995	1996	1997	1998	1999	2000
111	Micronesia, Federated States of	432	406	388	367	355	343	130	122	119	112	109	106	247	227	220	203	194	184
112	Monaco	1503	1583	1567	1668	1791	1877	946	974	845	879	883	883	752	792	783	822	871	902
113	Mongolia	63	80	83	105	109	120	15	16	14	16	14	16	44	51	52	68	72	85
114	Morocco	142	155	152	156	157	166	16	17	16	15	15	15	41	45	45	44	46	49
115	Mozambique	24	26	27	28	28	30	4	5	6	6	6	6	15	16	17	17	17	19
116	Myanmar	19	20	21	20	21	24	10	11	11	11	16	26	4	4	3	2	2	4
117	Namibia	373	344	353	366	362	366	104	82	84	79	85	80	213	175	182	189	214	217
118	Nauru	584	579	586	576	539	525	372	389	380	324	335	310	578	572	580	570	533	519
119	Nepal	51	54	60	63	63	66	3	3	4	4	3	4	13	14	18	21	18	19
120	Netherlands	1787	1816	1955	2038	2175	2255	1600	1451	1341	1381	1370	1283	1270	1202	1326	1381	1447	1523
121	New Zealand	1244	1267	1364	1450	1526	1623	929	992	1012	872	901	829	960	972	1054	1117	1183	1266
122	Nicaragua	133	130	117	110	111	108	40	39	24	27	23	22	104	96	63	67	59	56
123	Niger	20	21	21	23	22	22	3	3	3	3	3	2	9	9	9	10	10	10
124	Nigeria	23	21	20	22	20	20	1	1	1	1	2	2	3	3	3	4	5	4
125	Niue	833	997	1000	874	1092	1111	319	390	384	294	346	286	806	971	972	846	1060	1068
126	Norway	1865	2025	2193	2441	2558	2373	2265	2407	2358	2429	2584	2412	1571	1705	1848	2067	2179	2022
127	Oman	431	422	419	484	440	448	228	228	202	195	199	245	343	338	330	379	350	371
128	Pakistan	68	67	68	69	72	76	5	4	4	4	4	4	17	15	15	16	16	17
129	Palau	540	503	452	453	474	482	303	317	290	260	233	233	478	441	395	399	418	427
130	Panama	396	420	407	422	446	464	165	174	161	175	181	186	278	298	278	296	312	321
131	Papua New Guinea	105	106	118	135	153	147	29	29	31	29	28	27	96	95	105	123	137	130
132	Paraguay	320	296	320	304	324	323	40	50	47	45	45	43	88	106	105	114	128	124
133	Peru	197	200	212	220	236	238	58	61	62	62	60	59	110	116	122	127	141	141
134	Philippines	144	156	168	165	172	167	15	17	18	14	17	15	57	64	73	70	80	76
135	Poland	420	469	461	543	558	578	144	175	164	173	177	171	306	344	332	355	397	403
136	Portugal	1146	1210	1359	1344	1413	1469	556	620	597	635	681	614	707	782	880	907	1000	1045
137	Qatar	809	847	867	1034	964	849	563	636	638	645	693	729	598	648	661	792	746	658
138	Republic of Korea	536	614	661	635	766	909	185	221	215	164	210	258	196	238	271	294	330	401
139	Republic of Moldova	115	126	119	83	59	64	19	26	27	17	8	9	107	119	111	75	50	53
140	Romania	176	299	257	215	203	190	29	51	40	37	31	31	116	216	162	122	121	121
141	Russian Federation	369	355	390	382	379	405	103	119	122	77	46	66	300	277	284	263	245	293
142	Rwanda	42	46	44	39	41	40	8	8	9	8	8	6	20	23	21	20	22	20
143	Saint Kitts and Nevis	419	493	501	528	577	658	181	209	222	235	243	265	277	326	338	359	366	390
144	Saint Lucia	203	225	240	256	252	272	92	103	105	122	124	125	124	142	149	168	165	169
145	Saint Vincent and the Grenadines	269	271	307	315	344	374	92	96	103	105	111	124	178	182	196	196	212	244
146	Samoa	146	168	168	182	194	221	48	58	62	60	59	62	110	127	128	138	148	168
147	San Marino	2349	2410	2470	2723	2707	2805	1769	1978	1863	2111	2037	1822	2012	2039	2084	2341	2324	2402
148	Sao Tome and Principe	29	32	28	27	23	23	8	9	7	6	6	5	20	23	18	18	15	16
149	Saudi Arabia	681	649	652	729	683	684	312	318	322	306	313	354	536	506	512	576	542	541
150	Senegal	46	49	51	51	54	56	14	14	13	14	14	12	24	26	27	29	30	32
151	Seychelles	528	565	714	776	775	758	285	293	346	342	333	294	362	390	515	539	533	507
152	Sierra Leone	22	22	20	21	22	28	2	2	2	2	3	4	9	9	8	9	11	17
153	Singapore	737	780	824	915	936	913	368	374	364	374	326	290	308	314	325	385	363	326
154	Slovakia	596	695	608	641	649	690	196	225	211	215	191	188	489	564	558	587	580	618
155	Slovenia	1135	1163	1249	1282	1368	1462	667	662	643	671	687	621	887	923	991	1010	1076	1154
156	Solomon Islands	89	89	95	106	110	97	35	37	41	36	38	36	86	86	91	102	107	92
157	Somalia	15	13	13	11	9	7	2	2	3	3	8	13	6	6	8	7	7	5
158	South Africa	557	632	637	620	638	663	155	152	148	116	115	108	271	296	294	262	272	280
159	Spain	1168	1222	1278	1366	1451	1539	806	846	764	792	813	750	828	869	909	963	1019	1076
160	Sri Lanka	84	85	90	101	110	120	12	12	13	15	14	15	41	42	44	52	54	59
161	Sudan	30	29	29	39	41	51	3	3	3	3	3	3	9	8	6	9	10	11
162	Suriname	255	310	358	408	400	424	80	114	129	121	63	104	194	220	231	251	243	238
163	Swaziland	145	177	158	179	195	210	36	41	36	37	38	40	105	129	113	129	137	151
164	Sweden	1622	1714	1767	1746	2010	2097	1885	2096	1848	1797	1826	1685	1382	1453	1489	1464	1565	1622
165	Switzerland	2527	2588	2812	2927	3069	3229	2315	2339	2054	2127	2140	1988	1359	1415	1551	1606	1698	1796

Annex Table 5 Selected National Health Accounts indicators for all Member States, estimates for 1995 to 2000[a]

These figures were produced by WHO using the best available evidence. They are not necessarily the official statistics of Member States.

	Member State	Out-of-pocket expenditure % of total expenditure on health						Prepaid plans as % of private expenditure on health						Per capita total expenditure on health at average exchange rate (US$)					
		1995	1996	1997	1998	1999	2000	1995	1996	1997	1998	1999	2000	1995	1996	1997	1998	1999	2000
166	Syrian Arab Republic	23.9	28.1	31.2	33.4	35.2	36.6	0	0	0	0	0	0	18	21	24	26	28	30
167	Tajikistan	39.5	36.9	34	35	15.4	19.2	0	0	0	0	0	0	2	5	5	6	5	4
168	Thailand	44.7	42.6	36.9	32.7	35.3	36.2	7.6	7.8	8.6	9.7	9.7	9.6	97	110	93	71	73	71
169	The former Yugoslav Republic of Macedonia	9.4	13	16.1	12.9	15.9	15.5	0	0	0	0	0	0	119	129	114	135	107	106
170	Togo	52.4	58.4	51.5	44.8	42.9	45.7	0	0	0	0	0	0	10	9	11	10	9	8
171	Tonga	56.7	56.7	53.2	53.9	54.1	53.2	0	0	0	0	0	0	129	138	143	123	117	108
172	Trinidad and Tobago	43	44.4	45.6	42.6	42.4	42.7	6.4	6.3	6.5	6.6	6.5	6.5	189	207	220	250	259	268
173	Tunisia	38.1	27.1	17.3	16.3	16.8	17.6	13.2	16.6	22.8	21.9	20.5	19.5	137	142	133	145	155	145
174	Turkey	29.7	30.8	28.3	28	28.8	28.8	0.3	0.2	0.2	0.2	0.2	0.1	93	113	126	150	138	150
175	Turkmenistan	22.9	18.6	25.5	18.9	18.3	15.1	0	0	0	0	0	0	33	15	24	32	38	52
176	Tuvalu	29.1	31.3	30.2	29.3	29.3	28.6	0	0	0	0	0	0	110	130	131	117	127	120
177	Uganda	36.2	34.9	32.3	33.5	32.9	34.5	0.5	0.5	0.6	0.5	0.5	0.5	11	10	11	11	11	10
178	Ukraine	16	20.4	25	28.9	31.9	29.9	0	0	0	0	0	0	42	43	54	42	27	26
179	United Arab Emirates	13.1	13.4	13.7	13.1	14	15	19.5	19.2	19	19.9	19	18.3	619	631	729	752	758	767
180	United Kingdom	10.9	11	10.7	11	10.7	10.6	19.8	19.2	17	17.1	16.5	16.9	1357	1422	1531	1657	1753	1747
181	United Republic of Tanzania	36.7	43.3	44.5	44.4	47.2	44.1	0	0	0	0	4.5	4.2	7	9	10	10	11	12
182	United States of America	15.1	14.9	15.1	15.5	15.5	15.3	62	61.9	61.2	61.1	61.6	62.5	3621	3762	3905	4068	4252	4499
183	Uruguay	22.2	21.1	19.8	19.4	17	16.7	56.1	60.2	63.3	63.7	66.8	68.8	552	606	662	697	682	653
184	Uzbekistan	22.7	17.5	17.9	15.3	21.2	22.5	0	0	0	0	0	0	21	28	26	24	27	30
185	Vanuatu	33.9	42.4	35.8	34.6	39.7	39.1	0	0	0	0	0	0	47	40	46	43	47	44
186	Venezuela, Bolivarian Republic of	45.4	45	42.9	46	45	40.4	5	5.6	5.6	4.9	5.2	5.2	162	122	166	205	201	233
187	Viet Nam	55.2	60.3	63.5	65.6	70.1	68.7	0	0	0	0	0	0	11	15	16	17	21	21
188	Yemen	70.8	63.8	62.3	57.3	60.9	61.1	0	0	0	0	0	0	41	21	19	18	19	21
189	Yugoslavia	42.1	42.6	41.4	49.1	49.1	49	0	0	0	0	0	0	57	108	125	87	97	50
190	Zambia	32.3	33	31.9	31.9	30.5	28.6	0	0	0	0	0	0	20	20	24	20	18	18
191	Zimbabwe	30.9	30.1	27.4	33.2	23	22.2	23.4	20.9	21	16.4	39.6	46.5	44	54	67	60	36	43

[a] A zero does not always mean "not applicable"; when no information has been collated to estimate an entry, say private insurance and other prepaid plans, that entry is shown as zero.

[b] There is a break in the series for Japan between 1997 and 1998. Since 1998, data have been based on new Japanese national health accounts, estimated as a pilot implementation of the OECD manual *A System of Health Accounts*. Consequently, the comparability of data over time is limited. In addition, the data for the year 2000 have been largely developed by WHO and are not endorsed by the Government of Japan.

		Per capita total expenditure on health in international dollars						Per capita government expenditure on health at average exchange rate (US$)						Per capita government expenditure on health in international dollars					
		1995	1996	1997	1998	1999	2000	1995	1996	1997	1998	1999	2000	1995	1996	1997	1998	1999	2000
166	Syrian Arab Republic	43	39	43	47	51	51	14	15	16	17	18	19	33	28	30	31	33	32
167	Tajikistan	22	27	28	25	29	29	1	3	3	4	4	3	14	17	19	17	25	23
168	Thailand	210	237	242	227	228	237	47	56	53	44	43	41	103	121	138	140	133	136
169	The former Yugoslav Republic of Macedonia	213	242	263	339	277	300	108	112	95	118	90	90	193	210	220	295	233	254
170	Togo	34	31	39	35	36	36	5	4	5	5	5	4	16	13	19	20	20	19
171	Tonga	284	277	286	281	298	312	56	60	67	57	54	51	123	120	134	130	137	146
172	Trinidad and Tobago	298	320	352	409	440	468	95	101	104	127	132	136	150	156	167	208	225	237
173	Tunisia	332	347	361	400	442	472	77	96	103	115	122	113	186	234	280	316	348	369
174	Turkey	190	235	273	304	292	323	65	78	90	108	98	107	134	162	196	218	208	230
175	Turkmenistan	92	114	145	193	204	286	26	12	18	26	31	44	71	93	108	157	169	243
176	Tuvalu	725	839	885	918	924	860	78	90	91	83	90	86	514	577	617	648	654	614
177	Uganda	27	27	29	32	36	36	4	4	5	4	5	4	11	12	13	12	15	14
178	Ukraine	208	164	179	167	146	152	35	34	40	30	19	18	175	131	134	119	99	107
179	United Arab Emirates	663	651	783	816	769	761	495	502	578	600	596	596	530	518	621	651	604	591
180	United Kingdom	1315	1422	1482	1530	1672	1774	1138	1179	1223	1324	1405	1415	1103	1179	1184	1223	1340	1437
181	United Republic of Tanzania	20	20	21	21	24	27	4	4	5	5	5	6	11	10	10	10	10	13
182	United States of America	3621	3762	3905	4068	4252	4499	1639	1714	1767	1810	1883	1992	1639	1714	1767	1810	1883	1992
183	Uruguay	726	807	894	966	997	1005	273	285	304	324	332	304	359	379	411	449	486	468
184	Uzbekistan	95	95	94	86	88	86	16	23	21	21	22	24	74	79	77	73	70	66
185	Vanuatu	97	84	99	106	115	119	31	23	29	28	28	27	64	48	64	69	69	72
186	Venezuela, Bolivarian Republic of	270	228	267	310	266	280	84	64	91	106	106	134	141	119	146	160	140	160
187	Viet Nam	68	87	93	104	128	129	5	5	5	5	5	5	28	30	29	30	31	33
188	Yemen	62	54	60	69	68	70	9	6	6	6	6	7	14	15	18	25	22	22
189	Yugoslavia	205	243	251	217	228	237	33	62	73	45	49	26	119	140	147	111	116	121
190	Zambia	41	48	51	46	44	49	10	11	13	12	11	11	22	25	28	26	26	30
191	Zimbabwe	155	174	225	279	197	171	22	30	40	33	17	18	79	95	133	156	97	73

Annex Table 6 Summary prevalence of selected risk factors by subregion,[a] 2000[b,c]

Risk factor[d]	Prevalence criteria	AFR-D	AFR-E	AMR-A	AMR-B	AMR-D
Alcohol	Proportion consuming alcohol	38%	44%	67%	66%	62%
Blood pressure	Mean systolic pressure (mmHg)	133	129	127	128	128
Childhood sexual abuse	Proportion of adults with history of abuse	14%	33%	15%	9%	15%
Cholesterol	Mean cholesterol (mmol/l)[e]	4.8	4.8	5.3	5.1	5.1
Indoor smoke from solid fuels	Proportion using biofuel	73%	86%	1%	25%	53%
Iron deficiency	Mean haemoglobin level (g/dl)	10.6	10.6	12.5	11.2	11.2
Low fruit and vegetable intake	Average intake per day (g)	350	240	290	190	340
Overweight	Body mass index (kg/m²)	21.3	21.8	26.9	26.0	26.0
Physical inactivity	Proportion with no physical activity	12%	11%	20%	23%	23%
Underweight	Proportion less than 2 SD weight for age	32%	31%	2%	5%	12%
Unplanned pregnancies	Proportion not using modern contraception	91%	86%	33%	45%	68%
Unsafe health care injections	Unsafe injection(s) exposing to Hepatitis B each year	5%	4%	0%	0%	0%
Urban air pollution	Concentration of particles less than 10 micron (μg/m³)	23	16	13	15	20
Vitamin A deficiency	Proportion vitamin A deficient with night blindness	19%	23%	0%	9%	9%
Zinc deficiency	Proportion not consuming US recommended dietary intake	37%	62%	6%	26%	68%

[a] See the List of Member States by WHO Region and mortality stratum for an explanation of subregions.

[b] Estimates are age standardized to the WHO reference population most relevant to the risk factor:

alcohol, childhood sexual abuse, and physical inactivity: ≥15 years of age;

blood pressure, cholesterol, overweight, and low fruit and vegetable intake: ≥30 years of age;

iron deficiency, vitamin A deficiency, zinc deficiency, and underweight: children under 5 years of age;

unplanned pregnancies: women 15–44 years of age.

[c] This table reflects the latest available data and may differ slightly from information presented in Chapter 4.

[d] Many risk factors were characterized at multiple levels; here they are collapsed to show exposure or no exposure (or means).

[e] 1 mmol/l = 38.7 mg/dl.

EMR-B	EMR-D	EUR-A	EUR-B	EUR-C	SEAR-B	SEAR-D	WPR-A	WPR-B
10%	5%	87%	62%	86%	21%	14%	84%	57%
133	131	135	137	138	128	125	133	124
18%	18%	9%	18%	16%	6%	46%	16%	26%
5.0	5.0	6.0	5.1	5.8	4.7	5.1	5.2	4.6
6%	55%	0%	26%	7%	66%	83%	0%	28%
10.5	10.5	12.5	11.9	11.9	11.0	10.4	12.5	11.0
350	360	450	380	220	220	240	410	330
25.2	22.3	26.7	26.5	26.5	23.1	19.9	23.4	22.9
19%	18%	17%	20%	24%	15%	17%	17%	16%
8%	25%	2%	8%	3%	26%	46%	4%	16%
63%	82%	31%	66%	52%	45%	65%	46%	73%
0%	12%	0%	0%	1%	6%	10%	0%	8%
17	27	13	24	18	28	25	13	28
1%	16%	0%	0%	0%	28%	18%	0%	9%
25%	52%	4%	13%	6%	34%	73%	4%	9%

Annex Table 7 Selected population attributable fractions by risk factor, sex and level of development (% DALYs for each cause), 2000[a]

	World			High mortality developing AFR-D, AFR-E, AMR-D, EMR-D, SEAR-D		Low mortality developing AMR-B, EMR-B, SEAR-B, WPR-B		Developed AMR-A, EUR-A, EUR-B, EUR-C, WPR-A	
	Males	Females	Both sexes	Males	Females	Males	Females	Males	Females
Childhood and maternal undernutrition									
Underweight									
Diarrhoeal diseases	44	45	45	49	49	24	21	13	12
Low birth weight	10	11	10	12	12	3	3	2	2
Lower respiratory infections	40	40	40	46	46	23	25	7	8
Malaria	45	45	45	46	45	9	14	0	0
Measles	33	33	33	34	34	22	23	10	10
Protein–energy malnutrition	89	88	88	88	88	91	92	77	78
Iron deficiency									
Anaemia	100	100	100	100	100	100	100	100	100
Maternal mortality	...	11	11	...	13	...	6	...	1
Perinatal mortality	20	19	19	22	22	13	13	8	7
Vitamin A deficiency									
Diarrhoeal diseases	18	18	18	19	19	10	9	0	0
Malaria	17	16	16	17	17	5	7	0	0
Maternal mortality	...	10	10	...	12	...	5	...	0
Measles	15	15	15	15	15	12	13	0	0
Other infectious diseases	2	2	2	2	2	1	1	0	0
Zinc deficiency									
Diarrhoeal diseases	10	10	10	11	11	3	3	2	2
Lower respiratory infections	16	16	16	19	19	5	5	2	3
Malaria	18	18	18	19	18	3	4	1	1
Other diet-related risks and physical inactivity									
Blood pressure									
Cerebrovascular disease	61	62	62	56	56	57	60	72	72
Ischaemic heart disease	50	47	49	45	41	45	46	59	55
Other cardiovascular disease	14	13	14	11	10	12	12	20	18
Cholesterol									
Ischaemic heart disease	55	57	56	50	57	48	47	63	63
Ischaemic stroke	30	34	32	27	35	25	27	39	41
Overweight									
Diabetes mellitus	50	66	58	26	51	54	68	75	83
Ischaemic heart disease	21	22	21	8	14	22	23	34	33
Ischaemic stroke	21	25	23	9	14	20	23	34	35
Hypertensive disease	36	41	39	22	30	35	40	57	59
Breast cancer	...	8	8	...	4	...	6	...	12
Colon/rectum cancer	11	13	12	4	6	8	10	15	17
Corpus uteri cancer	...	42	42	...	29	...	36	...	49
Osteoarthritis	11	14	13	5	8	10	12	19	23
Low fruit and vegetable intake									
Ischaemic heart disease	30	31	31	32	34	31	31	29	27
Ischaemic stroke	19	20	19	20	21	19	20	18	18
Oesophagus cancer	19	21	20	22	23	19	20	17	17
Stomach cancer	19	20	19	20	22	19	20	18	18
Colon/rectum cancer	2	3	2	3	3	3	3	2	2
Trachea/bronchus/lung cancers	12	13	12	14	16	13	13	11	11
Physical inactivity									
Ischaemic heart disease	22	21	22	21	21	22	21	23	22
Ischaemic stroke	11	12	11	10	11	11	11	12	13
Breast cancer	...	10	10	...	9	...	10	...	11
Colon/rectum cancer	16	16	16	15	15	15	16	16	17
Diabetes mellitus	14	15	14	13	14	14	15	15	15

	World			High mortality developing AFR-D, AFR-E, AMR-D, EMR-D, SEAR-D		Low mortality developing AMR-B, EMR-B, SEAR-B, WPR-B		Developed AMR-A, EUR-A, EUR-B, EUR-C, WPR-A	
	Males	Females	Both sexes	Males	Females	Males	Females	Males	Females
Sexual and reproductive health									
Unsafe sex									
Cervix uteri cancer	...	100	100	...	100	...	100	...	100
HIV/AIDS	92	97	94	95	98	68	69	50	51
Sexually transmitted diseases	100	100	100	100	100	100	100	100	100
Lack of contraception									
Unsafe abortion	...	89	89	...	90	...	82	...	83
Unplanned pregnancies and maternal complications	...	17	17	...	19	...	13	...	10
Addictive substances									
Tobacco									
Chronic obstructive pulmonary disease	49	24	38	58	19	35	14	79	57
Mouth and oropharynx cancers	15	20	16	29	35	0	0	0	0
Trachea/bronchus/lung cancers	76	42	66	75	25	57	20	90	69
Other cancers	13	1	7	5	0	12	1	19	2
Other medical conditions	8	2	5	5	1	7	1	16	6
Cardiovascular disease	19	4	12	14	2	12	2	32	10
Alcohol									
Cirrhosis of the liver	39	18	32	19	7	45	13	63	49
Drowning	12	6	10	8	4	10	6	43	25
Epilepsy	23	12	18	14	7	27	13	45	36
Falls	9	3	7	5	1	8	3	21	8
Haemorrhagic stroke	18	1	10	7	2	21	2	26	0
Homicide	26	16	24	18	12	28	16	41	32
Ischaemic heart disease	4	-1	2	7	0	5	0	2	-3
Ischaemic stroke	3	-6	-1	1	0	3	0	5	-16
Unipolar depressive disorders	3	1	2	2	0	3	0	7	2
Liver cancer	30	13	25	23	10	32	11	36	28
Mouth and oropharynx cancers	22	9	19	11	4	28	10	41	28
Oesophagus cancer	37	15	29	17	6	42	16	46	36
Other cancers	6	3	4	2	1	5	2	11	8
Self-inflicted injuries	15	5	11	8	2	10	5	27	12
Poisoning	23	9	18	7	3	11	7	43	26
Other intentional injuries	13	7	12	7	3	20	11	32	19
Motor vehicle accidents	25	8	20	19	5	25	8	45	18
Other unintentional injuries	15	5	11	10	4	15	6	32	16
Illicit drugs									
Drug use disorders	100	100	100	100	100	100	100	100	100
HIV/AIDS	4	1	2	0	0	28	9	43	68
Self-inflicted injuries	5	2	4	10	2	1	0	5	9
Unintentional injuries	1	1	1	1	0	1	1	2	6
Environmental risks									
Unsafe water, sanitation and hygiene									
Diarrhoeal diseases	88	88	88	88	88	88	88	80	80
Urban air pollution									
Cardiopulmonary diseases[b]	2	2	2	1	1	4	4	2	2
Respiratory infections	1	1	1	1	1	1	2	0	1
Trachea/bronchus/lung cancers	5	6	5	5	4	8	9	3	3
Indoor smoke from solid fuels									
Chronic obstructive pulmonary disease	13	34	22	13	45	16	40	1	4
Lower respiratory infections	36	36	36	41	41	20	21	10	11
Trachea/bronchus/lung cancers	1	3	1	0	1	2	7	0	0
Lead exposure									
Cerebrovascular disease	4	2	3	4	3	3	2	4	2
Hypertensive disease	6	3	5	8	4	5	3	6	3

Annex Table 7 Selected population attributable fractions by risk factor, sex and level of development (% DALYs for each cause), 2000[a]

	World			High mortality developing AFR-D, AFR-E, AMR-D, EMR-D, SEAR-D		Low mortality developing AMR-B, EMR-B, SEAR-B, WPR-B		Developed AMR-A, EUR-A, EUR-B, EUR-C, WPR-A	
	Males	Females	Both sexes	Males	Females	Males	Females	Males	Females
Ischaemic heart disease	3	2	2	3	2	3	2	3	1
Other cardiovascular disease	1	0	1	1	0	1	0	1	0
Climate change									
Diarrhoeal diseases	2	2	2	2	3	2	2	1	1
Malaria	2	2	2	2	2	6	4	1	0
Other unintentional injuries	0	1	0	0	0	1	1	0	0
Protein–energy malnutrition	16	18	17	22	23	0	0	0	0
Occupational risks									
Risk factors for injury									
Drowning	1	0	1	1	0	1	0	1	0
Falls	18	3	12	22	3	17	3	12	2
Fires	4	0	2	3	0	11	1	2	0
Motor vehicle accidents	8	1	6	10	2	8	1	5	1
Poisoning	3	0	2	4	0	5	0	1	0
Carcinogens									
Leukaemia	3	2	2	2	1	2	2	3	3
Other malignant neoplasms	2	1	2	2	2	3	2	1	1
Trachea/bronchus/lung cancers	12	6	10	11	4	13	7	12	5
Airborne particulates									
Chronic obstructive pulmonary disease	17	2	10	10	1	20	2	17	4
Ergonomic stressors									
Low back pain	41	32	37	40	31	43	34	39	29
Noise									
Deafness	22	11	16	23	10	24	14	16	8
Other selected risks to health									
Unsafe health care injections									
Cirrhosis of the liver	23	26	24	32	35	24	27	4	5
HIV/AIDS	5	5	5	6	5	2	5	0	1
Hepatitis B	30	29	30	39	36	25	22	2	2
Hepatitis C	32	30	31	47	42	31	26	2	2
Liver cancer	29	27	28	20	22	36	35	2	2
Childhood sexual abuse									
Alcohol use disorders	5	7	5	8	11	5	5	2	7
Drug use disorders	5	8	6	7	11	4	5	2	8
Panic disorder	7	13	11	10	19	6	9	3	10
Post-traumatic stress disorder	21	33	30	27	43	22	26	10	28
Self-inflicted injuries	6	11	8	9	16	5	8	3	8
Unipolar depressive disorders	4	7	6	5	10	3	4	1	5

[a] The combined effects of any group of risk factors in this table will often be less than the sum of their separate effects.

[b] Selected cardiovascular and pulmonary diseases.

… Data not available or not applicable.

Annex Table 8 Distribution of attributable mortality and DALYs by risk factor, age and sex, 2000[a]

	Distribution of attributable deaths (% attributable events)						Distribution of attributable DALYs (% attributable events)					
	Age group				Sex		Age group				Sex	
	0-4	5-14	15-59	60+	Males	Females	0-4	5-14	15-59	60+	Males	Females
Childhood and maternal undernutrition												
Underweight	100	0	0	0	51	49	100	0	0	0	51	49
Iron deficiency	72	1	22	4	45	55	62	6	30	2	45	55
Vitamin A deficiency	85	1	14	0	43	57	86	1	12	0	44	56
Zinc deficiency	100	0	0	0	51	49	100	0	0	0	51	49
Other diet-related risks and physical inactivity												
Blood pressure	0	0	19	81	49	51	0	0	43	57	54	46
Cholesterol	0	0	22	78	48	52	0	0	50	50	55	45
Overweight	0	0	26	74	45	55	0	0	57	43	47	53
Low fruit and vegetable intake	0	0	23	77	53	47	0	0	49	51	57	43
Physical inactivity	0	0	21	79	50	50	0	0	48	52	53	47
Sexual and reproductive health risks												
Unsafe sex	16	1	77	6	47	53	18	1	79	2	46	54
Lack of contraception	0	0	100	0	0	100	0	0	100	0	0	100
Addictive substances												
Tobacco	0	0	30	70	79	21	0	0	61	39	82	18
Alcohol	1	1	65	33	91	9	1	3	87	9	85	15
Illicit drugs	0	0	100	0	80	20	0	2	98	0	77	23
Environmental risks												
Unsafe water, sanitation and hygiene	68	5	13	14	52	48	77	8	13	3	51	49
Ambient air pollution	3	0	16	81	51	49	12	0	40	49	56	44
Indoor smoke from solid fuels	56	0	5	38	41	59	83	0	8	9	49	51
Lead exposure	0	0	42	58	66	34	75	0	16	8	55	45
Climate change	86	3	6	5	49	51	88	5	6	1	49	51
Occupational risks												
Risk factors for injury	0	0	85	14	94	6	0	0	96	4	92	8
Carcinogens	0	0	28	72	81	19	0	0	52	48	80	20
Airborne particulates	0	0	11	89	89	11	0	0	54	46	91	9
Ergonomic stressors	0	0	0	0	0	0	0	0	95	5	59	41
Noise	0	0	0	0	0	0	0	0	89	11	67	33
Other selected risks to health												
Unsafe health care injections	10	2	53	35	63	37	16	3	67	13	61	39
Childhood sexual abuse	0	0	80	21	48	52	0	0	96	4	36	64

[a] The combined effects of any group of risk factors in this table will often be less than the sum of their separate effects.

Annex Table 9 Attributable mortality by risk factor, level of development and sex, 2000[a]

	High mortality developing countries AFR-D, AFR-E, AMR-D, EMR-D, SEAR-D		Low mortality developing countries AMR-B, EMR-B, SEAR-B, WPR-B		Developed countries AMR-A, EUR-A, EUR-B, EUR-C, WPR-A	
	Males	Females	Males	Females	Males	Females
	(000)	(000)	(000)	(000)	(000)	(000)
Childhood and maternal undernutrition						
Underweight	1 734	1 697	156	142	10	9
Iron deficiency	302	381	65	75	8	10
Vitamin A deficiency	314	420	20	25	0	0
Zinc deficiency	383	373	15	14	2	2
Other diet-related risks and physical inactivity						
Blood pressure	1 017	954	1 091	1 115	1 383	1 581
Cholesterol	682	723	434	416	996	1 165
Overweight	150	250	361	415	658	759
Low fruit and vegetable intake	491	437	432	354	527	487
Physical inactivity	312	285	240	236	410	439
Sexual and reproductive health risks						
Unsafe sex	1 284	1 383	71	92	15	41
Lack of contraception	...	132	...	16	...	1
Addictive substances						
Tobacco	1 031	185	1 048	217	1 814	612
Alcohol	356	72	729	115	552	- 21
Illicit drugs	66	14	53	8	44	20
Environmental risks						
Unsafe water, sanitation and hygiene	792	746	92	80	10	10
Urban air pollution	119	101	215	211	78	76
Indoor smoke from solid fuels	490	549	159	399	9	13
Lead exposure	60	33	46	23	49	23
Climate change	73	75	3	2	0	0
Occupational risks						
Risk factors for injury	141	9	122	8	28	2
Carcinogens	19	4	45	13	54	11
Airborne particulates	40	3	134	16	43	7
Ergonomic stressors	0	0	0	0	0	0
Noise	0	0	0	0	0	0
Other selected risks to health						
Unsafe health care injections	154	113	156	66	7	4
Childhood sexual abuse	19	21	12	15	6	5

[a] The combined effects of any group of risk factors in this table will often be less than the sum of their separate effects.

... Data not available or not applicable.

Annex Table 10 Attributable DALYs by risk factor, level of development and sex, 2000[a]

	High mortality developing countries AFR-D, AFR-E, AMR-D, EMR-D, SEAR-D		Low mortality developing countries AMR-B, EMR-B, SEAR-B, WPR-B		Developed countries AMR-A, EUR-A, EUR-B, EUR-C, WPR-A	
	Males	Females	Males	Females	Males	Females
	(000)	(000)	(000)	(000)	(000)	(000)
Childhood and maternal undernutrition						
Underweight	62 730	61 668	6 576	6 020	427	379
Iron deficiency	11 898	14 272	3 242	4 050	617	979
Vitamin A deficiency	10 919	14 218	675	823	1	1
Zinc deficiency	13 544	13 237	587	534	71	62
Other diet-related risks and physical inactivity						
Blood pressure	10 963	9 664	10 824	9 454	13 132	10 232
Cholesterol	7 794	7 808	4 879	3 730	9 463	6 764
Overweight	2 344	4 064	5 119	5 996	8 080	7 813
Low fruit and vegetable intake	5 505	4 963	4 550	3 319	5 062	3 262
Physical inactivity	3 596	3 336	2 697	2 477	3 866	3 120
Sexual and reproductive health risks						
Unsafe sex	39 324	45 240	2 685	2 994	591	1 035
Lack of contraception	…	7 495	…	1 181	…	137
Addictive substances						
Tobacco	14 206	2 477	13 808	2 486	20 162	5 942
Alcohol	11 106	2 059	21 830	3 690	16 462	3 176
Illicit drugs	3 236	796	2 743	570	2 689	1 183
Environmental risks						
Unsafe water, sanitation and hygiene	23 157	23 026	3 846	3 304	429	396
Urban air pollution	1 454	1 231	2 272	1 736	687	484
Indoor smoke from solid fuels	15 534	14 859	3 252	4 343	253	297
Lead exposure	3 206	2 747	3 020	2 564	886	502
Climate change	2 535	2 667	156	138	10	12
Occupational risks						
Risk factors for injury	6 266	485	4 686	463	1 118	106
Carcinogens	207	44	449	148	481	91
Airborne particulates	449	37	1 815	128	507	102
Ergonomic stressors	187	132	214	148	85	53
Noise	1 190	505	1 136	615	462	243
Other selected risks to health						
Unsafe health care injections	3 846	3 090	2 396	952	115	63
Childhood sexual abuse	1 425	2 932	1 118	1 415	391	954

[a] The combined effects of any group of risk factors in this table will often be less than the sum of their separate effects.

… Data not available or not applicable.

Annex Table 11 Attributable mortality by risk factor, sex and mortality stratum in WHO Regions,[a] 2000[b]

	WORLD			AFRICA				THE AMERICAS					
				Mortality stratum				Mortality stratum					
				High child, high adult		High child, very high adult		Very low child, very low adult		Low child, low adult		High child, high adult	
	Males (000)	Females (000)	Total (000)	Males (000)	Females (000)	Males (000)	Females (000)	Males (000)	Females (000)	Males (000)	Females (000)	Males (000)	Females (000)
Childhood and maternal undernutrition													
Underweight	1900	1848	3748	438	402	487	441	0	0	14	11	14	11
Iron deficiency	375	466	841	59	67	65	80	2	3	13	13	3	4
Vitamin A deficiency	333	445	778	90	112	120	151	0	0	2	3	2	2
Zinc deficiency	400	389	789	74	68	128	116	0	0	3	2	5	4
Other diet-related risks and physical inactivity													
Blood pressure	3491	3649	7141	87	128	79	116	179	191	170	162	20	20
Cholesterol	2112	2303	4415	34	52	36	53	161	189	88	79	10	9
Overweight	1168	1423	2591	14	19	21	35	135	137	117	144	15	18
Low fruit and vegetable intake	1449	1277	2726	21	31	33	41	92	79	81	58	7	7
Physical inactivity	961	961	1922	20	25	21	27	74	81	52	55	6	6
Sexual and reproductive health risks													
Unsafe sex	1370	1516	2886	198	234	805	923	8	8	22	27	17	11
Lack of contraception	…	149	149	…	16	…	33	…	0	…	5	…	4
Addictive substances													
Tobacco	3893	1014	4907	43	7	84	26	352	294	163	58	5	1
Alcohol	1638	166	1804	53	15	125	30	27	-22	207	39	22	6
Illicit drugs	163	41	204	5	1	1	0	10	7	7	4	1	0
Environmental risks													
Unsafe water, sanitation and hygiene	895	835	1730	129	103	207	169	0	1	16	15	13	10
Urban air pollution	411	388	799	11	11	5	5	14	14	16	14	3	2
Indoor smoke from solid fuels	658	961	1619	93	80	118	101	0	0	7	9	5	5
Lead exposure	155	79	234	5	4	4	3	2	1	14	7	2	1
Climate change	76	78	154	9	9	18	18	0	0	0	0	0	0
Occupational risks													
Risk factors for injury	291	19	310	14	1	18	1	3	0	17	1	2	0
Carcinogens	118	28	146	1	0	1	1	9	3	5	1	0	0
Airborne particulates	217	26	243	3	0	3	0	10	3	10	1	0	0
Ergonomic stressors	0	0	0	0	0	0	0	0	0	0	0	0	0
Noise	0	0	0	0	0	0	0	0	0	0	0	0	0
Other selected risks to health													
Unsafe health care injections	317	184	501	10	7	27	23	0	0	1	0	1	1
Childhood sexual abuse	38	41	79	0	0	2	1	1	1	1	0	0	0

[a] See the List of Member States by WHO Region and mortality stratum.

[b] The combined effects of any group of risk factors in this table will often be less than the sum of their separate effects.

… Data not available or not applicable.

EASTERN MEDITERRANEAN				EUROPE						SOUTH-EAST ASIA				WESTERN PACIFIC			
Mortality stratum				Mortality stratum						Mortality stratum				Mortality stratum			
Low child, low adult		High child, high adult		Very low child, very low adult		Low child, low adult		Low child, high adult		Low child, low adult		High child, high adult		Very low child, very low adult		Low child, low adult	
Males (000)	Females (000)	Males (000)	Females (000)	Males (000)	Females (000)	Males (000)	Females (000)	Males (000)	Females (000)	Males (000)	Females (000)	Males (000)	Females (000)	Males (000)	Females (000)	Males (000)	Females (000)
8	8	223	229	0	0	9	8	0	0	40	29	573	614	0	0	95	94
3	4	36	44	2	3	3	3	2	2	15	19	139	185	0	0	34	39
0	0	34	53	0	0	0	0	0	0	10	13	68	101	0	0	7	9
2	2	44	45	0	0	2	2	0	0	5	4	132	141	0	0	6	6
76	57	164	171	325	354	281	289	514	671	133	139	668	519	85	76	711	758
51	31	114	101	265	282	144	136	387	518	72	40	488	507	39	39	222	265
36	28	58	67	183	197	117	141	202	265	44	58	42	110	21	20	163	184
27	15	51	48	95	75	80	67	234	247	55	48	378	311	26	19	269	232
21	13	47	43	103	103	64	62	147	175	34	34	218	185	23	19	132	134
0	4	33	39	3	9	1	8	3	13	30	25	231	177	0	3	18	36
...	1	...	23	...	0	...	0	...	0	...	7	...	56	...	0	...	3
43	10	114	19	531	145	255	53	548	73	181	12	785	132	128	49	661	137
6	1	8	1	65	-85	100	25	338	88	51	9	148	21	23	-28	465	66
5	1	18	4	11	6	3	1	18	5	13	1	40	8	2	1	28	2
9	9	117	135	0	1	8	7	1	1	25	21	326	327	0	0	42	35
5	3	28	23	12	11	20	18	22	24	17	15	72	60	10	8	176	179
1	1	56	60	0	0	8	9	1	3	15	22	218	304	0	0	137	366
5	2	12	6	4	2	15	8	26	13	6	3	38	19	0	0	21	10
0	0	10	11	0	0	0	0	0	0	1	0	35	38	0	0	2	1
8	0	27	2	4	0	5	0	15	1	19	1	79	5	2	0	78	5
1	0	2	0	16	3	8	1	16	3	4	1	14	2	4	1	34	12
1	0	4	0	13	3	6	0	12	1	8	0	29	2	2	0	115	15
0	0	0	0	0	0	0	0	0	0	0	0	0	0	0	0	0	0
0	0	0	0	0	0	0	0	0	0	0	0	0	0	0	0	0	0
0	0	24	20	0	0	1	0	6	4	19	9	92	62	0	0	137	58
0	0	1	1	1	1	1	1	3	2	1	0	16	18	1	1	10	14

Annex Table 12 Attributable DALYs by risk factor, sex and mortality stratum in WHO Regions,[a] 2000[b]

	WORLD			AFRICA				THE AMERICAS					
				Mortality stratum						Mortality stratum			
				High child, high adult		High child, very high adult		Very low child, very low adult		Low child, low adult		High child, high adult	
	Males (000)	Females (000)	Total (000)	Males (000)	Females (000)	Males (000)	Females (000)	Males (000)	Females (000)	Males (000)	Females (000)	Males (000)	Females (000)
Childhood and maternal undernutrition													
Underweight	69 733	68 067	137 801	15 530	14 375	17 189	15 710	12	11	570	498	512	410
Iron deficiency	15 756	19 301	35 057	2 263	2 521	2 451	2 905	223	255	446	465	121	217
Vitamin A deficiency	11 596	15 042	26 638	3 178	3 856	4 208	5 167	0	0	79	103	53	68
Zinc deficiency	14 201	13 833	28 034	2 625	2 414	4 563	4 150	1	1	115	99	174	138
Other diet-related risks and physical inactivity													
Blood pressure	34 920	29 350	64 270	980	1 295	984	1 177	1 642	1 141	1 807	1 438	208	178
Cholesterol	22 136	18 301	40 437	395	563	456	578	1 451	1 012	1 070	803	109	87
Overweight	15 543	17 872	33 415	246	318	341	546	1 825	1 654	1 505	1 918	189	234
Low fruit and vegetable intake	15 117	11 544	26 662	253	354	434	471	833	536	896	581	72	67
Physical inactivity	10 159	8 933	19 092	225	280	262	309	691	576	582	585	61	68
Sexual and reproductive health risks													
Unsafe sex	42 600	49 269	91 869	6 205	7 753	24 059	29 664	281	235	843	912	521	310
Lack of contraception	...	8 814	8 814	...	997	...	1 732	...	2	...	375	...	203
Addictive substances													
Tobacco	48 177	10 904	59 081	591	97	1 311	367	3 567	2 606	2 190	813	51	14
Alcohol	49 397	8 926	58 323	1 441	393	3 621	785	2 925	702	7 854	1 443	789	170
Illicit drugs	8 669	2 549	11 218	543	156	495	163	797	410	758	323	199	71
Environmental risks													
Unsafe water, sanitation and hygiene	27 432	26 726	54 158	3 797	3 119	6 365	5 355	31	30	686	603	436	320
Urban air pollution	4 413	3 452	7 865	171	148	90	76	113	87	171	136	29	24
Indoor smoke from solid fuels	19 040	19 499	38 539	3 036	2 358	3 865	3 059	2	4	193	251	175	154
Lead exposure	7 112	5 814	12 926	512	488	460	433	68	49	907	789	140	125
Climate change	2 700	2 816	5 517	321	305	631	636	1	2	35	36	13	10
Occupational risks													
Risk factors for injury	12 071	1 054	13 125	662	55	773	68	116	14	745	74	92	9
Carcinogens	1 138	283	1 421	12	4	17	7	71	22	49	11	4	1
Airborne particulates	2 771	267	3 038	26	2	35	2	125	35	134	13	3	0
Ergonomic stressors	485	333	818	21	16	25	20	17	10	32	15	4	2
Noise	2 788	1 362	4 151	109	49	127	60	92	31	122	43	15	6
Other selected risks to health													
Unsafe health care injections	6 356	4 105	10 461	244	187	804	742	0	0	13	5	20	12
Childhood sexual abuse	2 934	5 302	8 235	49	102	167	238	98	320	147	118	46	27

[a] See the List of Member States by WHO Region and mortality stratum.
[b] The combined effects of any group of risk factors in this table will often be less than the sum of their separate effects.
... Data not available or not applicable.

EASTERN MEDITERRANEAN				EUROPE						SOUTH-EAST ASIA				WESTERN PACIFIC			
Mortality stratum				Mortality stratum						Mortality stratum				Mortality stratum			
Low child, low adult		High child, high adult		Very low child, very low adult		Low child, low adult		High child, high adult		Low child, low adult		High child, high adult		Very low child, very low adult		Low child, low adult	
Males (000)	Females (000)	Males (000)	Females (000)	Males (000)	Females (000)	Males (000)	Females (000)	Males (000)	Females (000)	Males (000)	Females (000)	Males (000)	Females (000)	Males (000)	Females (000)	Males (000)	Females (000)
324	312	8 203	8 407	10	9	367	324	32	29	1 634	1 239	21 297	22 766	6	6	4 048	3 972
239	277	1 449	1 746	87	211	166	271	110	161	681	847	5 614	6 883	31	81	1 876	2 462
9	8	1 159	1 758	0	0	1	1	0	0	347	406	2 321	3 368	0	0	241	306
66	63	1 547	1 574	0	0	65	56	5	4	197	152	4 635	4 961	0	0	208	219
840	570	1 781	1 698	2 624	1 828	2 699	2 180	5 386	4 632	1 394	1 402	7 010	5 316	781	451	6 783	6 044
605	320	1 273	1 051	2 062	1 317	1 461	996	4 109	3 211	828	412	5 562	5 528	380	227	2 376	2 195
534	456	882	1 027	1 922	1 735	1 420	1 445	2 578	2 684	650	818	686	1 939	334	295	2 430	2 804
322	172	607	550	785	413	777	511	2 431	1 684	614	524	4 139	3 521	237	118	2 718	2 042
265	164	559	492	852	654	636	494	1 461	1 236	414	409	2 489	2 186	228	160	1 436	1 318
30	162	1 125	1 508	114	202	50	240	134	295	1 009	925	7 413	6 004	12	65	804	995
...	119	...	1 210	...	3	...	83	...	47	...	397	...	3 354	...	1	...	290
593	197	1 780	379	4 991	1 464	3 381	715	7 230	832	2 712	180	10 474	1 621	994	325	8 313	1 296
162	22	328	36	3 103	416	2 183	446	7 543	1 570	1 793	284	4 927	675	708	43	12 020	1 941
449	78	624	147	764	365	179	82	717	225	427	41	1 376	260	231	101	1 109	129
314	315	3 797	4 506	33	33	287	262	64	57	734	506	8 762	9 725	14	13	2 112	1 879
55	36	345	291	91	60	197	141	217	153	184	155	820	693	70	44	1 862	1 410
32	32	1 817	1 691	0	0	233	244	18	49	458	532	6 641	7 596	0	0	2 569	3 528
238	187	606	504	75	43	304	189	424	211	379	337	1 489	1 198	15	10	1 496	1 251
10	10	357	391	1	2	5	5	2	2	19	15	1 213	1 325	0	1	92	77
287	25	1 224	96	180	22	243	19	495	41	715	63	3 517	258	85	10	2 939	301
15	2	24	5	131	21	82	12	166	31	43	8	150	27	31	6	342	127
22	1	44	4	140	42	79	6	132	10	101	7	341	29	31	8	1 558	107
9	3	25	16	21	11	18	12	21	14	26	19	111	78	9	5	146	110
60	21	142	88	117	47	92	50	136	92	219	185	799	303	26	22	735	365
0	0	437	390	0	0	8	5	106	59	356	156	2 341	1 759	0	0	2 028	791
41	83	85	225	61	175	72	158	132	205	42	56	1 079	2 340	29	96	888	1 158

Annex Table 13 Attributable years of life lost (YLL) by risk factor, sex and mortality stratum in WHO Regions,[a] 2000[b]

	WORLD			AFRICA				THE AMERICAS					
				Mortality stratum						Mortality stratum			
				High child, high adult		High child, very high adult		Very low child, very low adult		Low child, low adult		High child, high adult	
	Males (000)	Females (000)	Total (000)	Males (000)	Females (000)	Males (000)	Females (000)	Males (000)	Females (000)	Males (000)	Females (000)	Males (000)	Females (000)
Childhood and maternal undernutrition													
Underweight	64 119	62 766	126 885	14 780	13 660	16 428	14 980	2	2	458	389	475	375
Iron deficiency	11 891	13 967	25 858	1 906	2 128	2 108	2 553	30	27	378	361	83	101
Vitamin A deficiency	11 276	14 727	26 003	3 049	3 730	4 049	5 008	0	0	78	103	53	68
Zinc deficiency	13 459	13 167	26 626	2 473	2 284	4 319	3 942	0	0	92	77	163	128
Other diet-related risks and physical inactivity													
Blood pressure	30 206	25 342	55 548	873	1 152	874	1 038	1 336	900	1 536	1 226	186	156
Cholesterol	19 373	15 600	34 974	344	483	401	492	1 230	819	908	656	98	74
Overweight	11 276	11 868	23 143	177	229	267	416	1 174	921	1 138	1 321	142	166
Low fruit and vegetable intake	13 463	10 014	23 477	223	307	388	407	721	440	780	487	66	60
Physical inactivity	8 562	7 278	15 841	191	239	228	266	542	423	485	462	51	55
Sexual and reproductive health risks													
Unsafe sex	36 918	40 052	76 970	5 419	6 525	21 730	26 338	174	137	559	479	440	239
Lack of contraception	...	4 206	4 206	...	474	...	970	...	1	...	145	...	102
Addictive substances													
Tobacco	37 913	7 708	45 622	495	80	1 126	301	2 604	1 789	1 603	500	41	11
Alcohol	28 035	4 662	32 697	1 003	292	2 576	572	804	86	4 118	551	435	79
Illicit drugs	3 841	978	4 819	122	19	27	6	232	173	162	88	33	12
Environmental risks													
Unsafe water, sanitation and hygiene	24 917	24 315	49 232	3 612	2 937	6 148	5 139	3	3	467	387	395	280
Urban air pollution	3 533	2 871	6 404	153	132	80	67	87	65	133	99	24	20
Indoor smoke from solid fuels	17 341	17 805	35 146	2 948	2 329	3 760	3 028	1	2	136	137	159	139
Lead exposure	1 888	914	2 801	66	47	68	41	26	11	172	85	23	12
Climate change	2 415	2 530	4 945	301	285	583	589	1	1	11	11	10	8
Occupational risks													
Risk factors for injury	6 674	433	7 107	331	22	414	27	61	4	388	25	56	4
Carcinogens	1 105	271	1 376	12	4	17	7	68	21	47	11	4	1
Airborne particulates	1 344	143	1 487	21	2	28	2	50	16	56	4	1	0
Ergonomic stressors	4	1	5	0	0	0	0	0	0	0	0	0	0
Noise	0	0	0	0	0	0	0	0	0	0	0	0	0
Other selected risks to health													
Unsafe health care injections	5 504	3 675	9 179	223	174	757	702	0	0	10	4	16	10
Childhood sexual abuse	784	908	1 691	9	5	34	16	18	19	21	4	6	1

[a] See the List of Member States by WHO Region and mortality stratum.

[b] The combined effects of any group of risk factors in this table will often be less than the sum of their separate effects.

... Data not available or not applicable.

EASTERN MEDITERRANEAN				EUROPE						SOUTH-EAST ASIA				WESTERN PACIFIC			
Mortality stratum				Mortality stratum						Mortality stratum				Mortality stratum			
Low child, low adult		High child, high adult		Very low child, very low adult		Low child, low adult		Low child, high adult		Low child, low adult		High child, high adult		Very low child, very low adult		Low child, low adult	
Males (000)	Females (000)	Males (000)	Females (000)	Males (000)	Females (000)	Males (000)	Females (000)	Males (000)	Females (000)	Males (000)	Females (000)	Males (000)	Females (000)	Males (000)	Females (000)	Males (000)	Females (000)
268	258	7 523	7 777	1	1	318	276	9	7	1 352	984	19 329	20 885	1	1	3 176	3 172
95	108	1 164	1 368	20	19	94	82	46	39	402	468	4 459	5 455	4	3	1 103	1 256
9	8	1 149	1 748	0	0	1	1	0	0	344	403	2 306	3 354	0	0	239	304
58	55	1 485	1 519	0	0	62	54	5	4	174	129	4 439	4 773	0	0	188	201
764	490	1 582	1 490	2 170	1 484	2 396	1 930	4 850	4 099	1 225	1 231	6 176	4 619	582	338	5 657	5 191
560	274	1 148	915	1 768	1 107	1 308	877	3 747	2 862	731	356	4 927	4 722	295	172	1 908	1 791
419	289	648	721	1 317	1 040	1 130	1 075	2 139	1 975	448	565	486	1 273	175	122	1 616	1 753
299	149	548	481	692	350	705	453	2 236	1 507	549	455	3 699	3 054	196	94	2 363	1 770
232	125	477	409	705	511	559	424	1 319	1 070	342	330	2 135	1 811	167	109	1 130	1 043
4	47	917	1 030	75	114	22	117	79	172	810	511	6 188	3 779	4	31	498	533
...	31	...	639	...	1	...	12	...	10	...	175	...	1 551	...	0	...	95
448	133	1 416	282	3 856	858	2 786	489	6 270	580	2 066	135	8 660	1 403	752	200	5 792	948
132	16	139	22	1 223	19	1 383	296	5 524	1 050	1 156	189	2 936	462	309	- 60	6 299	1 087
110	22	430	92	266	136	63	32	424	113	313	16	924	194	58	18	676	59
261	266	3 633	4 350	3	4	247	223	39	30	640	414	8 212	9 209	2	2	1 254	1 072
47	30	305	253	73	44	170	118	191	129	154	128	718	594	53	31	1 343	1 161
27	27	1 736	1 614	0	0	224	211	16	24	386	390	6 324	7 140	0	0	1 625	2 764
83	40	163	83	40	14	180	81	316	122	73	42	443	226	5	2	230	107
7	7	317	354	0	0	4	3	1	1	15	10	1 105	1 223	0	0	59	37
179	12	620	41	88	6	117	8	335	22	443	29	1 812	118	34	2	1 795	116
15	2	23	4	126	20	80	12	162	30	42	8	146	24	30	6	332	122
8	1	35	3	60	11	45	2	90	3	57	4	263	22	9	1	621	71
0	0	0	0	1	0	0	0	1	0	0	0	0	0	0	0	0	0
0	0	0	0	0	0	0	0	0	0	0	0	0	0	0	0	0	0
0	0	351	346	0	0	7	4	86	48	301	136	1 957	1 556	0	0	1 796	696
10	11	29	33	15	15	18	11	62	30	12	10	359	461	10	15	180	276

Annex Table 14 Major burden of disease – leading 10 selected risk factors and leading 10 diseases and injuries, high mortality developing countries, 2000

Developing countries with high child and high or very high adult mortality (AFR-D, AFR-E, AMR-D, EMR-D, SEAR-D)

Risk factor	% DALYs	Disease or injury	% DALYs
Underweight	14.9	HIV/AIDS	9.0
Unsafe sex	10.2	Lower respiratory infections	8.2
Unsafe water, sanitation and hygiene	5.5	Diarrhoeal diseases	6.3
Indoor smoke from solid fuels	3.7	Childhood cluster diseases	5.5
Zinc deficiency	3.2	Low birth weight	5.0
Iron deficiency[a]	3.1	Malaria	4.9
Vitamin A deficiency	3.0	Unipolar depressive disorders	3.1
Blood pressure	2.5	Ischaemic heart disease	3.0
Tobacco	2.0	Tuberculosis	2.9
Cholesterol	1.9	Road traffic injury	2.0

[a] Iron deficiency disease burden is from maternal and perinatal causes, as well as direct effects of anaemia.

Annex Table 15 Major burden of disease – leading 10 selected risk factors and leading 10 diseases and injuries, low mortality developing countries, 2000

Developing countries with low child and low adult mortality (AMR-B, EMR-B, SEAR-B, WPR-B)

Risk factor	% DALYs	Disease or injury	% DALYs
Alcohol	6.2	Unipolar depressive disorders	5.9
Blood pressure	5.0	Cerebrovascular disease	4.7
Tobacco	4.0	Lower respiratory infections	4.1
Underweight	3.1	Road traffic injury	4.1
Overweight	2.7	Chronic obstructive pulmonary disease	3.8
Cholesterol	2.1	Ischaemic heart disease	3.2
Low fruit and vegetable intake	1.9	Birth asphyxia/trauma	2.6
Indoor smoke from solid fuels	1.9	Tuberculosis	2.4
Iron deficiency	1.8	Alcohol use disorders	2.3
Unsafe water, sanitation and hygiene[a]	1.7	Deafness	2.2

[a] Unsafe water, sanitation and hygiene disease burden is from diarrhoeal diseases.

Annex Table 16 Major burden of disease – leading 10 selected risk factors and leading 10 diseases and injuries, developed countries, 2000

Developed countries with very low or low child mortality levels (AMR-A, EUR-A, EUR-B, EUR-C, WPR-A)

Risk factor	% DALYs	Disease or injury	% DALYs
Tobacco	12.2	Ischaemic heart disease	9.4
Blood pressure	10.9	Unipolar depressive disorders	7.2
Alcohol	9.2	Cerebrovascular disease	6.0
Cholesterol	7.6	Alcohol use disorders	3.5
Overweight	7.4	Dementia and other central nervous system disorders	3.0
Low fruit and vegetable intake	3.9	Deafness	2.8
Physical inactivity	3.3	Chronic obstructive pulmonary disease	2.6
Illicit drugs	1.8	Road traffic injury	2.5
Unsafe sex[a]	0.8	Osteoarthritis	2.5
Iron deficiency[b]	0.7	Trachea/bronchus/lung cancers	2.4

[a] Unsafe sex disease burden is from HIV/AIDS and sexually transmitted diseases.

[b] Iron deficiency disease burden is from maternal and perinatal causes, as well as direct effects of anaemia.

Preventive fractions due to alcohol and cardiovascular disease in some regions are not shown in these tables.
NB. The selected risk factors cause diseases in addition to those relationships illustrated, and additional risk factors are also important in the etiology of the diseases illustrated.

- - - - - - - - - - - - - - -→ 1-24% population attributable fraction

————————→ 25-49% population attributable fraction

━━━━━━━→ 50%+ population attributable fraction

LIST OF MEMBER STATES BY
WHO REGION AND MORTALITY STRATUM

To aid in cause of death analyses, burden of disease analyses, and comparative risk assessment, the 191 Member States of WHO have been divided into five mortality strata on the basis of their levels of child mortality under five years of age (5q0) and 15 - 59-year-old male mortality (45q15). The classification of Member States into the mortality strata was carried out using population estimates for 1999 (UN Population Division 1998) and estimates of 5q0 and 45q15 based on WHO analyses of mortality rates for 1999.

Quintiles of the distribution of 5q0 (both sexes combined) were used to define a *very low child mortality* group (1st quintile), a *low child mortality* group (2nd and 3rd quintiles) and a *high child mortality* group (4th and 5th quintiles). Adult mortality 45q15 was regressed on 5q0 and the regression line used to divide countries with high child mortality into *high adult mortality* (stratum D) and *very high adult mortality* (stratum E). Stratum E includes the countries in sub-Saharan Africa where HIV/AIDS has had a very substantial impact.

Annex Figure 1. WHO Member States grouped by mortality strata, 1999

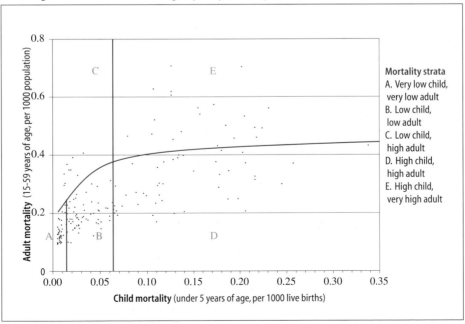

When these mortality strata are applied to the six WHO regions, they produce 14 epidemiological subregions, which are used throughout this report and in the Annex Tables to present results. The mortality strata to which WHO Member States are classified are listed below. This classification has no official status and is for analytical purposes only.

African Region

Algeria — AFR-D
Angola – AFR-D
Benin – AFR-D
Botswana – AFR-E
Burkina Faso – AFR-D
Burundi – AFR-E
Cameroon – AFR-D
Cape Verde – AFR-D
Central African Republic – AFR-E
Chad – AFR-D
Comoros – AFR-D
Congo – AFR-E
Côte d'Ivoire – AFR-E
Democratic Republic of the Congo – AFR-E
Equatorial Guinea – AFR-D
Eritrea – AFR-E
Ethiopia – AFR-E
Gabon – AFR-D
Gambia – AFR-D
Ghana – AFR-D
Guinea – AFR-D
Guinea-Bissau – AFR-D
Kenya – AFR-E
Lesotho – AFR-E
Liberia – AFR-D
Madagascar – AFR-D
Malawi – AFR-E
Mali – AFR-D
Mauritania – AFR-D
Mauritius – AFR-D
Mozambique – AFR-E
Namibia – AFR-E
Niger – AFR-D
Nigeria – AFR-D
Rwanda – AFR-E
Sao Tome and Principe – AFR-D
Senegal – AFR-D
Seychelles – AFR-D
Sierra Leone – AFR-D
South Africa – AFR-E
Swaziland – AFR-E
Togo – AFR-D
Uganda – AFR-E
United Republic of Tanzania – AFR-E
Zambia – AFR-E
Zimbabwe – AFR-E

Region of the Americas

Antigua and Barbuda – AMR-B
Argentina – AMR-B
Bahamas – AMR-B
Barbados – AMR-B
Belize – AMR-B
Bolivia – AMR-D
Brazil – AMR-B
Canada – AMR-A
Chile – AMR-B
Colombia – AMR-B
Costa Rica – AMR-B
Cuba – AMR-A
Dominica – AMR-B
Dominican Republic – AMR-B
Ecuador – AMR-D
El Salvador – AMR-B
Grenada – AMR-B
Guatemala – AMR-D
Guyana – AMR-B
Haiti – AMR-D
Honduras – AMR-B
Jamaica – AMR-B
Mexico – AMR-B
Nicaragua – AMR-D
Panama – AMR-B
Paraguay – AMR-B
Peru – AMR-D
Saint Kitts and Nevis – AMR-B
Saint Lucia – AMR-B
Saint Vincent and the Grenadines – AMR-B
Suriname – AMR-B
Trinidad and Tobago – AMR-B
United States of America – AMR-A
Uruguay – AMR-B
Venezuela, Bolivarian Republic of – AMR-B

Eastern Mediterranean Region

Afghanistan – EMR-D
Bahrain – EMR-B
Cyprus – EMR-B
Djibouti – EMR-D
Egypt – EMR-D
Iran, Islamic Republic of – EMR-B
Iraq – EMR-D
Jordan – EMR-B
Kuwait – EMR-B
Lebanon – EMR-B
Libyan Arab Jamahiriya – EMR-B
Morocco – EMR-D
Oman – EMR-B
Pakistan – EMR-D
Qatar – EMR-B
Saudi Arabia – EMR-B
Somalia – EMR-D
Sudan – EMR-D
Syrian Arab Republic – EMR-B
Tunisia – EMR-B
United Arab Emirates – EMR-B
Yemen – EMR-D

Mortality strata
A. Very low child, very low adult
B. Low child, low adult
C. Low child, high adult
D. High child, high adult
E. High child, very high adult

European Region

Albania – EUR-B
Andorra – EUR-A
Armenia – EUR-B
Austria – EUR-A
Azerbaijan – EUR-B
Belarus – EUR-C
Belgium – EUR-A
Bosnia and Herzegovina – EUR-B
Bulgaria – EUR-B
Croatia – EUR-A
Czech Republic – EUR-A
Denmark – EUR-A
Estonia – EUR-C
Finland – EUR-A
France – EUR-A
Georgia – EUR-B
Germany – EUR-A
Greece – EUR-A
Hungary – EUR-C
Iceland – EUR-A
Ireland – EUR-A
Israel – EUR-A
Italy – EUR-A
Kazakhstan – EUR-C
Kyrgyzstan – EUR-B
Latvia – EUR-C
Lithuania – EUR-C
Luxembourg – EUR-A
Malta – EUR-A
Monaco – EUR-A
Netherlands – EUR-A
Norway – EUR-A
Poland – EUR-B
Portugal – EUR-A
Republic of Moldova – EUR-C
Romania – EUR-B
Russian Federation – EUR-C
San Marino – EUR-A
Slovakia – EUR-B
Slovenia – EUR-A
Spain – EUR-A
Sweden – EUR-A
Switzerland – EUR-A
Tajikistan – EUR-B
The former Yugoslav
    Republic of Macedonia – EUR-B
Turkey – EUR-B
Turkmenistan – EUR-B
Ukraine – EUR-C
United Kingdom – EUR-A
Uzbekistan – EUR-B
Yugoslavia – EUR-B

South-East Asia Region

Bangladesh – SEAR-D
Bhutan – SEAR-D
Democratic People's
    Republic of Korea – SEAR-D
India – SEAR-D
Indonesia – SEAR-B
Maldives – SEAR-D
Myanmar – SEAR-D
Nepal – SEAR-D
Sri Lanka – SEAR-B
Thailand – SEAR-B

Western Pacific Region

Australia – WPR-A
Brunei Darussalam – WPR-A
Cambodia – WPR-B
China – WPR-B
Cook Islands – WPR-B
Fiji – WPR-B
Japan – WPR-A
Kiribati – WPR-B
Lao People's
    Democratic Republic – WPR-B
Malaysia – WPR-B
Marshall Islands – WPR-B
Micronesia, Federated
    States of – WPR-B
Mongolia – WPR-B
Nauru – WPR-B
New Zealand – WPR-A
Niue – WPR-B
Palau – WPR-B
Papua New Guinea – WPR-B
Philippines – WPR-B
Republic of Korea – WPR-B
Samoa – WPR-B
Singapore – WPR-A
Solomon Islands – WPR-B
Tonga – WPR-B
Tuvalu – WPR-B
Vanuatu – WPR-B
Viet Nam – WPR-B

ACKNOWLEDGEMENTS

Headquarters advisory group

Markus Behrend
Ruth Bonita
John Clements
Chris Dye
Joan Dzenowagis
Michael Eriksen
David Evans
Metin Gulmezoglum
Susan Holck
Christopher Murray
Thomson Prentice
Iqbal Shah
Kathleen Strong
Tessa Tan-Torres Edejer
Paul Van Look
Yasmin Von Schirnding
Maged Younes

Regional reference group

Billo Mounkaila Abdou
Sussan Bassiri
David Brandling-Bennet
Anca Dumitrescu
Myint Htwe
Soe Ynunt-U

Cost-effectiveness assessment

Taghreed Adam
Moses Aikins
Perihan Al-Husseini
Rob Baltussen
James K. Bartram
Robert E. Black
Ilja Borysenko
Cynthia Boschi-Pinto
Daniel Chisholm
Christina Ciecierski
Gerald Dziekan
Steeve Ebener
Sahra El-Ghannam
David Evans
Majid Ezzati
Valery Feigin
Laurence Haller
Chika Hayashi
Yunpeng Huang
Jose Hueb
Yvan Hutin
Raymond Hutubessy
Benjamin Johns
Jeremy Lauer
Carlene Lawes
Julia Lowe
Colin Mathers
Sumi Mehta
Christopher Murray
Pat Neff Walker

Louis Niessen
Kevin O'Reilly
Annette Pruess
Ken Redekop
Juergen Rehm
Anthony Rodgers
Nataly Sabharwal
Joshua Salomon
George Schmid
Bernhard Schwartlander
Anne-Marie Sevcsik
Mona Sharan
Kenji Shibuya
John Stover
Michael Sweat
Tessa Tan-Torres Edejer
Niels Tomijima
Mark Van Ommeren
Ying Diana Wu

Risk assessment

Alcohol
Ulrich Frick
Gerhard Gmel
Kathryn Graham
David Jernigan
Maristela Monteiro
Jürgen Rehm
Nina Rehn
Robin Room
Christopher T. Sempos

Urban air pollution
Ross Anderson
Aaron Cohen
Kersten Gutschmidt
Michal Krzyzanowski
Nino Künzli
Bart Ostro
Kiran Pandey
Arden Pope
Isabelle Romieu
Jonathan Samet
Kirk R. Smith

Work-related ergonomic stressors
Jim Leigh
Deborah Nelson
Sharonne Phillips
Annette Pruess

Blood pressure
Paul Elliott
Malcolm Law
Carlene Lawes
Stephen MacMahon
Anthony Rodgers
Stephen Vander Hoorn

Breastfeeding
Ana Pilar Betrán
Mercedes de Onis
Jeremy Addison Lauer

Work-related carcinogens
Carlos Corvalan
Tim Driscoll
Marilyn Fingerhut
Jim Leigh
Deborah Nelson
Annette Pruess

Childhood sexual abuse
Gavin Andrews
Justine Corry
Cathy Issakidis
Tim Slade
Heather Swanston

Cholesterol
Malcolm Law
Carlene Lawes
Stephen MacMahon
Anthony Rodgers
Stephen Vander Hoorn

Climate change
Diarmid Campbell-Lendrum
Sally Edwards
Sari Kovats
Paul Wilkinson

Fruit and vegetable intake
Louise Causer
Karen Lock
Martin Mckee
Joceline Pomerleau

Illicit drugs
Louisa Degenhardt
Wayne Hall
Michael Lynskey
Matthew Warner-Smith

Indoor smoke from solid fuels
Mirjam Feuz
Sumi Mehta
Kirk R. Smith

Unsafe health care injections
Gregory L. Armstrong
Yvan J. F. Hutin
Anja Hauri

Iodine deficiency
Robert E. Black
Stephen Fishman
Adnan Ali Hyder
Luke Mullany

Iron deficiency
Robert E. Black
Luke Mullany
Rebecca J. Stoltzfus

Lead exposure
José Luis Ayuso
Lorna Fewtrell
Philip Landrigan
Annette Pruess

Underweight
Robert E. Black
Stephen Fishman
Adnan Ali Hyder
Luke Mullany
Robert E. Black
Laura E. Caulfield

Work-related noise
Marisol Concha
Carlos Corvalan
Marilyn Fingerhut
Deborah Nelson
Robert Nelson

Work-related airborne particulates
Carlos Corvalan
Tim Driscoll
Marilyn Fingerhut
Jim Leigh
Deborah Nelson
Annette Pruess

Work-related risk factors for injuries
Marisol Concha
Carlos Corvalan
Marilyn Fingerhut
Jim Leigh
Deborah Nelson
Annette Pruess

Overweight
Rachel Jackson-Leach
W. Philip T. James
Eleni Kalamara
Cliona Ni Mhurchu
Chizuru Nishida
Neville J. Rigby
Anthony Rodgers
Maryam Shayeghi

Physical inactivity
Tim Armstrong
Fiona Bull
Tracy Dixon
Sandra Ham
Andrea Neiman
Mike Pratt

Poverty
Tony Blakely
Simon Hales
Charlotte Kieft
Nick Wilson
Alistair Woodward

Tobacco
Majid Ezzati
Alan D. Lopez

Unsafe sex
John Cleland
Martine Collumbien
Makeda Gerressu

Unsafe water, sanitation and hygiene
James K. Bartram
Lorna Fewtrell
David Kay
Annette Pruess

Vitamin A deficiency
Robert E. Black
Amy Rice
Keith P. West Jr

Zinc deficiency
Robert E. Black
Laura E. Caulfield

Text boxes

Causal web
Miguel A. Hernán
James M. Robins
Uwe Siebert

Collective violence
David Meddings

Coronary heart disease and work stress
Annette Pruess

Environmental tobacco smoke
Majid Ezzati
Alan D. Lopez
Kirk R. Smith

Genetics
Victor Boulyjenkov
Paul McKeigue
Pekka Puska

Housing and health
Carl-Gustaf Bornehag
Majid Ezzati
Yasmin von Schirnding

Interpersonal violence
Alex Butchart
Debarati Sapir

Life course
George Davey-Smith

Multiple causes
Robert Beaglehole

National nutrition campaigns
Rob Carter
Steven Crowley
Christine Stone
Theo Vos

Needlestick injuries
Annette Pruess

Nutritional transition
Barry Popkin

Occupational back pain
Supriya Lahiri
Charles Levenstein
Pia Makkanen

Patient safety
Itziar Larizgoitia
Silvester Yunkap Kwankam

Population-wide strategies for prevention
Robert Beaglehole
Malcom Law
Pekka Puska

Protective factors
Krishna Bose
Richard Jessor
Carol Ryff
Burton Singer

Road traffic injuries
Tony Fletcher
Emma Hutchison
Marge Peden
Ian Roberts

Tuberculosis
Chris Dye

Other contributors

Administrative assistance
Clarissa Gould-Thorpe

Data for figures
Malcom Law
Pekka Jousilahti
Hirotsugu Ueshima
Neville Young

Epidemiology input
Carlene Lawes
Patricia Priest

Statistical annex
Omar Ahmad
Christina Bernard
Carmen Dolea
Brodie Ferguson
Mie Inoue
Julie Levison
Dorothy Ma Fat
Colin Mathers
Chalapati Rao
Tanuja Rastogi
Joshua Salomon
Kenji Shibuya
Claudia Stein
Edward Tachie-Menson
Niels Tomijima
Thomas Truelsen
Sarah Wild

Mortality
Emmanuella Gakidou
Mollie Hogan

National health accounts
Patricia Hernandez
Chandika Indikadahena
Jean-Pierre Poullier
Nathalie Van De Maele

INDEX

Page numbers in **bold** type indicate main discussions.

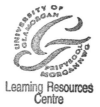